Self-Recovery: Treating Addictions Using Transcendental Meditation and Maharishi Ayur-Veda

Self-Recovery: Treating Addictions Using Transcendental Meditation and Maharishi Ayur-Veda

David F. O'Connell, PhD
Charles N. Alexander, PhD
Editors

The Haworth Press, Inc.
New York • London • Norwood (Australia)

Self-Recovery: Treating Addictions Using Transcendental Meditation and Maharishi Ayur-Veda has also been published as *Alcohol Treatment Quarterly*, Volume 11, Numbers 1/2 and 3/4 1994.

The Haworth Press, Inc., 10 Alice Street, Binghamton, NY 13904-1580 USA

Library of Congress Cataloging-in-Publication Data

O'Connell, David F.
Self-recovery : treating addictions using Transcendental Meditation and Maharishi Ayur-Veda / David F. O'Connell, Charles N. Alexander.
p. cm.
Includes bibliographical references and index.
ISBN 1-56024-454-2 (alk. paper).–ISBN 1-56023-044-4 (pbk. : alk. paper)
1. Substance abuse–Treatment. 2. Transcendental Meditation–Therapeutic use. 3. Medicine, Ayurvedic. I. Alexander, Charles Nathaniel. II. Title.
RC564.027 1994 94-3952
616.86'06–dc20 CIP

INDEXING & ABSTRACTING

Contributions to this publication are selectively indexed or abstracted in print, electronic, online, or CD-ROM version(s) of the reference tools and information services listed below. This list is current as of the copyright date of this publication. See the end of this section for additional notes.

- ***Abstracts in Anthropology***, Baywood Publishing Company, 26 Austin Avenue, P.O. Box 337, Amityville, NY 11701
- ***Abstracts of Research in Pastoral Care & Counseling***, Loyola College, 7135 Minstrel Way, Suite 101, Columbia, MD 21045
- ***ALCONARC Database***, Swedish Council for Information on Alcohol and Other Drugs, Box 27302, S-102 54 Stockholm, Sweden
- ***Cambridge Scientific Abstracts***, *Health & Safety Science Abstracts*, Cambridge Information Group, 7200 Wisconsin Avenue #601, Bethesda, MD 20814
- ***Criminal Justice Abstracts***, Willow Tree Press, 15 Washington Street, 4th Floor, Newark, NJ 07102
- ***Criminology, Penology and Police Science Abstracts***, Kugler Publications, P.O. Box 11188, 1001 GD Amsterdam, The Netherlands
- ***Excerpta Medica/Electronic Publishing Division***, Elsevier Science Publishers, 655 Avenue of the Americas, New York, NY 10010
- ***Index to Periodical Articles Related to Law***, University of Texas, 727 East 26th Street, Austin, TX 78705
- ***Inventory of Marriage and Family Literature (online and hard copy)***, National Council on Family Relations, 3989 Central Avenue NE, Suite 550, Minneapolis, MN 55421

(continued)

- ***Medication Use STudies (MUST) DATABASE***, The University of Mississippi School of Pharmacy, University, MS 38677
- ***Mental Health Abstracts (online through DIALOG)***, IFI/Plenum Data Company, 3202 Kirkwood Highway, Wilmington, DE 19808
- ***NIAAA Alcohol and Alcohol Problems Science Database (ETOH)***, National Institute on Alcohol Abuse and Alcoholism, 1400 Eye Street NW, Suite 600, Washington, DC 20005
- ***Psychological Abstracts (PsycINFO)***, American Psychological Association, P.O. Box 91600, Washington, DC 20090-1600
- ***Referativnyi Zhurnal (Abstracts Journal of the Institute of Scientific Information of the Republic of Russia)***, The Institute of Scientific Information, Baltijskaja ul., 14, Moscow A-219, Republic of Russia
- ***Social Planning/Policy & Development Abstracts (SOPODA)***, Sociological Abstracts, Inc., P.O. Box 22206, San Diego, CA 92192-0206
- ***Social Work Abstracts***, National Association of Social Workers, 750 First Street NW, 8th Floor, Washington, DC 20002
- ***Sociological Abstracts (SA)***, Sociological Abstracts, Inc., P.O. Box 22206, San Diego, CA 92192-0206
- ***SOMED (social medicine) Database***, Institute fur Dokumentation, Postfach 20 10 12, D-33548 Bielefeld, Germany
- ***Studies on Women Abstracts***, Carfax Publishing Company, P.O. Box 25, Abingdon, Oxfordshire OX14 3UE, United Kingdom
- ***The Brown University Digest of Addiction Theory and Application (DATA Newsletter)***, Project Cork Institute, Dartmouth Medical School, 14 S. Main Street, Suite 2F, Hanover, NH 03755-2015

SPECIAL BIBLIOGRAPHIC NOTES

related to special journal issues (separates) and indexing/abstracting

- ☐ indexing/abstracting services in this list will also cover material in the "separate" that is co-published simultaneously with Haworth's special thematic journal issue or DocuSerial. Indexing/abstracting usually covers material at the article/chapter level.
- ☐ monographic co-editions are intended for either non-subscribers or libraries which intend to purchase a second copy for their circulating collections.
- ☐ monographic co-editions are reported to all jobbers/wholesalers/approval plans. The source journal is listed as the "series" to assist the prevention of duplicate purchasing in the same manner utilized for books-in-series.
- ☐ to facilitate user/access services all indexing/abstracting services are encouraged to utilize the co-indexing entry note indicated at the bottom of the first page of each article/chapter/contribution.
- ☐ this is intended to assist a library user of any reference tool (whether print, electronic, online, or CD-ROM) to locate the monographic version if the library has purchased this version but not a subscription to the source journal.
- ☐ individual articles/chapters in any Haworth publication are also available through the Haworth Document Delivery Services (HDDS).

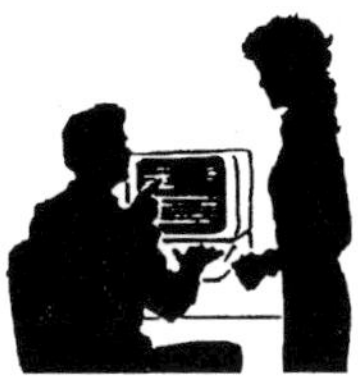

ABOUT THE EDITORS

David F. O'Connell, PhD, received his PhD in psychoeducational processes from Temple University. He is a licensed psychologist in private practice in Reading, PA. He is a consultant to the Caron Foundation, one of the nation's leading addictions treatment facilities. He is also an attending psychologist at St. Joseph's Hospital in Reading, PA. He holds a diplomate with the American Academy of Psychologists Treating Addictions and is listed in the National Register of Health Service Providers in Psychology. He has edited/co-authored two books on dual diagnosis, including *Managing the Dually Diagnosed Patient* (The Haworth Press, Inc., 1990) and has contributed articles to numerous addictions journals. He serves on the editorial board of the *Journal of Adolescent Chemical Dependency.* He is a member of the Society of Psychologists in Addictive Behavior in the American Psychological Association.

Charles N. Alexander, PhD, received his BA (magna cum laude, Phi Beta Kappa), MA and PhD in Psychology from Harvard University. He was a predoctoral fellow at Oxford University and a postdoctoral fellow at Harvard University in Psychology. He is Professor of Psychology, Director of the Division of Crime Prevention, Rehabilitation, and Drug Abuse in the Institute of Science, Technology and Public Policy, and Director of the Institute for Research on Higher States of Consciousness, at Maharishi International University, Fairfield, IA. He is the editor of three books, including *Higher Stages of Human Development* (Oxford University Press, 1990). He is Co-Principal Investigator on two major grants from the National Institutes of Health on the effects of the Transcendental Meditation program on physical and mental health and on risk factors such as alcohol and cigarette use. He has contributed over 60 articles to addictions, psychology, and health journals and books.

Self-Recovery: Treating Addictions Using Transcendental Meditation and Maharishi Ayur-Veda

CONTENTS

∞ ALL HAWORTH BOOKS & JOURNALS ARE PRINTED ON CERTIFIED ACID-FREE PAPER

About the Contributors

Authors are listed alphabetically, along with their highest academic degree and current professional appointments.

Charles N. Alexander, PhD, in Psychology, Harvard University. Professor of Psychology; Director, Division of Crime Prevention, Rehabilitation, and Drug Abuse in the Institute of Science, Technology and Public Policy; Director, Institute for Research on Higher States of Consciousness, Maharishi International University (MIU), Fairfield, IA.

Catherine Bleick, PhD, in Zoology, University of California, Berkeley. Coordinator of the Transcendental Meditation Program for Alcoholics in Los Angeles, CA.

Jim Brooks, MD, Wayne State University Medical School. Clinical Director, Mental Health Institute of Mount Pleasant, Mount Pleasant, IA; attending physician, College of Maharishi Ayur-Veda Health Center; adjunct clinical professor, MIU, Fairfield, IA.

Pat Corum, BA, in Business Administration, California State University, Hayward, CA. Drug-abuse counselor and attorney assistant, Kern County, California. Former inmate at San Quentin and Folsom prisons in California.

Michael C. Dillbeck, PhD, in Psychology, Purdue University. Professor of Psychology; Dean of the Graduate School, MIU, Fairfield, IA.

Susan L. Dillbeck, PhD, in Education, University of California, Berkeley. Professor, Department of Education; Dean of the Graduate School, MIU, Fairfield, IA.

George A. Ellis, PhD, in Criminology, Columbia Pacific University, CA. Chairman. Board of Directors. AGRO International, Inc., Guatemala/Costa Rica. Former National Program Director, Institute for Social Rehabilitation.

Jay Glaser, MD, University of Colorado Medical School. Director, Maharishi Ayur-Veda Health Center for Behavioral Medicine and Stress Management, Lancaster, MA.

John S. Hagelin, PhD, in Physics, Harvard University. Professor Chairperson, and Director of the Doctoral Program, Department of Physics; Director, Institute of Science. Technology and Public Policy, MIU, Fairfield, IA.

Linda Keniston-Dubocq, MD, Albert Einstein College of Medicine. Private practice in Family Medicine; Medical Director, Klearview Manor Nursing Home for the Developmentally Delayed, Waterville, ME.

Debra Levitsky, MS, PhD, candidate in Physiology, MIU, Fairfield, IA.

David O'Connell, PhD, in Psychoeducational Processes. Temple University. Licensed psychologist in private practice; consultant, Caron Foundation; attending psychologist, St. Joseph's Hospital, Reading, PA.

Diarmuid O'Murchu, BA (with Honors) in theology, Trinity College, Dublin, Ireland. Catholic priest and member of the Missionaries of the Sacred Heart; counselor and social psychologist working in London, England.

David W. Orme-Johnson, PhD, in Psychology, University of Maryland. Professor, Chairperson, and Director of the Doctoral Program, Department of Psychology; Dean of Research; Director of Research and Evaluation, Institute of Science, Technology and Public Policy, MIU, Fairfield, IA.

Maxwell Y. Rainforth, MS, in Mathematics, MA in Education, MIU. Lecturer in Statistics, Department of Psychology, MIU, Fairfield, IA.

Pat Robinson, PhD, in Psychology, University of Kansas. Postdoctoral Fellow in Psychology, MIU, Fairfield, IA.

Ann Royer, PhD, in Physiology, MIU. Independent researcher in the field of smoking cessation programs. Lac Beauport, Quebec, Canada.

David Sands, MD, University of Iowa. Assistant Professor of Physiology; clinical faculty, College of Maharishi Ayur-Veda; staff physician, Maharishi Ayur-Veda Medical Center, MIU, Fairfield, IA.

Hari M. Sharma, MD, King George's Medical College, Lucknow, India. Professor of Pathology; Director, Cancer prevention and Natural Products Research, Ohio State University, College of Medicine, Columbus, Ohio.

Frank Staggers, MD, Creighton University. Director, Haight-Ashbury Free Clinic Drug Detoxification, Rehabilitation, and Aftercare Program, San Francisco, CA.

Solomon S. Steiner, PhD, in Psychology, New York University. President, Pharmaceutical Discovery Corp., Elmsford, NY.

Edward Taub, PhD, in Psychology, New York University. Professor of Psychology, University of Alabama, Birmingham.

Kenneth Walton, PhD, in Chemistry, Vanderbilt University. Associate Professor of Neurochemistry; Director, Neurochemistry Laboratory; Associate Director, Division of Health, Institute of Science, Technology and Public Policy, MIU, Fairfield, IA.

Eric Weingarten, PhD, in Psychology, University of Kentucky. Supervising Psychologist, Tompkins County Mental Health Clinic, Ithaca, NY.

Preface

Over the past decade, researchers and clinicians have made important advances in the study of addictive diseases. Increasingly we have come to view chemically dependent patients as a heterogeneous population often with multiple addictions and showing concurrent psychiatric disorders. This knowledge has led to improved matching of clients with treatments, such as psychotherapy, pharmacotherapy, addictions counseling, and self-help group involvement. Significant advances have also been made in understanding the genetic and physiological basis of some forms of addiction which may lead to more effective biological treatments.

However, despite our best efforts to understand and treat addictions of all kinds, research shows that relapse rates remain unacceptably high and the formula for effectively controlling or eliminating addictive behaviors remains elusive. The present volume represents the culmination of over two decades of clinical and experimental research on a new, comprehensive approach to treating addiction: the Transcendental Meditation program and the other modalities of Maharishi Ayur-Veda. Research shows that this multistrategy approach produces lasting effects on addictive behavior and in many cases these changes are dramatic. Maharishi Ayur-Veda emerges as a natural biobehavioral approach that holistically addresses the psychological, physiological, and spiritual aspects of addictive behavior and could become a vital component of any program treating chemical dependency.

This is the first book on Transcendental Meditation, Maharishi Ayur-Veda, and addictions treatment. Its publication rests on the

[Haworth co-indexing entry note]: "Preface." O'Connell, David F., and Charles N. Alexander. Co-published simultaneously in the *Alcoholism Treatment Quarterly* (The Haworth Press, Inc.) Vol. 11, No. 1/2, 1994, pp. xvii-xviii; and: *Self-Recovery: Treating Addictions Using Transcendental Meditation and Maharishi Ayur-Veda* (ed: David F. O'Connell and Charles N. Alexander) The Haworth Press, Inc., 1994, pp. xvii-xviii. Multiple copies of this article/chapter may be purchased from The Haworth Document Delivery Center [1-800-3-HAWORTH; 9:00 a.m. - 5:00 p.m. (EST)].

dedication and arduous work done by the scientists, physicians, and clinicians who have pioneered the application of this new approach to addictive diseases. Their knowledge and enthusiasm is reflected in their inspired, original papers contributed to this volume. The book's structure and chapters are briefly summarized in the editors' introduction.

Producing a volume of this size and scope is a collective effort, and many individuals have generously contributed their knowledge and expertise. We especially thank Pat Robinson for her invaluable editorial contributions to every aspect of the book. Special thanks also to David Orme-Johnson and Susan Shatkin for their editorial advice and assistance. We also thank Paul Scholastico, Susan Kolson, Ken Walton, Gerry Geer, Steven Rector, Terry Bauer, Jim Gilmore, Craig Pearson, and Michael Dillbeck for their editorial assistance, and Dr. Alexander's doctoral students in psychology at Maharishi International University for their assistance in preparing the final manuscript. Appreciation also goes to Dr. John Hagelin for contributing the Foreword to this book, to Shepley Hansen for the book cover design, and to Mark Paul Petrick for the cover photo. Dr. O'Connell thanks his fiancee Barbara Rankin for her warm encouragement, and Dr. Alexander thanks his wife Vicki and son Nathaniel for their nurturing support. Finally, our deepest gratitude is offered to Maharishi Mahesh Yogi, the founder of Transcendental Meditation and Maharishi Ayur-Veda, for his selfless offering of this timeless knowledge at a time when the world is in such dire need of a path out of suffering.

We sincerely hope that this volume through its introduction of these holistic, natural approaches will have a profound impact on alleviating the problems of individuals with addictive diseases.

David F. O'Connell, PhD, West Lawn, Pennsylvania
Charles N. Alexander, PhD, Fairfield, Iowa
June 1993

Foreword

As a chronic debilitating disease, addiction affects, directly or indirectly, over 130 million Americans. It places a staggering burden on our health care system. In 1990, tobacco was the most prominent non-genetic contributor to mortality in the US (estimated 400,000 deaths) and alcohol was the third largest contributor (100,000 deaths). Currently, we spend more on addiction than we do on either cardiovascular disease or cancer. The total cost of addiction to society has been estimated to be over $550 billion per year including substance-related medical problems, crime, lost productivity, substance dependence treatment, and auto insurance losses paid (see Orme-Johnson, this volume). More than fifty percent of serious crimes committed in the United States are drug or alcohol-related. Personal suffering associated with drug and alcohol addiction is immeasurable. Thus, chemical addiction represents one of the greatest threats to our nation and world.

The response from treatment professionals and the medical and scientific communities has been vigorous. There are now dozens of treatment approaches to addiction, many of which have met with some level of success. However, relapse rates remain alarmingly high. Indeed, few would argue that we are winning the war on drugs. Although well-intended in their conception, development, and delivery, current approaches to the treatment of addiction are generally fragmentary and based on incomplete and often erroneous knowledge of health and full human potential.

John S. Hagelin, PhD, is Director, Institute of Science, Technology and Public Policy, Maharishi International University (MIU), Fairfield, IA.

[Haworth co-indexing entry note]: "Foreword." Hagelin, John S. Co-published simultaneously in the *Alcoholism Treatment Quarterly* (The Haworth Press, Inc.) Vol. 11, No. 1/2, 1994, pp. xix-xxi; and: *Self-Recovery: Treating Addictions Using Transcendental Meditation and Maharishi Ayur-Veda* (ed: David F. O'Connell and Charles N. Alexander) The Haworth Press, Inc., 1994, pp. xix-xxi. Multiple copies of this article/chapter may be purchased from The Haworth Document Delivery Center [1-800-3-HAWORTH; 9:00 a.m. - 5:00 p.m. (EST)].

Self-Recovery offers an entirely new, fresh perspective on the treatment of addictive diseases. It is the first book detailing the effects of the Transcendental Meditation program and Maharishi Ayur-Veda on addictions. Brought to light from the ancient Vedic tradition of India by Maharishi Mahesh Yogi, this natural, comprehensive approach to health care allows individuals to break negative habits that arise from an incomplete understanding of the relationship between mind, body, and environment. By *Self-Recovery*, the authors mean not only the restoration of individual self-esteem and self-worth, but the rediscovery of the Self as a silent, peaceful state of inner Being, a transcendental field of consciousness underlying individuality. Transcendental Meditation and the other approaches of Maharishi Ayur-Veda provide effortless technologies to experience the inner Self.

Self-Recovery details how, by purifying mind, body, and environment, these natural programs can achieve not only a drug-free life, but the ultimate goal of development–a complete awakening of individual potential and societal harmony. Only by experiencing the most basic, underlying level of existence, the transcendental Self, can all levels of life–physiological, psychological, spiritual, and social–be simultaneously nourished and healed from within. Such a holistic approach is critical to recovery from the devastating impact of addiction. With these approaches, the addict can emerge from the deep sleep of drug-induced functioning and awaken to the infinite possibilities of life.

The current crisis in health care demands the identification and implementation of innovative, life-supporting, cost-effective programs to prevent disease and promote health. According to a recent article in the *New England Journal of Medicine*, one-third of Americans have sought alternative medical treatment. Clearly, our society has become very serious about the need for more natural, prevention-oriented approaches to health, and is willing to expend the time and money necessary to stay healthy. There is growing interest among major health-care providers and policy makers in the applications of Transcendental Meditation and Ayurvedic medicine to disease prevention and health promotion. These programs offer an effective complement–or a comprehensive alternative treatment–to traditional treatment approaches to chemical dependency.

According to research in this volume by Dr. Alexander and colleagues, the effects of Transcendental Meditation are several times larger than standard treatments for reducing alcohol, cigarette, or illicit drug use. On a societal level, research by Orme-Johnson points to treating society as a whole, reducing crime and other negative social trends through the collective practice of advanced TM programs. These and other dramatic results of research on Transcendental Meditation and Maharishi Ayur-Veda establish these natural health care techniques as distinctively effective in the treatment of addictive diseases.

This book is essential reading for professionals treating those who are chemically dependent as well as for patients and their loved ones. Moreover, it offers a vital contribution to science and public welfare. Today, we look to science to create lasting solutions to the problems facing our nation. It is the mission of our MIU Institute of Science, Technology and Public Policy to identify, scientifically evaluate, and promote through public policy the most up-to-date, life-supporting solutions to problems confronting society. The programs outlined in this book offer scientifically validated, cost-effective, prevention-oriented programs that can benefit each individual and society as a whole. I encourage each reader to begin to study and implement the technologies outlined in this volume.

Self-Recovery brings a timeless, universal knowledge to the addictions field and revolutionizes our understanding of the addictive process and how it can be altered. Based on the holistic knowledge of natural law, this book offers great hope and vision for patients, therapists and all who seek a rediscovery of their Self and freedom from suffering. The profound knowledge of Transcendental Meditation and Maharishi Ayur-Veda presented in *Self-Recovery* can help eradicate this epidemic of human suffering, opening a new window for the field of rehabilitation that includes as its ultimate treatment goal, the attainment of the highest level of human potential.

John S. Hagelin, PhD
Fairfield, Iowa
September 1993

Introduction: Recovery from Addictions Using Transcendental Meditation and Maharishi Ayur-Veda

David F. O'Connell, PhD
Charles N. Alexander, PhD

Today, alcoholism and other chemical dependencies are recognized as chronic, often insidious, progressive conditions that, if untreated, can lead to devastating results for the individual and society. The financial, medical and personal costs of chemical dependence are reaching epidemic levels. The total cost for addiction is higher than any other health problem, including cardiovascular disease and cancer, in the United States.

Chemical dependencies are now believed to arise from multiple, interacting domains including biological, psychological, spiritual, and social factors. The addictions field recognizes the complex nature of chemical dependency and the need for a multidimensional approach that addresses the many components of the addictive process. Although many contemporary treatments for chemical dependency are described as holistic, few, if any, live up to this proclamation. Also, multimodal, intensive treatments are costly and remain plagued by high relapse rates. In contrast to conventional treatments, Transcendental Meditation (TM) and Maharishi Ayur-Veda

---

[Haworth co-indexing entry note]: "Introduction: Recovery from Addictions Using Transcendental Meditation and Maharishi Ayur-Veda." O'Connell, David F., and Charles N. Alexander. Co-published simultaneously in the *Alcoholism Treatment Quarterly* (The Haworth Press, Inc.) Vol. 11, No. 1/2, 1994, pp. 1-10; and: *Self-Recovery: Treating Addictions Using Transcendental Meditation and Maharishi Ayur-Veda* (ed: David F. O'Connell and Charles N. Alexander) The Haworth Press, Inc., 1994, pp. 1-10. Multiple copies of this article/chapter may be purchased from The Haworth Document Delivery Center [1-800-3-HAWORTH; 9:00 a.m. - 5:00 p.m. (EST)].

appear to provide a natural, comprehensive treatment approach that profoundly influences all levels of individual life that can impact on the addictive process.

This is the first book written on the application of TM and Maharishi Ayur-Veda to addictions treatment. It shares the pioneering experiences of clinicians using these holistic procedures as well as the striking findings of researchers who have investigated their effects. For those without prior introduction to this new approach, TM and Maharishi Ayur-Veda first will be briefly described followed by an overview of the book's structure and a preview of the contributing chapters.

TRANSCENDENTAL MEDITATION

The Transcendental Meditation program is a simple mental technique derived by Maharishi Mahesh Yogi (1969, 1986) from the ancient Vedic tradition of India, which has its source in the Rik Veda. It is easily learned, practiced for 20 minutes twice daily, and requires no change in lifestyle or beliefs. TM has been learned by four million people over the past thirty-five years.

In the early 1970's, the first empirical studies documenting the distinctive psychophysiological correlates of the TM technique were published by Robert Keith Wallace and his associates in *Science, Scientific American*, and the *American Journal of Physiology*. Since then, over 500 studies on TM conducted in over 200 research institutions worldwide have supported and extended these original findings, making it the most widely researched approach for the development of human consciousness. Also, several major grants have been awarded by the National Institutes of Health to study the biochemical correlates of TM, its effects on the treatment of chronic alcoholism and relapse prevention, hypertension, and the reduction of psychological stress and enhancement of self-concept in African-American adults.

Several meta-analyses, which quantitatively summarize the results of diverse studies in a field, suggest that TM has a significantly larger effect than other forms of meditation and relaxation in producing deep physiological rest (Dillbeck & Orme-Johnson, 1987), reducing psychological distress (Eppley, Abrams, & Shear, 1989), and promoting positive mental health (e.g., Alexander, Rainforth, & Gelderloos, 1991) in the general population.

To date there have been over 30 studies (see Alexander, Robinson, & Rainforth, this volume) specifically on the application of Transcendental Meditation to the treatment of substance abuse published in such journals as the *American Journal of Psychiatry, International Journal of the Addictions, Alcoholism Treatment Quarterly,* and *Addictive Behaviors*. This research has shown the often dramatic impact TM can have on the recovery process (for example, see Taub et al.'s study, this volume, with transient, chronic alcoholics).

During the practice of TM, the mind is said to settle down to increasingly quieter levels of mental activity, until even the subtlest level of thought is transcended, and consciousness becomes fully awake to itself alone, with no object of thought or perception. This silent unified state is held to be the direct experience of one's own innermost Self or Being, the transcendental foundation of individual life (Maharishi, 1969). This unique state of restful alertness, called transcendental consciousness, has been shown to be a fourth major state of consciousness, physiologically different on over 20 parameters from waking, dreaming or deep sleep (Alexander, Cranson, Boyer, & Orme-Johnson, 1987; Jevning, Wallace, & Beidebach, 1992).

Repeated experience of transcendental consciousness is said to lead to the unfoldment of higher states of consciousness in which the experience of inner, unbounded Self is maintained along with the ordinary waking, dreaming, and sleeping states of consciousness (Alexander et al., 1990).

MAHARISHI AYUR-VEDA

Ayurveda, which translates as "science of life," has its origins in the ancient Vedic civilization of India. Ayurveda has been recognized by the World Health Organization as a comprehensive system of natural medicine (Bannerman, Burton, & Ch'en Wen-Chieh, 1983). Over time and due to foreign influences, much of the knowledge of Ayurveda became misunderstood or was lost. In 1985, Maharishi, along with leading Ayurvedic physicians of India, restored those therapeutic approaches in accordance with the ancient Vedic understanding that the development of full human consciousness is the basis of ideal health and well-being. This modern reformulation of Ayurveda into a systematic form that can be investigated scientifically is known as Maharishi Ayur-Veda (Sharma, Triguna, & Chopra, 1991).

Maharishi Ayur-Veda provides a wide array of clinical and natural pharmacological procedures for the prevention of disease, the development of health, and promotion of longevity. In addition to the consciousness approach of TM which is described as the cornerstone of Maharishi Ayur-Veda, the twenty approaches include methods for physical purification, specialized herbal and fruit preparations, dietary and behavioral recommendations, and specialized breathing and physical exercises. Today, over sixty Maharishi Ayur-Veda medical centers have been opened in twenty-four countries and thousands of medical doctors and health-care professionals have received training in Maharishi Ayur-Veda.

There is a growing body of research on the physical approaches of Maharishi Ayur-Veda. This research has been sponsored, in part, by both the National Institutes of Health and the National Cancer Institute and published in such journals as *Journal of the American Medical Association; Neuropharmacology; Biochemistry Archives; Pharmacology, Biology, and Behavior,* and *Anticancer Research.* This research has documented significant antineoplastic, cardioprotective, immunomodulatory, antioxidant and other neurochemical effects of these treatments. For example, in laboratory animals, the effects of specialized herbal and fruit preparations include protection against and substantial regression of such cancers as lung and mammary carcinomas (Patel et al., 1992; Sharma et al., 1990). Clinical research has shown the positive effects of these modalities on such chronic conditions as rheumatoid arthritis, diabetes mellitus, and tension headaches (Sharma, 1993). Research has also demonstrated the effects of Maharishi Ayur-Veda on improving mental health and enhancing cognitive functioning. Of particular interest to addiction professionals is the finding that the herbal preparations of Maharishi Ayur-Veda result in the scavenging of free radicals, oxygen-rich molecules which damage the nervous system and are aggravated by the abuse of chemicals, particularly alcohol (Sharma, Dillbeck, & Dillbeck, this volume).

ORGANIZATION OF THIS VOLUME

This volume is truly interdisciplinary in scope, with original contributions by psychologists, physicians, physiologists, neurochemists, and other addictions professionals. Through these rich presentations of theory, research, and clinical case studies, the knowledge on Maharishi Ayur-Veda and the addictions comes alive. This book is divided into four sections. In the first section, researchers and clinicians examine the theoretical underpinnings and existing research on the TM program and its application to addictions treatment. Section two features two original, landmark research papers on the impact of TM on severe alcoholism and nicotine addiction. In section three, clinicians share case studies on the impact of TM on personal growth experienced during recovery from alcohol and other drug addictions. In section four, both theory and clinical application of the twenty approaches of Maharishi Ayur-Veda in chemical dependency treatment are presented.

Section one begins with a comprehensive review and quantitative meta-analysis of the research on TM and substance abuse by Charles Alexander (Director, Division of Crime Prevention, Rehabilitation, and Substance Abuse, MIU Institute of Science, Technology and Public Policy), research psychologist Pat Robinson, and statistician Maxwell Rainforth. Their statistical analysis suggests that the effects of TM on substance abuse are significantly larger than the effects of other relaxation techniques or even standard treatment approaches. They also introduce the theoretical framework of Maharishi's Vedic Psychology to explain TM's apparently holistic effect on four domains of life considered critical to addictions–physiological, psychological, spiritual, and social-environmental.

Three subsequent chapters address these domains of life: Walton and Levitsky examine the physiological level, O'Murchu the spiritual level, and Orme-Johnson the broader social/environmental level. In the final chapter of the book, O'Connell discusses the application of TM and Maharishi Ayur-Veda to the psychological domain of functioning.

The chapter by Kenneth Walton (Associate Professor, Department of Neurochemistry, Maharishi International University) and neurochemist Debra Levitsky addresses the neurochemical substrate of chronic stress and its contribution to the development of drug addiction. Exploring a neurochemical theory of addiction, they explain how TM normalizes physiological imbalances involved in addiction, leading to a state of improved balance and well-being.

Spirituality in recovery is the subject of Diarmuid O'Murchu's paper. A Catholic priest living in Ireland, Father O'Murchu clarifies several misconceptions about the relationship between meditation and spirituality. He explains how TM is compatible with the Twelve Steps program and can assist in achieving the highest goals of spirituality which are integral to recovery from addiction.

David Orme-Johnson (MIU Dean of Research and Director of Research and Evaluation for the MIU Institute of Science, Technology and Public Policy) focuses on the potential contributions of TM to resolving broader social problems associated with addiction. He proposes that drug and alcohol abuse are symptoms of a general stress-addiction-crime epidemic in society. He then reviews provocative sociological research findings showing how societal disorder–experienced as crime, drug abuse, political conflict, and economic instability–can be substantially reduced through the cost effective programs of TM and Maharishi Ayur-Veda.

Section two presents two seminal research studies that are among the most rigorous and significant thus far conducted on two major categories of chemical dependence–alcohol and nicotine addiction. A team of behavioral researchers comprising Edward Taub (Professor of Psychology at University of Alabama-Birmingham), Solomon Steiner, Ray Smith, Eric Weingarten, and neurochemist Walton present the results of their randomized, controlled trial using the TM program to treat severe, transient alcoholics. The subjects of this study–in the past referred to as skid-row-type alcoholics–are among the most treatment-refractory addicts. The impressive results of Taub et al. show that adding TM to usual in-patient care more than doubles the sobriety rate of severe alcoholics over an 18-month period. EMG biofeedback also showed favorable results.

Independent physiologist Ann Royer addresses the serious problem of nicotine addiction, reporting on the effects of TM on smoking behavior over almost two years. She found that the smoking quit rate for regular TM practitioners was over twice that of controls who attended an introductory lecture but did not start TM. Given the serious health consequences of nicotine abuse and its high prevalence among alcoholics and addicts, these findings have important implications for clinicians struggling to assist clients in recovery from multiple addictions.

Section three focuses on clinical applications and case studies of Transcendental Meditation. Catherine Bleick, clinician and pioneering researcher on the effects of TM on criminal recidivism, offers a detailed account of her experiences teaching TM to alcoholics and drug addicts participating in Twelve Steps programs in Los Angeles. Bleick presents several case studies of polymorphous abusers struggling against tremendous odds who used the TM program to gain not only sobriety but greater inner tranquillity. The next chapter is co-authored by George Ellis and Pat Corum. Clinician/researcher Ellis, who was the first to implement Transcendental Meditation programs in prisons and other rehabilitation facilities, gives a fascinating account of his experiences teaching TM in these settings. Co-author Pat Corum, a former prisoner and drug addict then serving a life sentence in Folsom and San Quentin prison, provides a powerful, personal account of the dramatic changes he experienced through the TM practice.

Next, physician Frank Staggers, Jr. (Director of the Haight Ashbury Free Clinic Drug Rehabilitation Program), along with researchers Alexander and Walton, discuss acute psychophysiological stress reactions and special problems that can arise during drug detoxification. They suggest that stress reduction through TM may be especially helpful in normalizing withdrawal symptoms and strengthening psychophysiological functioning during this critical first phase of recovery.

Section four features five physicians and two research psychologists who have pioneered the application of Maharishi Ayur-Veda in clinical settings. This section begins with David Sands' (Assistant Professor and staff physician, College of Maharishi Ayur-Veda Health Center at MIU in Fairfield, Iowa) presentation of issues relevant to the introduction of Maharishi Ayur-Veda into clinical practice. Dr. Sands also presents a case study of a middle-aged man suffering from alcohol abuse who was successfully treated using these natural clinical procedures. Next, physician Jay Glaser (Medical Director of Maharishi Ayur-Veda Health Center in Lancaster, Massachusetts) provides an overview of the theory of chemical dependence from the perspective of Maharishi Ayur-Veda. Dr. Glaser reviews its main treatment modalities and discusses case studies of patients involved in Twelve Steps programs who also benefited from this holistic approach.

In the following paper, psychiatrist Jim Brooks, who is Director of the Mental Health Institute of Mount Pleasant, Iowa shares his experience with the application of Maharishi Ayur-Veda in clinical settings. He presents the Ayurvedic view on the nature and diagnosis of mental illness and addictive behaviors, and illustrates, through several case studies, the practical application of Maharishi Ayur-Veda in clinical practice. Then, Linda Keniston-Dubocq, a family practice physician in Maine, presents a detailed case study of a 32-year-old woman suffering from alcoholism who was successfully treated using the modalities of Maharishi Ayur-Veda.

Finally is a paper written by physician Hari Sharma (Professor of Pathophysiology at Ohio State Medical School), and research psychologist Michael Dillbeck and Susan Levin Dillbeck (MIU Professors of Psychology and Education, respectively). They review research on Maharishi Ayur-Veda and propose a model clinical program for the prevention of substance abuse among high risk juveniles that includes an experimental design to test its effectiveness.

The book concludes with an article by counseling psychologist and addictions treatment specialist David O'Connell on the integration of Maharishi Ayur-Veda with more conventional treatments of chemical dependence. The process of recovery through this new approach is considered in the context of a developmental perspective on the stages of recovery, and in relation to self-psychology theory and practice. Also, the implications of TM and Maharishi Ayur-Veda for spiritual development in recovery are considered.

This volume was conceived with two main goals in mind. The first was to present a totally new paradigm for the understanding and treatment of addiction based on this ancient holistic system of natural medicine. The second was to demonstrate the distinctive efficacy of this approach through the presentation of research and case studies on its application to chemical dependence. It is our hope that this volume will succeed in awakening the addictions field to this viable new approach that is complementary to conventional treatments for substance abuse.

This book, however, is not just about recovery from addiction. It is about recovery of the Self–the transcendental foundation of individual existence–the loss of which has rendered contemporary life less than fulfilling for us all. Rediscovery of our own essential Being is vital not only to recovery from addiction but to the blossoming of full human potential in higher states of consciousness, which lie latent within everyone.

REFERENCES

Alexander, C.N., Cranson, R.W., Boyer, R.W., & Orme-Johnson, D.W. (1987). Transcendental consciousness: A fourth state of consciousness beyond sleep, dreaming, and waking. In J. Gackenbach (Ed.), *Sleep and dreams: A sourcebook* (pp. 282-315). New York: Garland.

Alexander, C. N., Davies, J. L., Dixon, C. A., Dillbeck, M. C., Druker, S. M., Oetzel, R. M., Muehlman, J. M., & Orme-Johnson, D.W. (1990). Growth of higher stages of consciousness: Maharishi's Vedic psychology of human development. In C. N. Alexander & E. J. Langer (Eds.), *Higher stages of human development: Perspectives on adult growth* (pp. 286-340). New York: Oxford University Press.

Alexander, C. N., Rainforth, M.V., & Gelderloos, P. (1991). Transcendental Meditation, self-actualization, and psychological health: A conceptual overview and statistical meta-analysis. *Journal of Social Behavior and Personality, 6* (5), 189-247.

Alexander, C. N., Robinson, P., & Rainforth, M. (this volume). Treating and preventing alcohol, nicotine, and drug abuse through Transcendental Meditation: A review and statistical meta-analysis. *Alcoholism Treatment Quarterly.*

Bannerman, R. H., Burton, J., & Ch'en Wen-Chieh (Eds.) (1983). *Traditional medicine and health care coverage.* Geneva, Switzerland: World Health Organization.

Dillbeck, M. C. & Orme-Johnson, D. W. (1987). Physiological differences between Transcendental Meditation and rest. *American Psychologist, 42*, 879-881.

Eppley, K. R., Abrams, A. I., & Shear, J. (1989). Differential effects of relaxation techniques on trait anxiety: A meta-analysis. *Journal of Clinical Psychology, 45*, 957-974.

Jevning, R., Wallace, R. K., & Beidebach, M. (1992). The physiology of meditation: A review. A wakeful hypometabolic integrated response. *Neuroscience and Biobehavioral Reviews, 16*, 415-424.

Maharishi Mahesh Yogi. (1969). *On the Bhagavad-Gita: A translation and commentary, Chapters 1-6*. Baltimore: Penguin Press.

Maharishi Mahesh Yogi. (1986). *Life supported by natural law*. Washington, DC: Age of Enlightenment Press.

Patel, V. K., Wang, J., Shen, R. N., Sharma, H. M., & Brahmi, Z. (1992). *Nutrition Research, 12*, 51-61.

Sharma, H. (1993). *Freedom from disease*. Toronto: Veda Publishing.

Sharma, H. M., Dillbeck, M. C., & Dillbeck, S. L. (this volume). Implementation of the Transcendental Meditation program and Maharishi Ayur-Veda to prevent alcohol and drug abuse among juveniles at risk. *Alcoholism Treatment Quarterly*.

Sharma, H. M., Dwivedi, C., Satter, B. C., Gudehithlu, K. P., Abou-Issa, H., Malarkey, W., & Tejwani, G. A. (1990). Antineoplastic properties of Maharishi-4 against DMBA-induced mammary tumors in rats. *Pharmocology, Biochemistry, and Behavior, 35*, 767-773.

Sharma, H. M., Triguna, B. D., & Chopra, D. (1991). Maharishi Ayur-Veda: Modern insights into ancient medicine. *Journal of the American Medical Association, 265*, 2633-2637.

Wallace, R.K. (1970). Physiological effects of Transcendental Meditation. *Science, 167*, 1751-1754.

Wallace, R.K. & Benson, H. (1972). The physiology of meditation. *Scientific American, 226*, 84-90.

Wallace, R.K., Benson, H., & Wilson, A.F. (1971). A wakeful hypometabolic physiologic state. *American Journal of Physiology, 221*, 795-799.

SECTION I: THEORY AND RESEARCH ON TRANSCENDENTAL MEDITATION AND ADDICTIONS

Treating and Preventing Alcohol, Nicotine, and Drug Abuse Through Transcendental Meditation: A Review and Statistical Meta-Analysis

Charles N. Alexander, PhD
Pat Robinson, PhD, OTR
Maxwell Rainforth, MS, MA

Decades of efforts in the treatment of substance abuse have failed to yield a comprehensive treatment strategy that successfully addresses the multidimensional nature of chemical addiction. The current paper proposes that the Transcendental Meditation (TM) program provides a holistic, natural, and effective approach that positively impacts a constellation of factors–social, environmental, physiological, psychological, and spiritual–that influence addictive behavior.

This article is divided into three sections. Section one describes the scope of the problem of substance dependence and the limitations of current drug treatment approaches. Section two provides a

---

Charles N. Alexander, Pat Robinson, and Maxwell Rainforth are all affiliated with the Psychology Department of Maharishi International University in Fairfield, IA 52557.

The authors wish to thank Francine Greenstein for her research and editorial assistance and Mike Robinson for his technical assistance.

[Haworth co-indexing entry note]: "Treating and Preventing Alcohol, Nicotine, and Drug Abuse Through Transcendental Meditation: A Review and Statistical Meta-Analysis." Alexander, Charles N., Pat Robinson, and Maxwell Rainforth. Co-published simultaneously in the *Alcoholism Treatment Quarterly* (The Haworth Press, Inc.) Vol. 11, No. 1/2, 1994, pp. 13-87; and: *Self-Recovery: Treating Addictions Using Transcendental Meditation and Maharishi Ayur-Veda* (ed: David F. O'Connell and Charles N. Alexander) The Haworth Press, Inc., 1994, pp. 13-87. Multiple copies of this article/chapter may be purchased from The Haworth Document Delivery Center [1-800-3-HAWORTH; 9:00 a.m. - 5:00 p.m. (EST)].

theoretical framework–the Vedic Psychology of Maharishi Mahesh Yogi–and supporting research for understanding how TM may address the multiple causes of addiction. Section three begins with a qualitative review of 19 studies on the effects of TM on the use of alcohol, cigarettes, and illicit drugs. It then features a statistical meta-analysis that quantitatively compares the effects of TM with those of relaxation and standard treatments on substance use and its time course.

I. THE PROBLEMS OF SUBSTANCE DEPENDENCE

Scope of the Problem

The toll of chemical dependency on human health and happiness is staggering. Approximately 15 percent of the American population is chemically addicted to alcohol or drugs (Yoder, 1990). If family members of addicts are included, it is estimated that as many as three to four times this percentage is either addicted or directly affected by someone else's addiction (Yoder, 1990). Considering only alcohol related problems, the financial drain to society including reduced productivity, crimes, accidents, and health care services is projected to be $150 billion a year by 1995 (Health and Human Services, 1986). The U.S. Department of Health and Human Services (1992) has used heroin as an example of the costs associated with illicit drug use. The typical heroin addict commits an average of 178 crimes per year, costing society approximately $55,000 per year for *each* heroin user's criminal activities (Johnson et al., 1985).

However, financial burdens pale in comparison to human loss and suffering. According to a recent report issued by the Department of Health and Human Services (1992), cocaine-related medical emergencies in the United States rose 34.8% in the first quarter of 1992. Alcohol and other drugs are estimated to account for 52% of all traffic fatalities and 54% of violent crimes in the United States (in Hazelden, 1991). Furthermore, smoking remains the leading cause of avoidable death in America, estimated at 1,000 deaths a day; and, since 1987, lung cancer has replaced breast cancer as the leading cancer killer among women (Surgeon General, 1988). Even this partial list of statistics on the deleterious effects of substance abuse underscores the dire need of successful rehabilitation and prevention programs.

Causes, Treatments, Limitations

Rehabilitation involves not only the treatment of specific symptoms, but it also addresses the underlying causes of the problem. Therefore, the etiology of addiction is considered important to treatment planning. What factors account for chemical dependence? The reductionistic view that categorized chemical dependence as having a single cause producing a single effect has been replaced by the broader concept of addiction as a progressive behavior pattern that is the product of multiple, dynamically interacting domains (Health & Human Services, 1991; Klitzner, 1987; Marlatt, 1988). For example, the biopsychosocial model posits that addictive behaviors emerge from complex transactions among physiological, psychological, and social factors operating within a person's life (Brownell, 1982; Donovan, 1988; Orford, 1985; Schwartz, 1982). Environmental (Clarke & Saunders, 1988; Shoemaker & Sherry, 1991) and spiritual (Brown & Peterson, 1990; Rokeach, 1981; Whitfield, 1985) factors have also been suggested as significant contributors to the addictive process.

Although there are many forms of chemical dependence and abusers are a heterogeneous population, there appear to be a number of commonalities inherent in the etiology of addiction (Donovan & Marlatt, 1988). Within four domains–physiological, psychological, social/environmental, and spiritual–key processes and characteristics have been identified which may underlie a wide range of addictive behavior.

Physiological Factors

Donovan (1988) discusses three general categories of physiological factors which may be important precursors or contributors to addiction: constitutional predisposition; the immediate physiological effects of the addictive substance on the individual (such as the depletion of certain neurotransmitters: Saunders, 1988; Tennant,

1985); and development over time of tolerance, dependence and withdrawal symptoms in response to the addictive substance.

Psychological Factors

Extensive investigations into the psychological aspects of chemical dependence indicate that various aspects of personality, mood, and expectations are involved in the addictive process. Psychological factors consistently identified with addictive behavior include low self-esteem (Steffenhagen, 1980); lack of maturity (Rush, 1979); negative affect (Spotts & Shontz, 1991); impulsiveness (Solomon, 1977); rebelliousness (Jones, 1968); external locus of control (Hawkins, Lishner, & Catalano, 1985; Jurich & Polson, 1984); inadequate coping skills (Wills & Shiffman, 1985), cognitive distortions (Chatlos, 1989), and overlearned or stereotypic cognitive response patterns (Langer, Perlmutter, Chanowitz, & Rubin, 1988).

Barbara Yoder (1990), addressing the origins of addiction, emphasizes the key role of such psychological processes: "The process of addiction begins with shame and low self-esteem . . . . It's based on a fallacy–the notion that something outside of us can make us whole" (p. 3). In an effort to diminish low self-esteem and accompanying negative affect (including anxiety, depression and anger), individuals may turn to outside means, such as the addictive behavior, to compensate for lack of inner psychological resources. In the short term, recourse to addictive substances may provide an illusory sense of well-being, power, and control, but over the long term it undermines both the functioning of the nervous system and the ability to interact effectively with others. Thus, the addictive behavior which at first appeared to make life less painful and more controllable, itself becomes uncontrollable and debilitating (Donovan, 1988; Rodin, Maloff, & Becker, 1984). Individuals possessing such suboptimal psychological characteristics may be particularly vulnerable to social and environmental stressors and thus be all the more prone to turn to drugs in a maladaptive attempt to cope with stress (Oetting & Beauvais, 1987).

Social/Environmental Factors

Social and environmental factors are considered in one category because these variables together are considered forces extrinsic to the individual. Social factors are those proximal aspects of one's surroundings that involve relationships with other people. How a person reacts to friends, co-workers, and family and how others respond to the individual form the hub of social interactions. Some key social factors thought to impact substance dependence include poor family relations, peer pressure, and lack of immediate social support (Beckman & Bardsley, 1986; Clarke & Saunders, 1988; Health & Human Services, 1991; Oetting & Beauvais, 1989). Cultural/environmental variables comprise more distal, overarching and enduring factors that may negatively impact drug use, such as lack of societal cohesion, crime, poverty, unemployment, racism, poor education, and inadequate health care access (Clarke & Saunders, 1988; Elliot, Huizinger, & Ageton, 1985; Health & Human Services, 1991; Long & Scherl, 1984).

Spiritual Factors

It has also been postulated that spiritual problems are a bedrock of addictive and other destructive behaviors (Jung, 1933). Moore (1992, p. xii) remarks that, "The great malady of the twentieth century, implicated in all our troubles and affecting us individually and socially is 'loss of soul.' When soul is neglected, it doesn't just go away; it appears symptomatically in obsessions, addictions, violence, and loss of meaning." Soul is described, "not as a thing," but as a subtle dimension of one's existence that deals with a person's essential value, "personal substance," connectedness to others and existence as a whole.

Moore (1992, p. xvi) hypothesizes that the plethora of complaints of modern living which drive people to seek outside help–emptiness, vague depression, disillusionments about marriage and family, loss of values, and a yearning for spiritual fulfillment–all are symptoms of spiritual deficiency. This spiritual malaise may arise from loss of contact with one's ultimate source or foundation, whether conceived of as an inner soul (Moore, 1992; Whitfield, 1985) or as a "Higher Power" (Alcoholics Anonymous World Services, 1981). (From the perspective of Maharishi's Vedic Psychology, "spirit" or "soul" refers ultimately to the transcendental level, or universal Self, at the basis of individual life–see later *Spiritual Factors* subsection of Section II).

Spiritual aspects figure prominently in some formulas for recovery from chemical dependence, such as the Twelve Steps programs (Gorski, 1989) and the Hazelden (1991) program. However, there have been only a few empirical studies explicitly documenting the effects of spiritual factors on chemical dependence (e.g., Brown & Peterson, 1990; Padelford, 1974; Shoemaker & Sherry, 1991).

It may be that a profound sense of well-being only arises naturally from the healthy functioning of all aspects of individual life–body, mind, spirit, social interaction, and environment. When one or more dimensions of life are deficient, people experience lack of personal fulfillment, placing them at risk for seeking to restore a sense of wholeness through chemical substances.

Thus if treatment is to be successful and sustainable, it must be capable of addressing all the levels potentially involved in the addictive process (Donovan, Kivlahan, & Walker, 1986).

Treatments

For the purposes of this paper, four general treatment categories are identified which share commonalities with the approaches outlined by Brickman et al. (1982) and Marlatt (1988). Each category addresses a major factor thought to underlie addictive behavior. Contemporary treatment of chemical dependence may typically involve at least two treatment categories (Alford, Koehler, & Leonard, 1991; Schroeder, 1991).

1. The *medical* approach focuses on the physiological aspects of addiction. Addiction is viewed primarily as a disease of the body, and experts treat the disease by employing pharmacological agents. Each prescription typically acts upon a single arena of physiological functioning (Dongier & Schwartz, 1989).
2. The *psychological* approach is utilized primarily by professional therapists. It usually addresses the cognitive and/or emotional domains. Techniques employing the cognitive restructuring approach, such as Ellis' rationale emotive therapy or Beck's cognitive therapies, emphasize self management skills and target the correction of faulty intellectual discriminations (such as, "I should retaliate every criticism directed

toward me"), and misinformation (such as, "Alcoholism really only occurs in the population of derelicts") (Clarke & Saunders, 1988). Therapeutic interventions directed toward resolving the emotional problems of addicts include the approach of psychodynamic self psychology (see O'Connell, this volume).

3. The *spiritual* approach addresses spiritual shortcomings related to addiction. Self-help groups, including the widely proliferated and popular Twelve Steps programs include this approach. The Twelve Steps hold that addicts cannot solve their problems alone and positive change is possible only by surrendering control to a "Higher Power." Also incorporating this approach are professional therapeutic programs designed to realign core values, such as Brown and Peterson's (1991) values clarification procedures.
4. The *social/environmental* category focuses on changing social interaction and broader sociocultural processes that underlie addictive behavior. Community-based programs complement the other three general treatment approaches and may include behavioral or attitudinal training to encourage abstinence or prevention. For example, the Twelve Steps "group" provides strong social support that may include modeling, where the addict is expected to emulate an abstinent member's behavior (Gorski, 1989). Some community-based rehabilitation programs focus on proximal social relations strongly impacting on substance use, such as the family (Stanton & Todd, 1979) or same-age peers (Kofoed, Tolson, Atkinson, Toth, & Turner, 1987). Broader prevention-oriented programs encompassing educational, social, and job training activities are also included in this category.

Limitations of Treatment

Despite the availability of medical, psychological, spiritual, and social/environmental approaches, the effects of treatment have been neither uniform nor widely successful in any of these categories (McLellan, Alterman, Cacciola, Metzger, & O'Brien, 1992).

The medical approach has yet to find a "cure" for addiction or provide side-effect free medications. While pharmacology can be effective in coping with the physical symptoms, it still involves reliance upon an external (albeit more acceptable) chemical agent and thus cannot empower healing from within.

Despite the billions of dollars spent yearly on psychological treatment in the United States (Hollister, 1990), evidence suggests that different types of professional counseling for alcoholism as well as various settings (residential versus out-patient, longer versus shorter in-patient programs) do not differ significantly in terms of outcome (Hester & Miller, 1989). Emrick (1975) has reported that untreated alcoholics often improve as much as those receiving formal treatment. Treatment for chemical dependence is dogged by high drop-out rates, and, for those completing treatment, formidable relapse rates. For substance abuse programs, including alcohol, Stark (1992) reported an attrition of greater than 50% within the first month of treatment. Of those adults actually completing treatment for alcohol and drug dependence, nearly two-thirds relapse within 90 days of discharge from treatment (Surgeon General, 1988). Adolescent recidivism rates for drug rehabilitation are similarly elevated (Catalano, Hawkins, Wells, & Miller, 1990-91).

While the spiritual/social approach of Twelve Steps programs is widely used, low in cost, and provides useful social support, several limitations have been noted. Statistics on outcomes involving the Twelve Steps have been sparse by virtue of its tradition of anonymity (Hollister, 1990). However, self-report data reported on the AA Twelve Steps program indicates that 50%-60% of those attending meetings who do not receive concurrent professional help drop out within 90 days of their first meeting (Gorski, 1989). On a practical level, some people report difficulty believing in and/or contacting a Higher Power (Christopher, 1988; Levin, 1987; Rachel V., 1992). Also, some members note a lack of peace of mind despite achievement of abstinence (Hazelden, 1991).

More distal environmental approaches to solving and preventing substance abuse, such as prevention-oriented education of parents and abusers, have made substantial progress in increasing public awareness of the problems to be solved, but, to date, have been insufficient to curb epidemic levels of serious substance abuse (U.S. Dept. of Health & Human Services, 1991).

Regardless of the general treatment approach, relapse rates remain unacceptably high. What causes relapse? Not surprisingly, factors exacerbating relapse are similar to those components thought to underlie addictive behavior itself, including physical withdrawal distress, negative emotional states, interpersonal conflicts, social pressure, and stressful environments (Cronkite & Moos, 1980; Cummings, Gordon, & Marlatt, 1980; Gorski & Miller, 1986; Shiffman 1979). Unfortunately, current treatments, even when they involve aspects of all major treatment categories, typically fail to effectively address the complex phenomenon of addiction. What alternative strategies could be envisioned for the comprehensive treatment of addiction?

Alternative Treatment Recommendations

Greaves (1980) suggests that treatments for addiction have generally failed because "We want the person to give up something that gives him pleasure and/or relieves stress while offering little in return except vague, distant promises of a better life and improved self-esteem" (p. 26). Consistent with Greaves' recommendations, several replacement behaviors have been suggested that aim to relieve stress and enhance happiness, while promoting self-sufficiency rather than dependence on external agents. These nonpharmacological, self-directed approaches include meditation, relaxation training, expressive art therapy, and exercise (Greaves, 1980; Friedman & Glickman, 1986; Clarke & Saunders, 1988; Marlatt & George, 1984).

While broadly recommending meditation and relaxation, many programs do not delineate specific means to achieve the desired benefits. For example, the eleventh step of the Twelve Steps program recommends meditation or contemplation exercises but does not suggest a specific approach (Gorski, 1989). However, scientific methods can provide useful tools for objectively determining the relative efficacy of different treatment approaches, including meditation and relaxation techniques.

The most widely researched method of meditation is the Transcendental Meditation (TM) program, a simple mental technique which is practiced twenty minutes twice daily. This technique was brought to light by Maharishi Mahesh Yogi (1966) from the Vedic tradition of India which has its source in the ancient Rik Veda. More than 500 studies on TM have been conducted at over 200 research centers worldwide. The TM program is appropriate for diverse populations because it requires no change in lifestyle or beliefs, is taught in a simple, standardized course, and is reported to be effortless to practice (Alexander & Sands, 1993; Denniston, 1986; Maharishi, 1969). Moreover, research indicates that TM may be distinctively effective in producing substantive, holistic changes across the major domains of life believed to be significant for the treatment and prevention of substance dependence (Alexander, 1993; Eppley, Abrams, & Shear, 1989; Gelderloos, Walton, Orme-Johnson, & Alexander, 1991).

What mechanism allows this simple technique to provide multidimensional effects for the individual? The mechanics of TM may be explained in the context of Maharishi's Vedic Psychology (Maharishi, 1969, 1986; Orme-Johnson, 1988).

II. A THEORETICAL FRAMEWORK FOR UNDERSTANDING THE EFFECTS OF TM ON SUBSTANCE DEPENDENCE: MAHARISHI'S VEDIC PSYCHOLOGY

Maharishi's Vedic Psychology recognizes that individual life is composed of multiple domains. However, unlike the biopsychosocial model and other systems theories, it sequentially orders these domains in terms of depth and comprehensiveness of functioning. In Maharishi's explanation (Maharishi, 1972), the mind is hierarchically structured in layers that are progressively more subtle, abstract, and more unified. At the most active and concrete level of mental functioning are the faculties of action and the senses (see Figure 1). The senses are said to be the interface between the body (the physiological domain) and the deeper levels of the mind. Guided by the senses, the body performs actions. More subtle is the level of the thinking mind which gives direction to the senses and behavior through the processes of thought and memory. The thinking mind is in turn directed by the intellect which makes decisions about the contents of the mind. Deeper still is the level of feeling and intuition which informs and guides decision-making. At the subtlest level of the mind is the individual ego (the "I"), or active experiencer who knows the world through all the other levels

FIGURE 1. Levels of the mind according to Maharishi's Vedic Psychology.

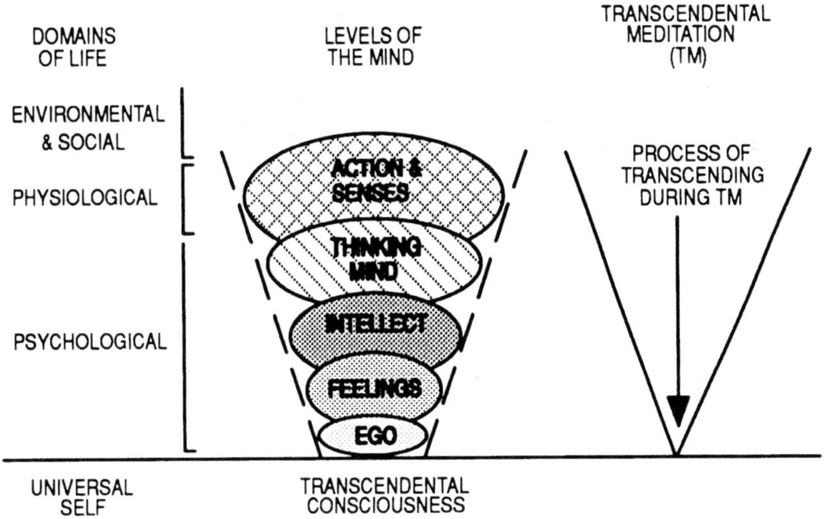

of mental functioning. These four levels of mind are said to constitute the individual self (comprising the psychological domain).

Finally, according to Vedic Psychology, underlying the subtlest level of functioning of the individual is the transcendental Self or Being, an abstract, silent, unified field of pure consciousness, identified as the self-sufficient source of all mental processes. Maharishi (1969) explains:

> Self has two connotations: lower self and higher Self. The lower self is that aspect of the personality which deals only with the relative [i.e., changing] aspect of existence . . . the mind that thinks, the intellect that decides, the ego that experiences. This lower self functions only in the relative states of existence–waking, dreaming, and deep sleep. . . . The higher Self is that aspect which never changes [i.e., unchanging], absolute Being, which is the very basis of the entire field of relativity, including the lower self. (p. 339)

Contemporary psychological perspectives on spirituality deal primarily with the deeper aspects of the individual self experienced in the waking state (cf. Moore, 1992). But, according to Maharishi's Vedic Psychology, deeper than the individual self is the transcendental Self which is described as the common origin of all minds, the "Self of all Beings" (Maharishi, 1969, p. 338). This non-changing level lies transcendental to the "lower self," which deals only with the changing values of the world–perceptions, thoughts, values, and feelings. Research indicates that very few people "actualize" the deepest levels of their own individual nature (e.g., Alexander, Rainforth, & Gelderloos, 1991; Chandler, 1991) much less realize their universal nature or higher Self which is said to provide the foundation for all aspects of individual life.

If the higher Self or Being is the essential nature of the mind, why does the experience of Self remain outside the realm of daily experience? Maharishi (1966) explains this seeming discrepancy using the process of vision as an example:

> Since the mind ordinarily remains attuned to the senses, projecting outwards towards the manifested realms of creation, it misses or fails to appreciate its own essential nature, just as the eyes are unable to see themselves. Everything but the eyes themselves can be seen through the eyes. Similarly, everything is based on the essential nature of the mind . . . and yet, while the mind is engaged in the projected field of manifested diversity, Being [pure consciousness] is not appreciated by the mind, although it is the very basis and essential constituent. (p. 30)

If the mind is to experience its subtler levels and ultimately the inner Self, then somehow the outward march of the mind through the senses must be reversed. The TM technique is described as a means of reversing the ordinary thinking process by allowing awareness to settle down to deeper, quieter levels until the finest level of the individual ego or "I" is transcended and the mind experiences its source. This is the experience of pure consciousness–consciousness alone without thoughts or fluctuations–the silent Self or Being (Maharishi, 1986).

In the ancient traditions of both East and West, it was maintained that the deepest desire of man is to "Know the Self" or to experience one's own essential Being. It could be said we all "crave" the experience of our own ultimate nature. If it is the case that the ordinary activity of waking state denies us the experience of our Self, just as the "eyes are unable to see themselves" (Maharishi, 1966, p. 30), then how do we know ourselves? If we want to see our eyes, we must turn to their reflection in a mirror. Likewise, when the deep desire to know the Self is unfulfilled, we typically look to things outside of ourselves, confirming our identity through the reflection of other people's opinions and our accomplishments or possessions. Thus we become dependent upon means extrinsic to ourselves to fulfill ourselves and to identify who we are. However, ownership of things is a poor substitute for ownership of the Self. When taken to an extreme, this process of "object-referral"–referring to objects or others outside of ourselves to know who we are–places us at risk for chemical dependence as we search for increasingly potent external substitutes for the lost, inner experience of the Self.

In providing a natural, "self-referral" experience of the Self alone, undisturbed by sensory or mental activity, TM gratifies this craving for direct Self-knowledge. Maharishi (1969, p. 424) describes this rediscovery of the "Being of the Self" as fulfilling because "having come home, the traveler finds peace. . . . This state of self-sufficiency leaves one steadfast in oneself, fulfilled." The experience of one's inherent Self is not only immediately gratifying, but is said to holistically nourish all the more manifest levels of life (ego, feelings, thought and action) that spring from this source. Thus, "watering the root" of Being through TM (as one waters the root of a tree) is predicted to simultaneously benefit all levels of functioning potentially related to problems of substance abuse. Evidence supporting this prediction is presented below.

Effects of TM on Physiological, Psychological, Spiritual, and Social/Environmental Factors

Physiological Factors

Individuals at risk for drug addiction typically cope poorly with environmental and interpersonal stressors, which leads to a chronic state of physiological overarousal and mental anxiety. Such individuals may seek drugs as a path of relief from tension and negative feelings. While the immediate effects of the drug may temporarily ameliorate mental distress, the drug itself further disrupts the equilibrium of the body, creating more imbalance and distress which in turn causes the individual to seek relief through ingestion of more addictive substances. Chronic substance abuse results in the depletion of key neurotransmitters such as serotonin that are involved in the regulation of homeostasis, and in the overproduction of cortisol, a hormone triggered in the "stress response" (see Walton & Levitsky, this volume).

TM appears to provide a natural antidote to this cycle of addiction. Each experience of TM provides the body deep rest which neutralizes accumulated stress and restores psychophysiological balance (Wallace, 1993). A statistical meta-analysis (see Section III for a definition) of 31 physiological studies found that during TM there is a significantly greater reduction in physiological arousal as indicated by lower respiration rate, skin conductance level, and plasma lactate (a stress hormone) compared to simply resting with eyes closed (Dillbeck & Orme-Johnson, 1987). Also, TM subjects showed significantly lower baseline levels of arousal than controls, suggesting that a cumulative effect was being maintained outside the meditation experience as well (Dillbeck & Orme-Johnson, 1987). Moreover, opposite to the effects of stress leading to addiction, experiments indicate that TM significantly increases serotonin and reduces cortisol (indicating reduced arousal) in as short a time as four months of practice (MacLean et al., 1992). Other studies also have demonstrated enhanced serotonin function in both disabled (Subrahmanyam & Porkodi, 1980) and nondisabled populations through TM (Bujatti & Riederer, 1976).

Research indicates that TM also enhances resistance to stress during daily activity by promoting more rapid mobilization, habituation, and stability of autonomic response to stressful stimuli (Brooks & Scarano, 1985; Goleman & Schwartz, 1976; Orme-Johnson, 1973) than various control conditions.

Because of the severity and complexity of the physiology of addiction, the mental approach of TM may be complemented by use of natural physical approaches provided by Maharishi Ayur-Veda to purify and balance physiological functioning (see Glaser, and also Sands, in this volume, on the multiple strategies of this traditional, prevention-oriented health care system).

According to Maharishi's Vedic Psychology, it is changes in

mental functioning, through the enlivening of pure consciousness during TM, that underlie the physiological benefits described above. The following section details these positive changes.

Psychological Factors

There have been a large number of empirical investigations on the influence of TM on psychological factors associated with addiction. This research will be presented according to the levels of the mind (described above), beginning with action or behavior; followed by the thinking and discriminatory levels; then, the more delicate feelings and individual ego levels. Emphasis will be placed on the deeper levels of feeling and ego because Maharishi's Vedic Psychology views these as the most influential.

Action/behavior level. Action is said to be initiated through the senses and motor functions, which, in turn, are directed by deeper mental levels. A tendency toward impulsive and rebellious behavior is associated with individuals at risk for substance abuse. Because impulsive responses typically lack effective direction from deeper, more powerful levels of mental functioning (such as reasoning), they are often maladaptive and consequently unsuccessful. Maharishi (1966) explains that the inability to fulfill desires in appropriate ways may lead to more extreme antisocial responses, such as crime and chemical dependence.

The TM program has been shown to reduce impulsive and rebellious behaviors in prison inmates, as measured by reduced aggression, hostility, rule infractions, and substantially reduced recidivism (criminal relapse) for up to six years after release (Abrams & Siegel, 1978; Alexander, 1982; Bleick & Abrams, 1987). Also, TM has been shown to reduce impulsivity and aggressiveness in the normal population (Penner, Zingle, Dyck, & Truch, 1974), to enhance positive social behaviors such as academic performance in school (Kember, 1985), and productivity on the job (Alexander, Swanson, Rainforth, Carlisle, & Todd, 1993, Frew, 1974). Vedic Psychology holds that such improvements in behavior spontaneously result from positive changes at the deeper levels of mind.

Thinking/intellectual level. Chemical dependence has been linked to a wide range of cognitive dysfunctions, including disorganized thinking, poor coping skills, inadequate decision-making, and inflexible cognitive response patterns. The focus of current cognitive treatment methods on retraining the addict's style and content of thinking has dominated the field, at least in part, because of the assumption that while the *contents* of the mind can be altered, the fundamental *capacity* of the mind tends to be fixed by adolescence (Cattell, 1946). TM offers a complementary approach to current treatment strategies by focusing on unfoldment of deeper, latent capacities of the mind itself.

A number of longitudinal studies have shown growth of fluid intelligence in TM practitioners compared to matched control groups at an age (young adulthood) when such changes do not typically occur (e.g., Aron, Orme-Johnson, & Brubaker, 1981; Cranson et al., 1991; Dillbeck, Assimakis, Raimondi, Orme-Johnson, & Rowe, 1986). Related aspects of mind and intellect have also shown improvement through TM, including cognitive flexibility (Alexander et al., 1989; Dillbeck, 1982); choice reaction time (Cranson et al., 1991); learning and memory (Dillbeck, Orme-Johnson, & Wallace, 1981); creativity (Travis, 1979); and moral reasoning (Chandler, 1991).

While decision-making guides behavior, Maharishi's Vedic Psychology proposes that the deeper level of feeling, in turn, strongly impacts on the quality and direction of decisions.

Feeling level. Numerous studies indicate that substance dependence is associated with negative emotions, such as depression, anxiety, and anger. Because drugs alter mood, it is widely recognized that a substantial portion of substance abuse revolves around the creation of a temporary positive mood and escape of negative feelings. However, as tolerance to drugs increase, greater amounts are required to create a momentary "high," which is followed by the inevitable crash to negative feelings. Conversely, extensive research indicates that TM alters mood naturally, reducing negative emotions and increasing positive affect. This change is immediate during TM and quickly generalizes to activities outside of meditation (Gelderloos, Hermans, Ahlstrom, & Jacoby, 1990). Thus, one's emotions become progressively more positive and stable, the opposite of the affective sequelae of addiction.

In an exhaustive statistical meta-analysis, Eppley, Abrams, and Shear (1989) analyzed anxiety outcomes of 146 meditation and relaxation treatment groups. TM was compared to a wide variety of treatments, including progressive muscle relaxation, the relaxation response, concentration meditation, EMG biofeedback, and various placebo techniques. The results indicated that TM reduced trait anxiety (i.e., chronic stress) significantly more than the other meditation or relaxation techniques studied. Other techniques (including the placebos) produced more modest effect sizes, except for concentration meditation which appeared to produce no effects on anxiety. These overall conclusions were sustained even after controlling for possible confounding factors such as type of population, age, sex, experimental design, researcher bias, duration and hours of treatment, pretest anxiety, expectation, and attrition.

Similar differential reductions in depression and anger have been shown for TM practitioners compared to treated and untreated controls (Alexander, 1982; Abrams & Siegel, 1978). For example, over a three-month period, a random assignment study found TM to be more effective than psychotherapy in decreasing depression, anxiety, and emotional numbness in Vietnam veterans suffering from post-traumatic stress disorder (Brooks & Scarano, 1985).

Other research indicates that TM practitioners also experience significant improvements in positive affect, including increased happiness, well-being (Gelderloos, 1987; Weiss, 1990), and emotional stability (Overbeck, 1982; Penner et al., 1974). A recent statistical meta-analysis (Alexander, Rainforth, & Gelderloos, 1991) showed that TM also produced a significantly larger effect on the growth of positive affect than other forms of meditation and relaxation studied, as indicated by enhanced capacity for intimate contact, openness to one's feelings, and spontaneity.

According to Maharishi's Vedic Psychology, emotional well-being, in turn, depends upon development, at a deeper level, of a strong and secure "I" or ego.

Individual ego level. Vedic Psychology views the ego as the subtlest level of the individual mind. The ego, or "I" actively experiences the world through the senses, thinking, and feelings–coordinating information from all the more manifest levels of the mind. Thus, the "I" forms the basis of the "self" (with a small "s") which is held to be composed of the ego, feelings, intellect, and mind (Maharishi, 1969). A strong ego or "I," then, provides the foundation for an integrated self, because when the ego is strengthened, all levels of the mind are positively influenced.

Unfortunately, although the ego has an enormous impact on thought and feelings, research indicates that it typically becomes "set" in its mode of functioning by late adolescence (Loevinger, 1976; Loevinger et al., 1985). Moreover, once solidified, ego development has proven highly recalcitrant to change by treatment interventions (Cook-Greuter, 1990). This poses a significant challenge for recovery from chemical dependence because, as reported earlier, low self-esteem appears to be at the very bedrock of the addictive process. Individuals with low self-esteem look "outside the self" (Yoder, 1990, p. 3) for support and fulfillment, placing them at risk for chemical dependence. In contrast, through TM, one effortlessly accesses the most refined level of the individual "I," and thereby strengthens the integrity of the ego from within. Maharishi (1969, p. 423) explains how, during TM, the status of the "pure individuality of the 'I'" is gained en route to the experience of the universal status of Self or Being: "In the process of transcending, the mind retires from the experience of multiplicity and gains the experience of . . . its own individual nature. Then, transcending its individual status, it expands into cosmic Being, . . . the state of transcendental consciousness."

Each time awareness experiences the subtlest level of the "I" and then merges into transcendental Self-consciousness, the individual self is said to be profoundly nourished from its foundation. Thus, ego development would be predicted to be substantially influenced through TM practice.

Indeed, self-esteem, as measured by psychological instruments such as the Tennessee Self-concept Scale, the Netherlands Personality Inventory, and the Repertory Grid, has been shown to significantly improve after only 1-3 months of TM practice (Nystul & Garde, 1977; Van Den Berg & Mulder, 1976; Turnbull & Norris, 1982). Similar gains in self-reliance (Gelderloos et al., 1991), internal locus of control (Hjelle, 1974) and field independence (Pelletier, 1974) have been evidenced in TM practitioners compared to matched or random assignment controls.

According to the humanistic psychologist Abraham Maslow (1968), the apex of personal development is a state of "self-actualization" in which the unique potential of the individual is realized. Self-actualizers are said to be characterized by high self-esteem, ego integration, creativity, moral vision, and respect for others and nature (Maslow, 1968, p. 26). Not surprisingly, research indicates that very few individuals, less than 1% of the general population, appear to achieve a mature level of self-actualization (Cook-Greuter, 1990). (The perspective of Maharishi's Vedic Psychology on the ultimate goal of human development is described below).

Results of a recent comprehensive meta-analysis suggest that contact with the deepest levels of mind, through TM, may be distinctively effective in promoting self-actualization (Alexander, Rainforth, & Gelderloos, 1991: 42 separate treatment groups evaluated). In contrast to other forms of meditation and relaxation which showed only a modest influence on self-actualization, TM produced a marked effect (controlling for duration of interventions and strength of experimental design). After only a three-month average intervention, TM subjects increased by 30% on the major composite scale of the most widely used measure of self-actualization, the Personal Orientation Inventory. Longer treatment time resulted in larger effect sizes for TM (but not for other techniques), suggesting this practice has a cumulative influence.

Two additional longitudinal studies of college graduates and prison inmates indicate that TM promotes advanced ego development (as measured by Loevinger's scale, 1976) beyond late adolescence. A ten-year study indicated that alumni of Maharishi International University (MIU) who practiced TM markedly increased in ego development compared to alumni from three control universities over the same period who were matched for age, gender, and pretest year (Chandler, 1991; Chandler & Alexander, in review: total N = 136). Moreover, the MIU alumni had a higher percentage achieve the two highest levels (indicative of self-actualization) than any of the 40 other groups surveyed in the extant literature.

Another longitudinal study (Alexander, 1982) examined self-development in 133 adult maximum-security prisoners with a known history of drug abuse, a population viewed as highly resistant to further developmental progress (Martin, Sechrest, & Redner, 1981). Over a 13-17 month period, the TM group increased by one full stage in ego development compared to wait-list controls and four other treatment programs. This growth in psychological maturity would appear to account for the one-third lower criminal relapse (recidivism) rate found for TM parolees over a 3.5-year period compared to random samples from the other four programs. This latter study suggests that regardless of the starting point–even in adults with serious anti-social problems–TM can cultivate the inner development of the ego. Thus TM appears to holistically improve psychological functioning at all levels of the individual self, correcting tendencies that can lead to addiction.

Whereas the pure individuality of the "I" or ego constitutes the subtlest level of the individual self, Maharishi's Vedic Psychology proposes that the ultimate spiritual foundation of life is the universal Self or pure consciousness at the source of the individual mind. The unfoldment of pure consciousness–which is also referred to as transcendental consciousness–will be explored more fully in the following section.

Spiritual Factors

A few visionary psychologists have recognized the possibility of experiencing a purely transcendental or universal level of the mind (James, 1902/1958; Jung, 1933; Maslow, 1964). Although such experiences are almost always described as "ineffable" and fleeting in nature, these thinkers held that they can still profoundly impact the quality and meaning of life. For example, Maslow (1964, p. 75) once remarked that just one "peak" experience–described as a moment of "transcendent ecstasy"–can promote self-actualization and alter the course of addiction and other self-destructive behaviors. Some of the experiences Maslow described bear similarity to those reported by TM practitioners. Several case studies subjectively report the profound effect of even the initial experience of transcendental consciousness through TM on the lives of drug abusers (Bleick, this volume; Ellis & Corum, this volume; O'Connell, 1991).

Until recently, transcendental experiences have occurred spontaneously with such rarity that they could not be systematically studied in the laboratories. Hence, their proposed existence and potential benefits lay outside the realm of objective verification through scientific research. However, since TM is said to systematically promote the experience of transcendental consciousness–even under laboratory conditions–it has enabled direct scientific investigation of the psychophysiology of transcendence. Consistent with both subjective experience and the prediction of Vedic Psychology, transcendental consciousness experienced through TM has been shown to be a distinctive state of "restful alertness," differing from ordinary waking, dreaming and sleeping on over 20 psychophysiological parameters (Alexander, Cranson, Boyer, & Orme-Johnson, 1987).

Two striking findings particularly support this claim. When subjects were requested to press a button immediately after experiencing transcendental consciousness during TM, their button presses were found to be highly correlated with a period of natural breath suspension up to one minute in length, indicating a profound state of physiological rest. Also these button presses were correlated with heightened EEG coherence across frequency band and cortical location, suggesting a simultaneous state of heightened alertness (Badawi, Wallace, Orme-Johnson, & Rouzere, 1984; Farrow & Hebert, 1982). This interpretation is bolstered by the finding that elevated EEG coherence during TM is also significantly correlated with several indicators of mental alertness outside of the practice, including enhanced neural reaction time, fluid intelligence, concept formation, creativity, and moral reasoning (e.g., Dillbeck, Orme-Johnson, & Wallace, 1981; Orme-Johnson & Haynes, 1981).

If this profound state of restful alertness simultaneously nourishes all levels of functioning, then it follows that those TM practitioners who experience transcendental consciousness with greater frequency and clarity should display even more marked holistic improvements. Indeed, this has been shown to be the case for measures of all levels of mental functioning–including sensory-motor speed and flexibility; non-verbal intelligence and creativity; reduced emotional distress and greater well-being; and enhanced internal locus of control, ego development, and self-actualization (see review by Alexander, Gerace, Rainforth, & Beto, in press). These findings thus lend objective support to Maslow's claim that transcendental or peak experiences can profoundly impact on the quality of individual life.

According to Vedic Psychology, however, the purpose of spiritual growth is not temporary experience of transcendence but a stable state of enlightenment in which the full potential of the mind is permanently realized. Maharishi (1969) predicts that repeated experience of transcendental consciousness during TM provides the foundation for the sequential unfoldment of three stable higher states of consciousness. He explains that the first stable state of enlightenment, termed cosmic consciousness, is realized when the nervous system is entirely free of stress and transcendental consciousness is permanently experienced along with waking, dreaming, and sleeping. Only at this level is true freedom from craving and dependence achieved because awareness is now permanently established in the self-referral state of Being (pure consciousness), and remains completely fulfilled, undisturbed by changes on the active, surface levels of life.

Just as the development of individual identity provides the foundation for personal relationships (cf. Erikson, 1968), the development of a cosmic identity, or the universal Self, would appear to provide the natural basis for developing profound intimacy not only with other individuals but with all of life. Through continued practice of TM and the other approaches of Maharishi Ayur-Veda (Glaser, this volume), a sixth state of consciousness–termed refined cosmic consciousness or God consciousness–is said to dawn, in which feelings and perceptions are optimally developed and one comes to fully appreciate the creator and creation (Maharishi, 1969).

Maharishi (1969) states that this intimacy between the inner Self and outer creation experienced in the sixth state naturally culminates in complete union of Self and world in the seventh state of consciousness, termed unity consciousness. Whereas pure consciousness was initially experienced as the inner, transcendental foundation of subjective experience, in unity consciousness, it is experienced as permeating all of outer, objective existence as well. Thus, all of existence, external and internal, is now realized to be nothing but the Self functioning within itself.

Thus growth of complete self-sufficiency and inner contentment in higher states of consciousness is predicted to lead to satisfying relationships based on mutual appreciation and on sharing of abundant inner resources rather than on the need for approval from others. The following section discusses the effects of TM not only on social relationships but on the environment as a whole.

Social and Environmental Factors

Contemporary psychology acknowledges that social milieus profoundly influence individual functioning (Murphy, 1992; Whitehead, 1978). Adverse social contexts characterized by poor family cohesion, low social support, or negative peer pressure all contribute to a poor self-concept and the need to seek well-being and peer recognition through substance abuse. However, the individual need not be victimized by these circumstances. Because of the reciprocal relationship between the individual and social environment, when the individual is profoundly nourished from within through TM, this provides a natural basis for giving more and receiving more from others.

Several studies suggest that TM improves capacity for warm personal relationships, sociability, and appreciation of others (Alexander et al., 1991; Geisler, 1978; Gelderloos et al., 1987), thus leading to enhanced marital and job satisfaction and better relations with co-workers (Aron & Aron, 1982; Broome, 1989; Alexander, Swanson, Rainforth, Carlisle, & Todd, 1993).

But what can be done to influence the broader environment, including pervasive factors such as violence, poverty, and racism—that burden already vulnerable individuals and families, placing them at greater risk for chemical dependence? As stated earlier, Vedic Psychology holds that Being, or the Self, is a unified field of consciousness underlying and connecting all of humanity. If this is the case, then contacting and enlivening this underlying field by a critical mass of people practicing TM could create a positive influence throughout society (Maharishi, 1988).

In fact, over 40 sociological studies now indicate that as little as 1% of a population practicing TM, or even the square root of that number practicing the advanced TM and TM-Sidhi program in a group, significantly decreases negative social trends and improves quality of life in the whole society (Orme-Johnson, this volume).

Significant societal changes include reductions in crime, auto accidents, homicides, suicides, and political violence, along with improvements in economic indicators and political cooperation in the populations studied (e.g., Cavanaugh, King, & Ertuna, 1989; Dillbeck, 1990; Orme-Johnson, Alexander, Davies, Chandler, & Larimore, 1988).

Although only a few of these studies have directly assessed reduction of substance abuse in society, more than 20 have documented substantial reduction in violent crimes and traffic accidents, a substantial proportion of which are recognized to occur under the influence of alcohol or other substances. This provides intriguing indirect evidence that this collective influence not only reduces negative societal factors (such as crime) contributing to drug abuse but may also reduce the incidence of substance abuse itself in the larger society. Thus, TM may be useful, not only in treating individual addicts, but in preventing broader negative conditions in society that otherwise foster drug abuse and other forms of anti-social behavior.

Summary

Research indicates that TM produces a wide range of physiological, psychological, spiritual, social, and environmental effects opposite those associated with the causes of addiction. Moreover, these effects occur naturally as a by-product of neutralizing stress and experiencing greater inner fulfillment, with no attempt made to manipulate behavior, beliefs, or attitudes. As inner contentment and fulfillment grow, the need to seek gratification outside of one's self naturally subsides and addictive behavior falls off.

If TM is capable of holistically strengthening all levels of individual life, then it offers (1) *primary prevention* (Skinner, 1981) by inoculating individuals against the stress and dissatisfaction leading to initial substance use; (2) *secondary prevention* (Skinner, 1981) through stemming the downward spiral of growing dependence that can turn a casual user into an addict; (3) *treatment* of addictions by reversing long-standing weaknesses and imbalances; and (4) *relapse prevention* since factors exacerbating relapse are similar to those leading to initial chemical dependence (Brownell, Marlatt, Lichtenstein, & Wilson, 1986).

TM's capacity to reduce substance abuse in the general population (preventing addiction) and to promote abstinence in heavy users (thereby treating addiction and preventing relapse) will be directly assessed in the next section.

III. THE EFFECTS OF TM ON SUBSTANCE ABUSE

This section presents both a narrative review and a quantitative summary called a meta-analysis, on the effects of TM on alcohol, cigarettes, and illicit drugs (which include cannabis products, hallucinogens, and narcotics). This review includes consideration of legal substances–nicotine and alcohol–not only because of their dire health consequences but because initial adolescent experimentation with these substances has been shown to expand to the use of illicit drugs (Surgeon-General, 1988).

In an earlier narrative review on TM and substance abuse, Gelderloos et al. (1991) described 24 studies, 12 of which provided sufficient data on drug use outcomes to compute statistical effect sizes for the current meta-analysis. To locate further studies on TM, a systematic search of five computer data bases–PsycINFO, DrugINFO, MEDLINE, Sociological Abstracts, and Social Work Abstracts–was executed as well as hand searches of references appearing in relevant review articles. These searches located 12 more studies on the effects of TM on substance abuse, seven of which provided sufficient data to compute effect sizes. Thus, of the 36 studies located on TM and substance abuse, 19 studies with a total of 4,524 subjects, of which 3,249 were TM participants and 1,275 were controls or other treatment participants, met criteria for inclusion in the current meta-analysis.

First the 19 studies will be summarized in narrative fashion, with three particularly rigorous studies featured in detail. Then, a meta-analysis comparing the magnitude of effects for TM with the results of other meta-analyses on drug outcomes will be presented.

Narrative Summary

Table 1 summarizes the 19 TM studies that are included in the meta-analysis on drug use outcomes, including information on each study's population, research design, total number of subjects, interval between pretest and last follow-up (in the case of retrospective and cross-sectional surveys which lack pretests, it represents length of TM practice), types of substances included in the study, and major findings. Because the studies vary substantially in rigor, the table is organized according to strength of research design, with the weaker studies presented first and the strongest studies at the end.

The first three studies were retrospective surveys of a total of 2,500 people, mostly students, who had learned TM. Study 1 was a large retrospective study of TM participants without controls while Studies 2 and 3 included "yoked" peer controls who were non-meditating friends (and Study 3 used random sample survey methods). These three studies showed a large effect on reduced usage for all classes of substances in TM meditators, including a 75%-90% reduction for illegal drugs during a time-period averaging 20 months for the largest study. The controls in Studies 2 and 3 showed no reduction in substance abuse over the same period. It should be noted that because retrospective surveys must rely on memory and are not longitudinal, their reliability and validity may be constrained.

Studies 4 and 5 are cross-sectional studies of the general population. Study 5 compared smoking and drinking in long-term meditators averaging 2 years of TM practice, new meditators, and non-meditating working adults. Because new meditators had only been practicing TM for 2 weeks or less, they were also considered as a control group. Long-term meditators showed significant reductions in alcohol and tobacco consumption compared to new meditators and non-meditators. Also, significant correlations were found between length of time of regular TM practice and reduced alcohol and cigarette consumption in the long-term meditating group. The new TM group and non-meditating controls were comparable in drinking and smoking levels, suggesting that the positive effect was due to long-term TM practice and not to the type of person who started TM (i.e., self-selection).

The next eight studies (6-13) are longitudinal investigations of 3 to 20 months duration; except for Studies 6 and 7, all included untreated control groups. One study (6) followed prisoners and one

(Study 8) followed young out-patient drug users, while the others were composed of the general population, mostly students. Study 8 showed rapid and sustained reductions in illicit drugs in young German drug users who learned TM while controls indicated no consistent change. Studies 7, 9, 10, and 11 showed similarly marked reductions in the use of alcohol and illicit drugs in high school and college students who regularly practiced TM. Non-meditating controls in these studies showed no consistent change. Study 11 also reported significant primary drug prevention in the TM group relative to controls: only 10.5% of TM subjects who were initially nonusers of cannabis subsequently starting using it after 6 months compared to 35% of initial nonuser controls. Studies 12 and 13 also showed significant decreases in alcohol and/or tobacco consumption in adults who regularly practiced TM relative to well-matched controls, with Study 12 conducted at 2 different work sites in the U. S. automotive industry.

The remaining 6 longitudinal studies (14-19) are rigorous experiments. In these studies, self-selection (e.g., the possibility of more highly-motivated people choosing TM) is eliminated by random assignment of subjects to TM or other treatment/control groups, although two of the studies (15 & 17) had limited sample size. Two studies (16 & 18) used college students, and one study (14) followed elderly African-Americans. The other three were composed of heavy users–young Swedish drug addicts (Study 15), Vietnam veterans suffering from Post-Traumatic Stress disorder (Study 17), and skid-row-type alcoholics (Study 19). The results of these well-designed studies replicate the other TM studies, with TM participants showing significant reductions in substance abuse compared to controls. For example, young institutionalized addicts from low socioeconomic backgrounds in Sweden (Study 15) who were randomly assigned to learn TM deceased significantly in hashish, LSD, and opiates over a three-month period, compared to controls assigned to group therapy. In Study 17, meditating Vietnam veterans significantly reduced alcohol consumption compared to non-meditating controls who received psychotherapy. In Study 18, conducted for the U.S. Army Research Institute for the Behavioral and Social Sciences, students from a community college who learned TM

TABLE 1. Studies on TM and Substance Abuse Included in Narrative Review and Meta-Analysis

Author	Population	Research Design	Total N TM/ Control	Interval between Pretest & Last Follow-up*	Types of Drugs	Major Findings For TM Group
1. Benson & Wallace (1972)	General, mostly 19-28 yrs., USA	Retrospective Survey	1862	20 months average	Alcohol, tobacco, cannabis, hallucinogens, narcotics	After 20 months, 90% stopped using/selling substances
2. Shafii et al. (1974 & 1975)	General, 75% under 30 yrs., USA	Retrospective Survey with untreated controls	216 126/90	range: 1-39 months	Alcohol tobacco, cannabis	Significant reduction in alcohol, marijuana & cigarettes, compared to controls
3. Monahan (1977)	General, USA	Retrospective Survey with untreated controls	415 263/152	20 months average	Alcohol, tobacco, cannabis, hallucinogens, narcotics	Significant decline in all categories, compared to controls
4. Farinelli (1989)	General, Italy	Cross-Sectional with untreated controls	207 107/100	2 years	Alcohol, tobacco	Lower use of cigarettes and alcohol, compared to controls
5. Friend (1975)	General, employed adults, USA	Cross-Sectional with untreated controls	193 128 long-term TM 27 new TM 38 controls	2 years	Alcohol, tobacco	Long term TM: significant decreases in alcohol and tobacco consumption compared to new TM subjects and controls
6. Abrams (1989)	Prisoners, USA	Longitudinal with subjects as own controls	14	9 months	Tobacco	No significant changes in smoking
7. Lazar et al. (1977)	General, USA	Longitudinal with subjects as own controls	36 13/1mo. TM 9/2mo. TM 14/3mo. TM	range: 1-3 months	Alcohol, tobacco, cannabis, hallucinogens, narcotics	Significant reduction in substance use for all categories compared to controls

TABLE 1 (continued)

Author	Population	Research Design	Total N TM/ Control	Interval between Pretest & Last Follow-up	Types of Drugs	Major Findings For TM Group
8. Schenk-luhn & Geisler (1977) Geisler (1978)	High-school/ college-age drug users, West Germany	Longitudinal, with TM plus drug rehabilitation vs. drug rehabilitation alone	115 76/39	18 months	Cannabis, hallucino-gens, narcotics	50% discontinued all classes of drugs by 4 mos.; 89% ceased using any substance by 18 mos.
9. Nidich (1989)	College students, USA	Longitudinal, with TM vs. personal adjustment class	51 15/36	2.25 months	Alcohol, cannabis	Significant reduction in marijuana and alcohol compared to controls
10. Throll (1989)	General, 15-20 yrs., New Zealand	Longitudinal, with untreated controls	46 30/16	3-4 months	Alcohol, tobacco, cannabis, hallucino-gens	Significant reduction in all categories compared to controls
11. Katz (1977)	High school/ college students, USA	Longitudinal, with untreated controls	467 269/198	8 months	Alcohol, cannabis	Significant reduction in marijuana, hashish, and alcohol use, compared to controls
12. Alexander et al. (1993)	Adults at industrial work site, USA	Longitudinal, with untreated controls	86 45/41	3 months	Alcohol, tobacco	Significant reduction in cigarette and alcohol use compared to controls
13. Royer (this volume)	General, USA	Longitudinal, with untreated controls	324 110/214	range: 20-24 months	Tobacco	Significant (81%) decrease or cessation of smoking in regular meditators compared to controls (33%)
14. Schneider et al. (1992)	Elderly African-Americans, USA	Experiment with random assignment to TM, progressive muscle relaxation, or lifestyle counseling	112 37 TM 37 PMR 38 LC	3 months	Alcohol, tobacco	No significant differences found between groups

TABLE 1. (continued)

Author	Population	Research Design	Total N TM/ Control	Interval between Pretest & Last Follow-up	Types of Drugs	Major Findings For TM Group
15. Brautigam (1977)	Drug users, 17-24 yrs. low income, Sweden	Experiment with random assignment to TM or untreated control	20 10/10	3 months	Cannabis (hashish), hallucinogens, narcotics	Significant decrease in use of alcohol, cannabis, & hallucinogens, compared to controls
16. Ottens (1975)	College Students, USA	Experiment with random assignment to TM, self-control, or untreated control	54 18 TM 18 Self-Cntrl 18 controls	10 weeks	Tobacco	Significant decrease in smoking, compared to controls; Self-Control group also showed significant decrease
17. Brooks & Scarano (1985)	Vietnam Vets with Post-Traumatic Stress Disorder USA	Experiment with random assignment to TM or psychotherapy	18 10/8	3 months	Alcohol	Significant reduction in degree of alcohol problem compared to controls
18. Myers & Eisner (1974)	Male college students, USA	Experiment with random assignment to TM, karate, or untreated control	180 60 TM 60 karate 60 control	4 months	Alcohol; cannabis, hallucinogens, narcotics	Significant reduction in hallucinogens & hard drugs compared to Karate & controls
19. Taub et al. (this volume)	Skid-row (80% black) alcoholics, IQ at least 80, and generally no brain damage, USA	Experiment with random assignment to TM, EMG biofeedback, neurotherapy or routine therapy alone**	108 33 TM 20 EMG 28 neurotherapy 27 routine therapy	18 months	Alcohol	After 18 months, significant number (65%) were abstinent compared to neurotherapy (28%) and controls (25%). EMG group also showed significant abstinence.

*Initial training for TM takes place in seven sessions. For Studies 1-5 (with no pretest), this column represents length of TM practice.
**All experimental subjects in Taub et al. also received routine therapy.

showed significant reductions in illicit drug use compared to those assigned to karate or the untreated control group.

In the above 19 studies, substance usage was consistently associated with (1) total length of time practicing TM, and (2) regularity of TM practice each day. While only five studies were exclusively composed of high-users or addicts, even studies of the general population typically identified and documented significant reductions in serious abuser subgroups, suggesting that TM provides secondary prevention. The three studies (4, 6, 14) that did not reach significance all shared a common factor: a restricted number of actual users at pretest (e.g., only 17 smokers out of 107 in the TM group in Study 4; 9 smokers out of 14 in Study 6; and, 11 drinkers out of 37 in the TM group and only 4 drinkers out of 38 in the control group in Study 14). In Studies 4 and 6, only the *total* TM samples had been analyzed; thus, the average smoking levels at pretest were very low (diluted because of inclusion of nonsmokers), and the presence of floor effects made detection of significant changes highly unlikely. In Study 14, only the heavy drinkers were analyzed, so the sample size (and hence statistical power) was quite small, also making it unlikely to detect the presence of relatively large effects in the data set. (Study 6 was also hindered by a small total sample size.)

Because the studies reviewed above vary in strength of research design, the greatest confidence should be placed in the longitudinal and experimental investigations which provide the most scientific rigor. Below are detailed descriptions of three of these studies (8, 13, and 19). Each study provides an example of the effects of TM on one major substance category–illicit drugs, cigarettes, or alcohol.

Illicit Drugs

For 18 months, Geisler and Schenkluhn (Geisler, 1978; Schenkluhn & Geisler, 1977) followed 115 high school and college-aged drug users who attended an out-patient drug rehabilitation center in Germany. All were serious drug users with the majority of these young people reporting multiple usage of illicit drugs, including cannabis products, hallucinogens, amphetamines/barbiturates, and opiates. The experimental group consisted of 76 subjects who learned TM in addition to receiving standard out-patient drug counseling while the control group comprised 39 students of comparable age, gender, and severity and type of drug consumption who received only standard out-patient drug counseling. A retrospective survey determined drug usage 2 years prior to the study, and prospective usage was obtained monthly during the first year of the study and at 18 months. TM subjects showed significant, positive changes in both drug usage and psychological health relative to controls; the rate of change increased with regularity and length of time practicing TM. After 4 months of TM practice, 50% of the experimental group had stopped taking illicit drugs; by 18 months, 89% had discontinued using drugs. The TM participants also displayed enhanced psychological health on multiple measures of the Freiburger Personality Inventory relative to controls after only 2 months of TM practice.

Cigarettes

Royer's prospective study on smoking cessation (this volume) surveyed 324 smoking adults who attended a TM introductory lecture and were recontacted 18 months later. Before the lecture, each person completed a questionnaire on smoking habits, motivation to quit, and demographics. Subsequently, 110 people started TM, forming the experimental group, while 214 who did not begin TM agreed to comprise the control group. Although TM is not specifically a smoking cessation program, and at no time were the TM participants admonished to quit, significantly more (51%) of the experimental group who were regular in their TM practice quit compared to controls (21%). When reduction of smoking (at least 5 cigarettes less per day, which was a 25% average decrease) was considered along with cessation, 81% of regular TM practitioners quit or decreased smoking compared to 33% for non-meditating controls. While it could be argued that those who started TM were more motivated to stop smoking, data collected before the people chose to learn TM showed the TM group (including regular and irregular meditators) and the control group to be comparable in demographic characteristics, smoking habits, and motivation to quit.

Alcohol

In a study funded by the National Institute of Alcohol Abuse and Alcoholism, 108 transient, chronic alcoholic inpatients (80% African-American) were randomly assigned to one of four treatments: TM, EMG biofeedback, neurotherapy, or regular drug counseling alone (which served as an active control) (Taub, Solomon, Smith, Weingarten, & Walton, this volume). Participants were followed for 18 months using sophisticated monthly interviews and cross-validation of self-reports of drinking via breath tests, dates of reported incarcerations/hospitalizations, and information from friends/family. After 18 months, 65% of the TM group were abstinent compared to 55% of the EMG muscle relaxation group, 28% of the neurotherapy group, and 25% of those receiving standard counseling. TM subjects also improved significantly on five of the six subscales of the Profile of Mood States (POMS), showing reduced negative affect and enhanced positive mood more than the other three groups. Because of the favorable results observed in the TM participants, at the request of hospital unit supervisors, 104 project-ineligible patients (due to conditions including severe brain damage, serious medical problems, or IQ below 80), also learned the TM technique. It was anecdotally noted that these patients, many with brain damage, successfully practiced TM and reported benefits of relaxation and subjective experiences similar to those noted in other studies, suggesting that even severe alcoholics with additional handicapping conditions can benefit from this technique.

Earlier reviews have suggested that meditation may provide an effective, holistic treatment for chemical abuse (Clarke & Saunders, 1988; Friedman & Glickman, 1986; Greaves, 1980; Marlatt & George, 1984). The above narrative review supports this conclusion, at least in the case of TM. However, our findings contrast with one other narrative review (Klajner, Hartman & Sobell, 1984) concluding that there is insufficient evidence to support the contention that meditation or relaxation techniques are effective in reducing substance abuse or even anxiety. However, the conclusion drawn by this latter review may be due, in part, to its limited consideration of TM studies (less than 5% of TM studies on anxiety and less than

25% of TM studies on substance abuse were included). The difference in its conclusion from the above may also be due to the subjective nature and potential imprecision of applying the narrative review method itself. A quantitative meta-analysis which overcomes such limitations and analyzes the effects of all TM studies on substance abuse is presented below

The Advantages of Statistical Meta-Analysis

Narrative reviews lack quantitative methods to accurately estimate and compare the relative magnitude of treatment effects produced in different studies. Lacking an objective means to estimate and integrate findings, the reviewer must rely on subjective judgment and less than precise qualitative techniques, such as simply counting significant positive findings. However, such results may be misleading because studies with large samples may be statistically significant even though their treatment effects are relatively small (Hedges & Olkin, 1980). As a result, discrepancies in study conclusions often reflect differences in sample sizes. Meta-analysis provides more reliable conclusions by taking into account the influence of sample size on statistical significance level (Glass, McGaw, & Smith, 1981; Hunter & Schmidt, 1990). An additional advantage of meta-analysis is that strength of research design and types of population can be coded and statistically controlled for their potential influence. In meta-analysis, the basic computational step is to express all findings across studies in the same metric–a quantitative index called an "effect size." Effect sizes measure the difference in means at posttest between experimental and control conditions in standard deviation (Z-score) units, adjusting for pretest differences in the case of longitudinal studies with control groups. Use of effect sizes thus permits synthesis of evidence across studies using different measurement scales, research designs, and number of subjects (Cohen, 1977). In the behavioral sciences, an effect size of .80 standard deviation units is considered large while .50 suggests a medium treatment effect and .20 a small effect (Cohen, 1977).

Meta-Analysis on Psychological Outcomes of Heavy Abusers Practicing TM vs. Typical Populations Practicing Other Forms of Meditation and Relaxation

Since Maharishi's Vedic Psychology holds that everyone has the capacity to transcend, it follows that TM should be universal in its application. Thus it is predicted that the psychological benefits for TM practitioners relative to controls in the general population (see Section II) will also be found in substance abuse populations. To test this hypothesis, the effects of TM relative to controls on psychological outcomes are assessed in studies on known serious substance abusers. Because it is important to evaluate whether the psychological effects of TM are also distinctive relative to other forms of meditation and relaxation, these TM outcomes for heavy users also are compared to those for practitioners of other forms of meditation and relaxation reported in prior meta-analyses.

Nineteen TM studies were located that measured psychological outcomes in subjects with a history of substance abuse; only three studies (Brautigam, 1977; Brooks & Scarano, 1985; and Geisler, 1978) overlapped with the 19 TM studies used in the current quantitative reviews. With the exception of these three studies of out-patient drug users, all other studies investigated prison inmates (see Dillbeck & Abrams, 1987, for a listing of these 16 studies). While virtually all of these prisoners had a history of heavy substance abuse, and many continued to abuse substances in the prison setting, it was not feasible to directly assess current substance abuse levels because admission of such behavior would result in punitive action by prison officials. Although it would be ideal to include results from diverse samples, at this time the majority of psychological findings are available only for inmates/substance abusers. On the other hand, if this high risk population shows positive psychological changes, it is likely that less high risk abusers may also experience positive changes.

Psychological Outcomes in Heavy Abusers Practicing TM vs. Controls

Fourteen of the studies on heavy abusers reported on negative psychological outcomes, such as depression, anger, hostility, and anxiety. In these studies, the average effect size for TM relative to controls in reducing overall negative psychological functioning was .64. A subset of 12 of these studies evaluated trait anxiety separately. The average effect size for reducing anxiety for heavy abusers practicing TM was almost identical, at .63. This reduction is comparable to the decrease in trait anxiety reported in Eppley et al.'s (1989) meta-analysis for the general population practicing TM (.70, N = 35 studies).

Ten of the TM studies on heavy abusers reported on positive psychological outcomes, such as self-concept and internal locus of control. In these studies, the average effect size for TM relative to controls in enhancing overall positive psychological function was .51 ($t(9) = 9.85$, $p = .000002$). Although this enhancement was highly significant statistically, it was somewhat smaller than the average effect size of .78 (N = 18 interventions) for self-actualization reported in Alexander et al.'s (1991) TM meta-analysis for the general population. However, this discrepancy may be due to a difference in the positive outcomes being assessed: none of the prison studies included measures of self-actualization.

Psychological Improvements in Heavy Abusers vs. the General Population Practicing Other Forms of Meditation and Relaxation

The reduction in anxiety among heavy abusers practicing TM (effect size = .63) is almost twice that for other meditations and relaxation techniques among the general population (effect size = .35, based on 111 studies in Eppley et al., 1989). This difference is statistically significant ($t(121) = 2.46$, $p = .008$, one-tailed). Also, effect size for heavy users who practice TM (.51) is significantly larger than that found in the general population (.21) practicing other meditation/relaxation methods ($t(27) = 2.17$, $p = .02$).

Thus, as initially predicted, heavy abusers who start TM also show significant improvements in psychological functioning relative to untreated controls and compared to practitioners of other forms of meditation and relaxation in the general population. These changes may mediate (in part) the reductions in substance use shown for TM compared to other treatments reported below.

First, a meta-analysis will be presented on the effects of TM relative to control conditions for substance use. Next, effect sizes for TM will be compared to effect sizes of other standard treatments in reducing substance use. Finally, the time course of TM treatment outcomes will be explored relative to those of other programs to determine if these effects fall off, are maintained, or even increase over time.

Meta-Analysis on Effects of TM in Reducing Substance Use Compared to Control Conditions

All TM studies were included which reported sufficient data on levels of drug usage for an effect size to be calculated. Based on Glass et al.'s (1981) methods, this calculation required knowledge of either means and standard deviations, t or F statistics, or frequency distributions on Likert scales.[1] Also, where quit rates or percentages using drugs were reported for both TM and control groups, effect sizes were calculated using a probit transformation (Glass et al., 1981).

For each TM study, effect sizes are shown in Table 2 by class of substance, indicating change in usage levels for the TM group relative to the control conditions. Although usually untreated, some studies had more "active" controls (e.g., Studies 8, 9, 14, 17, 19). All effect sizes are only for subjects (or the subset of subjects) reporting substance usage at pretest in the TM or control condition, except for 3 studies (Abrams, 1989; Farinelli, 1989; Nidich, 1989) where only change in consumption patterns for the entire sample was reported. Where data were also available for the subgroup of regular TM practitioners versus controls, effect sizes are shown in Table 2 in parentheses. In the case of illicit drugs, results on cannabis products, LSD and other hallucinogens, and narcotics were combined under a single effect size because there were too few outcomes in any sub-category (except cannabis, reported separately below) for statistical analysis. Because long term outcomes are most clinically meaningful, all effect sizes were based on the last available follow-up data. The average follow-up across substance categories was 9.7 months. (Initial training in TM takes place in 7 sessions over a one-week period.)

As in Table 1, studies are listed in order of increasing design strength which was coded on a scale from 1 (weakest) to 6 (strongest). Scores on this scale along with total number of subjects for each study were used to calculate weights used in averaging effect sizes across studies (see bottom of Table 2), since studies with small sample sizes or weak design may provide less reliable results.[2] The average sample size was 116 for longitudinal studies. Simple averaging yielded results that were highly similar to the weighted averages. Weighted averages across studies are reported for each kind of substance category for the following: all studies, well-designed studies only (longitudinal and experimental), observational studies (using cross-sectional or retrospective designs), general population studies, and studies with populations at risk for high consumption of alcohol and illicit drugs. (None of the cigarette studies exclusively targeted heavy users or separated them out for subgroup analysis.)

One-sample t-tests (one-tailed) were used to examine whether mean effect sizes were significantly greater than zero, indicating consistent differences between TM and the control condition. For the 14 studies reporting alcohol consumption, the average TM effect size was .55 ($t(13) = 3.97$, $p = .0008$); the average effect size for the 12 TM studies reporting cigarette usage relative to controls was .87 ($t(11) = 6.26$, $p = .00003$); and the average effect size for TM in the 10 studies reporting illicit drug consumption relative to controls was .83 ($t(9) = 8.85$, $p < .000005$). For cannabis, the average effect size of .70 was also highly significant ($t(9) = 7.10$, $p < .00003$). Among casual users of alcohol and illicit drugs in the general population, average effect sizes (.42 and .74 respectively) were also significant ($t(11) = 4.56$, $p = .0004$; $t(7) = 6.43$, $p < 0002$). For serious users of these substances, average effect sizes were considerably larger (at 1.35 and 1.16 respectively), but based on too few studies to permit statistical inferences to be made.

It is encouraging to note that for each of the three major substance categories, better-designed TM studies (i.e., longitudinal and experimental) produced at least the same or higher average effect sizes (.55 for alcohol; .97 for cigarettes; .91 for illicit drugs) than studies based on cross-sectional and retrospective survey designs (.54 for alcohol; .79 for cigarettes; .64 for illicit drugs). These findings, and also the larger TM effect sizes for serious users of alcohol and drugs, suggest that the pattern of positive treatment

TABLE 2. Meta-Analysis on Effects of the Transcendental Meditation Program vs. Control Conditions on Substance Use

Study	Study Characteristics		Effect Size by Category of Substance (regular TM only in parentheses)		
	Research Design Code*	Total Sample Size	Alcohol Use	Cigarette Use	Illicit Drug Use
1. Benson & Wallace (1972)	1	1862	0.51	1.03	0.74
2. Shafii et al. (1974 & 1975)	2	216	0.43	1.14	0.75
3. Monahan (1977)	2	415	0.33 (0.41)	0.69 (0.73)	0.42
4. Farinelli (1989)	3	207	0.58	0.67	
5. Friend (1975)	3	193	0.84	0.42	
6. Abrams (1989)	4	14		0.69	
7. Lazar et al. (1977)	4	36	0.35	0.38	0.64 (0.81)
8. Schenkluhn & Geisler (1977); Geisler (1978)	5	115			1.10 (1.52)
9. Nidich (1989)	5	51	0.41		1.00
10. Throll (1989)	5	46	0.37	1.78	1.25
11. Katz (1977)	5	467	0.20 (0.47)		1.36
12. Alexander et al. (1993)	5	86	0.89	2.29	
13. Royer (this volume)	5	324		0.48 (0.86)	
14. Schneider et al. (1992)	6	112	0.62	0.28	
15. Brautigam (1977)	6	20			1.23
16. Ottens (1975)	6	54		1.34	
17. Brooks & Scarano (1985)	6	18	2.28		
18. Myers & Eisner (1974)	6	180	−0.45		0.39
19. Taub et al. (this volume)	6	108	0.54		
Weighted Mean Effect Sizes:					
All studies			0.55	0.87	0.83
Well-designed studies			0.55	0.97	0.91
Cross-sectional studies			0.54	0.79	0.64
General population			0.42	0.89	0.74
Populations at risk for alcohol/drug abuse			1.35		1.16

Research Design Code: 1 = retrospective survey; 2 = survey with controls; 3 = cross-sectional with controls; 4 = longitudinal; 5 = longitudinal with controls; 6 = random assignment experiments effects for TM cannot be attributed to the inclusion of studies with weak designs or studies focusing on more casual users.

Comparing Results of TM Meta-Analysis with Results of Meta-Analyses on Other Treatments for Reducing Substance Abuse

To assess the clinical relevance of the above results, average effect sizes of TM were compared to average effect sizes of other treatments for reducing alcohol, cigarette and illicit drug use.

Because TM is generally classified as a relaxation technique (e.g., Klajner et al., 1984), it is first compared to studies on relaxation. Also TM is likely to be similar to relaxation approaches on such non-specific treatment factors as degree of self-directedness, time spent in practice, and expectations of outcome. Although no published meta-analyses on relaxation treatments could be found, 10 primary studies were located in which the effects of relaxation were compared to treated or untreated controls on alcohol abuse. Only published studies on relaxation were evaluated because they tend to be strongest in design and were more readily available. For purposes of comparison to TM, this was also a conservative approach because journals are more likely to accept studies with significant findings for publication (e.g., Hedges, 1984).

Average effect sizes for TM were then compared to results for conventional treatments reported in published meta-analyses. The advantage of focusing on published meta-analyses is that they provide independent calculation of effect sizes for other treatments without requiring additional exhaustive search of primary studies. The relaxation studies and meta-analyses on conventional treatments were located in the same way as the TM studies, through hand and computer searches. Meta-analyses on other treatments for alcohol, cigarettes, or illicit drugs were included that (1) reported effect sizes or results that could be converted to effect sizes;[3] and (2) comprised 10 or more primary studies (10 is considered the minimum number of cases per group for performing statistical analyses, such as t-tests (Gay, 1981). When there were less than 10 cases, outcomes were pooled with the data for the most similar treatment category to allow at least minimal statistical power for meta-analytic comparisons.[4] When overlap of primary studies was very high between meta-analyses, only results for the more comprehensive meta-analyses were incorporated.[5]

For each substance category, first the average effect size and major characteristics for the meta-analyses are presented, and then these effect sizes are statistically compared with the average effect size for TM via analysis of variance planned comparisons.[6]

Alcohol

Relaxation Meta-Analysis. A total of 10 primary studies with 11 relaxation treatment groups were located. Three of the studies employed biofeedback, five used muscle relaxation techniques other than biofeedback (such as progressive muscle relaxation), and two investigated meditation (clinically standardized meditation, the relaxation response), and one used a cognitive-affective approach for anxiety reduction. The subjects in all studies were either heavy social drinkers or alcoholics. The mean length of initial training in relaxation methods was approximately 5 weeks.

Table 3 presents the sample characteristics and treatment effect sizes (relative to controls) for each primary study. The average sample size was 57 participants. The mean interval between pretest and the last follow-up for relaxation treatments was 11.3 months. (For the TM studies specifically on alcohol consumption, the interval between pretest and Posttest averaged 10.6 months.) All studies, except one, were random-assignment experiments or longitudinal investigations with either untreated controls or more "active" controls (e.g., Studies 3,5,6,9,11). Effect sizes were calculated in the same way as for the TM studies.

As seen at the bottom of Table 3, the average effect size for all 11 interventions was .15. A one-sample t-test (1-tailed) found no significance between relaxation treatments and control conditions ($t(10) = 1.24$, $p = .12$). By contrast the average effect size for TM was .55 ($N = 14$ cases). Although the average effect size for relaxation was small, the effect in the three biofeedback studies on heavy drinkers was larger (but still less than half the average effect in the two TM studies of heavy drinkers).

The mean effect size findings (and standard deviations) of previously published meta-analyses on standard treatments are featured in Table 4 (along with the results of meta-analyses on TM and

TABLE 3. Meta-Analysis of Effects of Relaxation Treatments vs. Control Conditions on Alcohol Use

Author	Population	Research Design Code**	N per group: Relax./Controls	Interval between Pretest & Last Follow-up	Relaxation vs. Control Condition	Effect Size
1. Denney, Baugh, & Hardt (1991)	Alcoholics, male, 22-72 yrs., USA	2	119/114	Training*–8 session; Follow-up–12 mos.	Biofeedback-assisted relaxation training vs. standard inpatient care	0.11
2. Marlatt & Marques (1977)	High volume drinkers, male, 23.5 yrs., USA	5	10/9	Training–6 wks., Follow-up–7 wks.	Relaxation Response vs. placebo	–0.12
3. Marlatt & Marques (1977)	High volume drinkers, male, 23.5 yrs., USA	5	8/9	Training–6 wks., Follow-up–7 wks.	Progressive muscle relaxation vs. placebo	0.00
4. Murphy, Pagano, & Marlatt (1986)	Heavy social drinkers, male, 21-30, USA	6	18/13	Training–8 wks., Follow-up–6 wks.	Clinically Standardized Meditation vs. untreated controls	0.61
5. Miller & Taylor (1980)	Alcoholics, 45 yrs., USA	6	18/23	Training–10 wks., Follow-up–12 mo.	Behavioral self-control training, with & without relaxation	0.00
6. Olson, Devine, Ganley, & Dorsey (1981)	Alcoholics, male & female, 21-73 yrs., USA	6	37/35	Training–33 days, Follow-up–4 yrs.	Progressive muscle relaxation & covert desensitization vs. multimodal group therapy	–0.02
7. Rohsenow, Smith, & Johnson (1985)	Heavy drinkers, male, 20-22 yrs., USA	6	15/21	Training–1 mo., Follow-up–5.5 mo.	Relaxation & anxiety management training vs. untreated controls	0.11
8. Ormrod & Budd (1991)	Alcoholics, USA	6	18/18	Training–4 wks., Follow-up–3 mo.	Relaxation & anxiety management training vs. untreated controls	0.20
9. Peniston & Kulkosky (1989)	Alcoholics, 40-50 yrs., USA	6	10/10	Training–28 days, Follow-up–13 mo.	EEG Biofeedback/autogenic training vs. group therapy	0.92
10. Schneider et al. (1992)	Elderly hypertensive blacks	6	37/38	Training–3 mo.	Progressive muscle relaxation vs. lifestyle counseling	0.37
11. Taub et al. (this volume)	Alcoholics USA	6	20/27	Training–1 mo., Follow-up–18 mo.	EMB Biofeedback plus routine therapy vs. routine therapy alone	0.71
Weighted mean effect size						0.15

* Length of initial training for relaxation treatment.

** Research Design code: 1 = retrospective survey; 2 = survey with controls; 3 = cross-sectional with controls; 4 = longitudinal; 5 = longitudinal with controls; 6 = random assignment experiments on relaxation): the first meta-analysis addresses primary and secondary prevention programs for all substance categories (Tobler, 1986); the second focuses on driving-under-the-influence treatment programs (Wells-Parker & Bangert-Drowns, 1990); the third meta-analysis concerns smoking cessation treatments (Kottke, Battista, Defriese, & Brekke, 1988); the fourth and fifth summarize the results of the meta-analyses on relaxation and TM reported above.

Results of Meta-Analyses on Standard Alcohol Treatments. Tobler (1986) examined 91 studies of 143 primary and secondary drug prevention programs for adolescents (grades 6-12) in mostly urban and suburban areas (conducted between 1972 and 1984). The majority of these programs were school-based with 12.6% targeting special populations, including students with school problems, minority students, and delinquents. Five basic program modalities were studied: (1) programs promoting knowledge about drug consequences; (2) programs facilitating intrapersonal growth; (3) strategies for resisting peer pressure, including training in refusal skills or teaching social and life skills; (4) combined programs providing knowledge about drug consequences and enhancing intrapersonal skills; and (5) alternative programs, including a wide range of community activities or activities to enhance individual competence, such as reading skills or job skills. The duration of these programs ranged from 1-41 hours with the majority lasting from 1-20 hours. All treatment groups were compared either to a health class or to a no-treatment group. The total number of participants per program varied widely. (For example, in the peer influence resistance programs, participants per program ranged from 20 to 902 participants for random assignment experimental studies and 10 to 389 for longitudinal studies with control groups.) Substance use outcomes were derived from self-report measures. The average interval between pretest and posttest for all the Tobler studies (on alcohol, cigarettes, and drugs) was 3.8 months.

Tobler's data indicates an overall effect size of .17 for the 27 programs specifically targeting alcohol consumption relative to control conditions. From posthoc analysis, Tobler identified programs for resisting peer pressure as the most effective, which showed an effect size of .33 (N = 13 interventions). She then combined all other prevention programs, with an average effect size of

TABLE 4. Mean Effect Sizes for all Meta-analyses on Substance Abuse Treatment

Meta-analysis	Target substances	Population	Total Number of studies	Sample Size per Study	Interval Between Pretest and Last Follow-up	Treatment Categories	Mean Effect Size $\pm$ S.D. (Number of treatment groups)
1. Tobler (1986)	Alcohol	Adolescents	91	Range: 10-902	Mean 3.75 months	Educational prevention programs– Counteracting peer influence;	0.33 ± 0.11 (13)
						Other prevention approaches (didactic, personal development, alternative activities enhancing competence):	0.07 ± 0.37 (20)
	Cigarettes					All prevention programs:	0.38 ± 0.31 (40)
	Illicit drugs					Counteracting peer influence:	0.47 ± 0.22 (15)
						Other prevention approaches:	0.13 ± 0.37 (45)
2. Wells-Parker & Bangers-Drowns (1990)	Alcohol	Driving under the influence offenders	39		Range: 2 wks-2 yrs	Most educational; also substance abuse therapies; therapeutic probation; mixed modalities	0.10 ± 0.16 (39)

Meta-analysis	Target substances	Population	Total Number of studies	Sample Size per Study	Interval Between Pretest and Last Follow-up	Treatment Categories	Mean Effect Size ± S.D. (Number of treatment groups)
3. Kottke et al. (1988)	Cigarettes	Adult smokers–patients & general	39	Median: 190	13 months	Counsling/advice: Pharmacological treatment* (e.g., nicotine chewing gum, clonidine): Printed self-help materials: Unconventional treatments** (e.g., acupuncture, sensory deprivation, hypnosis, and relaxation.):	0.18 ± 0.42 (24) 0.29 ± 0.33 (20) 0.08 ± 0.14 (11) 0.39 ± 0.46 (24)
4. Relaxation studies (Table 3)	Alcohol	Alcoholics & heavy drinkers	10	Mean: 57	Mean: 12.2 months	Relaxation training, biofeedback, meditation, anxiety management training	0.15 ± 0.41 (11)
5. TM studies (Table 2)	Alcohol Cigarettes Illicit drugs	General & special populations	19	Mean: 116+	Mean: 9.7 months	The Transcendental Meditation program	0.55 ± 0.51 (14) 0.87 ± 0.48 (12) 0.83 ± 0.30 (10)

* 5 studies on clonidine were added (see footnote[4])
** 5 studies on relaxation were added (see footnote[4])
\+ Mean sample size for longitudinal studies (N=15)

.07 (N = 20 interventions: of these remaining 20 interventions, alternative programs were the most effective for all substance categories combined). By contrast, the average effect size for TM was .55 (N = 14 interventions).

The second meta-analysis (Wells-Parker & Bangert-Drowns, 1990), funded by the National Institute on Alcohol Abuse and Alcoholism, is an on-going examination of 187 treatment interventions to reduce driving-under-the-influence (DUI) recidivism. Over 60% of the treatment programs analyzed were primarily alcohol abuse educational programs, while 23% primarily involved psychotherapy, and for 17% probation was the treatment for DUI. The population for this study is DUI offenders–the profile for repeat offenders suggests 95% are men, and 80% are unmarried with a median age of 32 (Yoder, 1990). Although the database for this study is large, they found that studies with weaker designs showed inflated results and increased variability. Thus, only experiments and longitudinal studies with control groups were included (N = 39 interventions). The effect sizes presented are preliminary data for these strong studies (Wells-Parker, personal communication, 1993). The typical interval between pretest and posttest was 1 year, with a range from 2 weeks to 2 years. Outcomes were usually measured in DUI arrests, or in some cases, car accidents or other traffic safety violations. All studies included control groups comprising either punitive treatment or no intervention. Initial findings show an 8%-13% proportional reduction in DUI arrests relative to controls, resulting in a small but robust effect size of .10, significant at $p < .01$, two-tailed (Wells-Parker, personal communication, 1993).

TM Effects on Alcohol Compared to Effects for Relaxation and Other Treatments. Figure 2 displays the effect sizes for TM, relaxation and the other treatment modalities on reduced alcohol consumption.

Planned comparisons for ANOVA on independent samples (Maxwell & Delaney, 1990) indicated that the average effect for TM was significantly larger than each treatment modality, including: relaxation programs ($t(12) = 5.27$, $p = .0001$); programs to resist peer pressure ($t(13) = 3.73$, $p = .0013$); other prevention programs combined ($t(14) = 8.51$, $p = .0000033$); and DUI interventions ($t(13) = 10.27$, $p = .00000007$).[7]

Cigarettes

Meta-Analysis on Standard Treatments. Two meta-analyses on smoking cessation treatments were located. The most comprehensive was Kottke et al.'s (1988) examination of 108 interventions from 39 controlled trials. They analyzed outcomes for a variety of treatment approaches, most of which incorporated multiple modalities. The primary component of these treatments was one of four intervention types: nicotine replacement therapies such as nicotine gum (N = 15 studies); individualized face-to-face counseling by a physician or counselor (N = 24 studies); bibliotherapy–self-help kits consisting of printed materials (N = 11 studies); or unconventional treatments (such as acupuncture, sensory deprivation, and hypnosis, N = 18 studies). Data on nicotine replacement therapies were supplemented by results from five clinical trials (Covey & Glassman, 1991) on the longer-term effects of the drug clonidine, increasing the total number of studies on pharmacological treatments to 20 (see note [4]); also 6 published relaxation studies, located through hand and computer searches, were added to the unconventional treatment category, increasing its total to 24 studies (see note [4]).

The number of participants in each study varied widely, from 26 to 935, with a median of 190. Duration of treatment interventions ranged from 0-6 months with an average of 1.2 months. Outcomes were measured as smoking quit rates over a follow-up period ranging up to 12 months. At 12 months, the average proportional difference in quit rates between intervention and control groups was 5.8%. For each primary study (data provided by Kottke, personal communication, March 1993), percentage quit rates at 12 months were converted via probit transformation to effect size units, yielding an average effect size of .26 for all interventions versus controls. Broken down by primary intervention, the effect sizes were: nicotine replacement–.29 (including the 5 clonidine studies); counseling/advice–.18; bibliotherapy–.08, unconventional treatments–.39 (including the 6 relaxation studies). By comparison, the overall effect size for TM on cigarettes was .87 (N = 12 studies), with an average pre-post interval of 12.7 months.

Tobler's (1986) meta-analysis (see above) also included 40 educational programs focusing on smoking prevention. Almost all

FIGURE 2. Average effect size for reduction in alcohol use, comparing TM with relaxation programs, preventive education programs and driving-under-the-influence treatment programs.

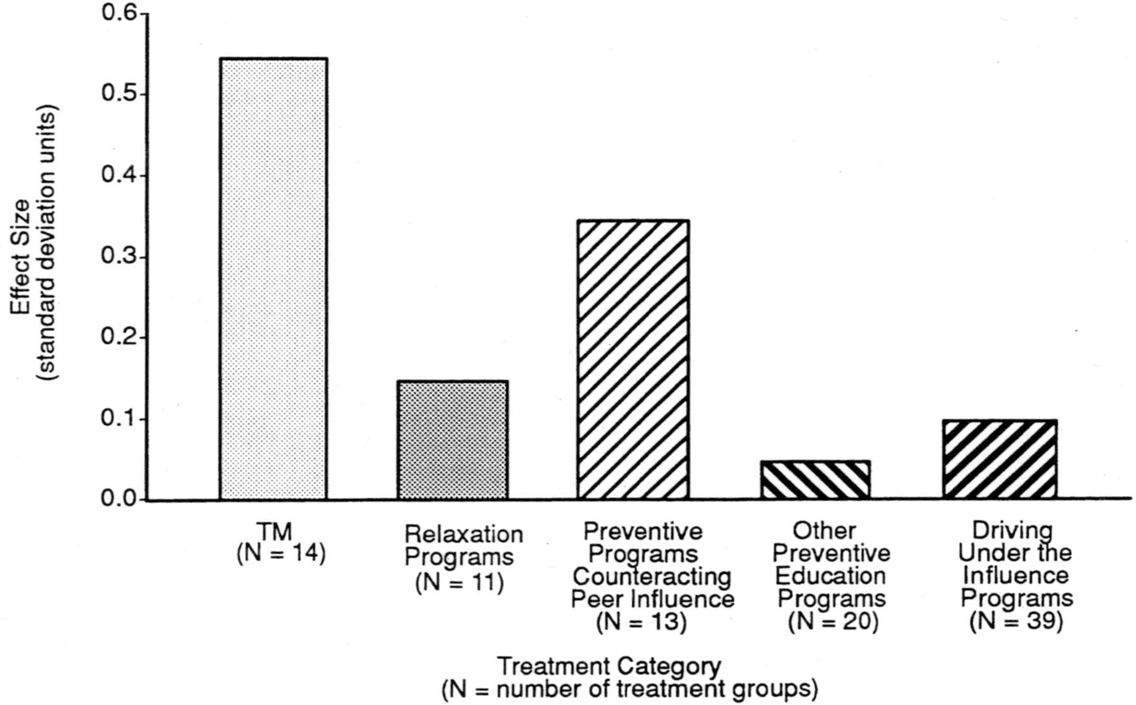

of those were teaching resistance to peer pressure (N = 38); their average effect size relative to controls was .38. Only two treatment programs involved other educational programs; their average effect size was .45.

TM Effects on Smoking Compared to Effects of Other Standard Treatments. Figure 3 shows average effect sizes for TM and the other smoking cessation programs. Planned comparisons (all one-tailed) showed that the effect of TM was significantly larger than for each treatment modality, including: educational prevention programs ($t(11) = 10.07$, $p = .00000034$); pharmacological treatments ($t(11) = 10.17$, $p = .0000003$); individual counseling ($t(35) = 5.40$, $p = .0000025$); bibliotherapy ($t(11) = 13.02$, $p = .000000025$); and unconventional treatments ($t(12) = 10.06$, $p = .0000002$).[7]

Illicit Drugs

Tobler's (1986) meta-analysis also included 60 interventions for illicit drug usage. There was an average effect size of .47 (N = 15 interventions) for the programs teaching resistance to peer pressure relative to control conditions, and an effect of .13 for the other combined prevention programs (N = 45 interventions). The average effect for TM on illicit drug use was .83 (N = 10 studies). Figure 4 shows the effect sizes for TM and for drug prevention programs.

Planned comparisons (all one-tailed) indicated the effect of TM was significantly larger then the effects of programs to resist peer pressure ($t(9) = 7.98$, $p = .00001$); and of other drug prevention programs combined ($t(10) = 18.34$, $p = .0000000025$).[7]

Time Course of Standard Treatments and TM on Reducing Substance Abuse

Because high relapse rates seriously undermine the effectiveness of treatments for substance abuse, it is important to specifically investigate how TM compares to other treatment programs in sustaining abstinence rates over the long-term.

Time Course for Standard Treatments

Data on cumulative abstinence/relapse rates at different time points were not consistently available for the meta-analyses re-

FIGURE 3. Average effect size for reduction in cigarette use, comparing TM with preventive education programs and smoking cessation programs.

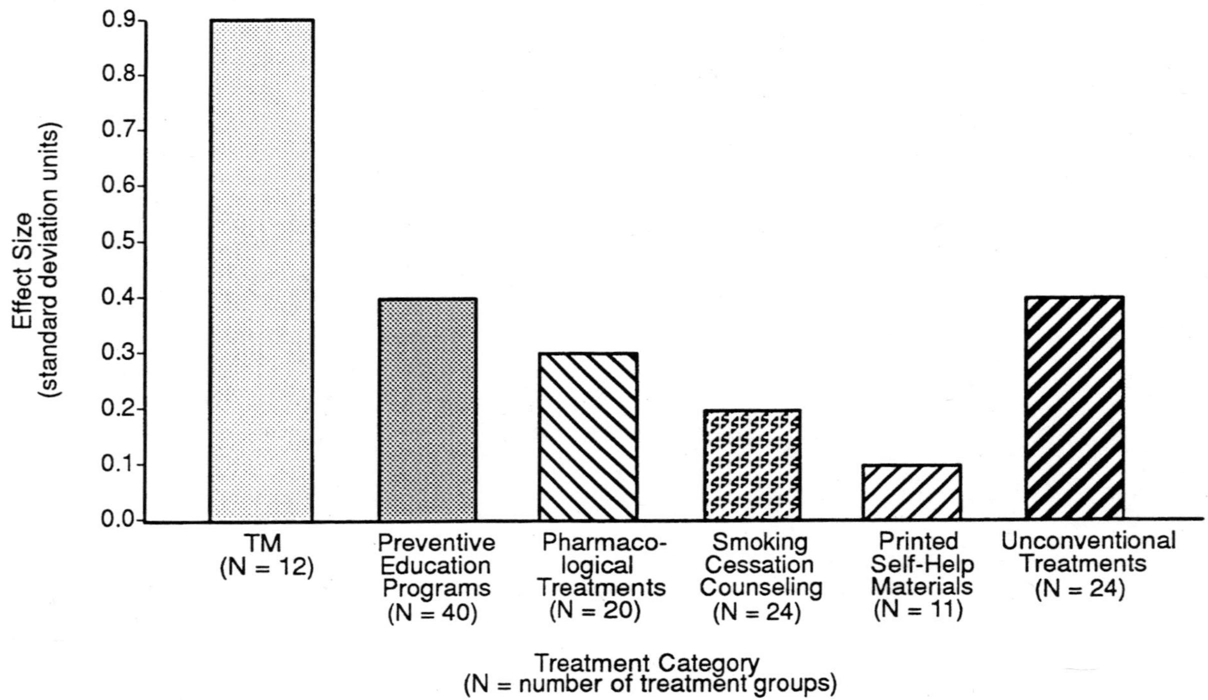

FIGURE 4. Average effect size for reduction in use of illicit drugs, comparing TM with preventive education programs.

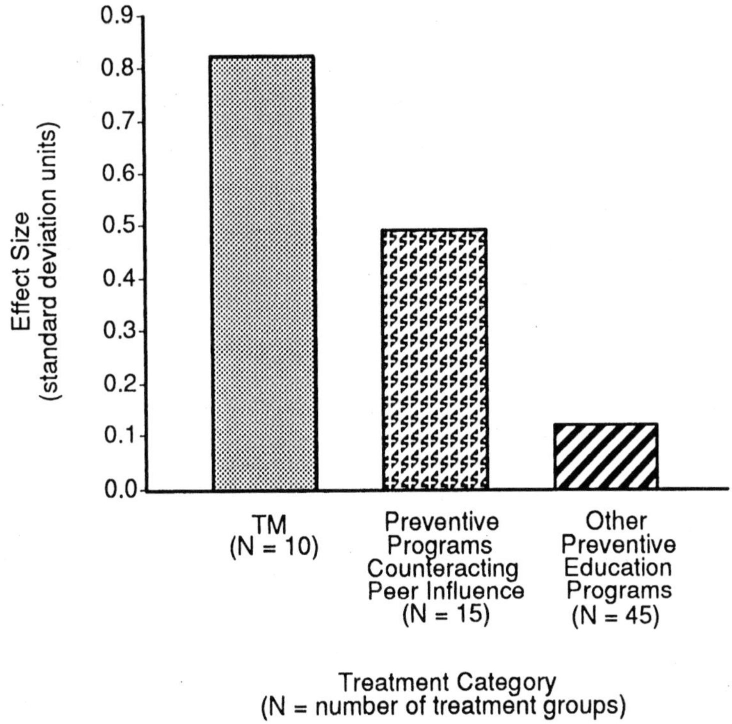

ported in Table 4. Fortunately, however, typical relapse rates over time for standard treatments are assessed in Hunt, Barnett, and Branch's (1971) classic review of 84 studies of individuals successfully completing cigarette, heroin, or alcohol treatment programs. Subsequent research has supported the general pattern observed in this review, although no quantitative synthesis of relapse rates has been published in recent years (Surgeon General, 1988). The relapse patterns from Hunt et al. are displayed in Figure 5.

Because these data are only for clients who successfully completed treatment, the first measurement point begins at 100% abstinence. Since an attrition rate of 50% typically occurs during the first

FIGURE 5. Relapse rates over time after successful completion of standard substance abuse treatment programs. (Source: Hunt et al., 1971; © 1971 Clinical Psychology Publishing Co., Inc., Brandon, Vermont.)

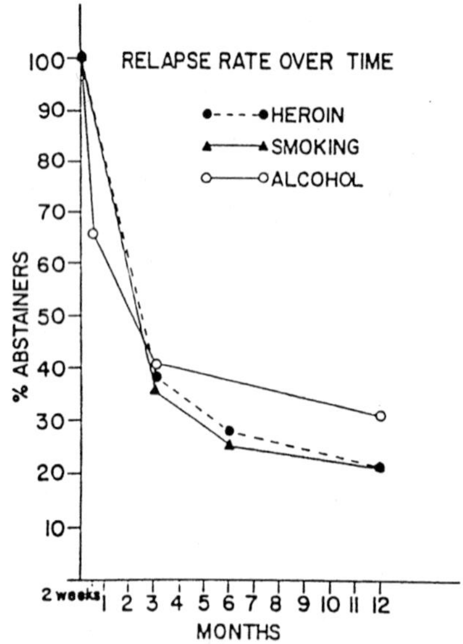

month of treatment (Stark, 1992), Hunt et al.'s samples represent a highly self-selected (motivated) group of individuals. Nonetheless, even for these selected subjects, abstinence rates fall off precipitously in the first three months following completion of treatment and continue to gradually decline in the succeeding months up to one year. Across substances as diverse as cigarettes, alcohol, and heroin, Hunt et al. observed a strikingly similar relapse pattern. This suggests that the key processes underlying relapse may be similar, and it underscores the difficulty of long-term quitting of legal as well as illicit substances.

Time Course for TM

Figure 6 graphically summarizes the time course of the effects of TM on alcohol, cigarette, and illicit drug consumption.[8]

The TM time course over an 18-month time period was calculated differently from the Hunt et al. time course. Hunt et al.'s first measurement point is the end of treatment (at 100% abstinence).

Since TM is self-directed and self-sustaining (i.e., once learned it is practiced by oneself), this "treatment" has no defined end point, Therefore, assessing abstinence rate from the end of treatment is not an appropriate stating point for measuring the TM time course. Also, because TM results were reported in different outcome variables (e.g., total abstinence in some cases, reduced level of consumption in others), effect size is used as a common metric for measuring reduced substance consumption rather than the abstinence rates used by Hunt et al. Further, because total abstinence (or reduced use), at least for alcohol and cigarettes, is not required for starting TM, initial high effect sizes for TM would not be expected for these substances.

Since this analysis examines changes in effect size over time, it necessitated including only studies reporting outcomes for the baseline as well as two post-intervention time points so that at least two effect sizes could be calculated. This criterion led to the inclusion of seven studies with four outcomes for alcohol, five outcomes for cigarettes, and four for illicit drugs.

Hunt et al. arbitrarily chose 3, 6, and 12 months for their time points. Because TM outcomes are reported for a variety of times including those that extend beyond 12 months, more time points were incorporated for Figure 6–1.5, 3, 6, 9, 12, and 18 months. Within each study, effect sizes were estimated for each of these points, either by interpolation (for longitudinal studies on the same subjects) or by linear trend fitting (for studies in which time point was a between-groups factor). In every case, however, effect sizes were not estimated beyond the last time point investigated in the study.

Finally, in averaging effect sizes across all studies at each time point, it was necessary to take account of missing data points due to the shorter duration of some studies. Because of the confounding influence of differing sample and design characteristics, failure to do so may distort the picture of changes in effect size over time. Therefore a multiple regression was performed on the set of all effect sizes from all time points of all studies, using the regression model to compensate for each study's tendency for stronger or weaker effect sizes. It is the estimated average effect sizes over time obtained from the fitted regression equation that are plotted in Figure 6.

FIGURE 6. Magnitude of the effect of TM on reducing alcohol, cigarettes, and illicit drug use as a function of time.

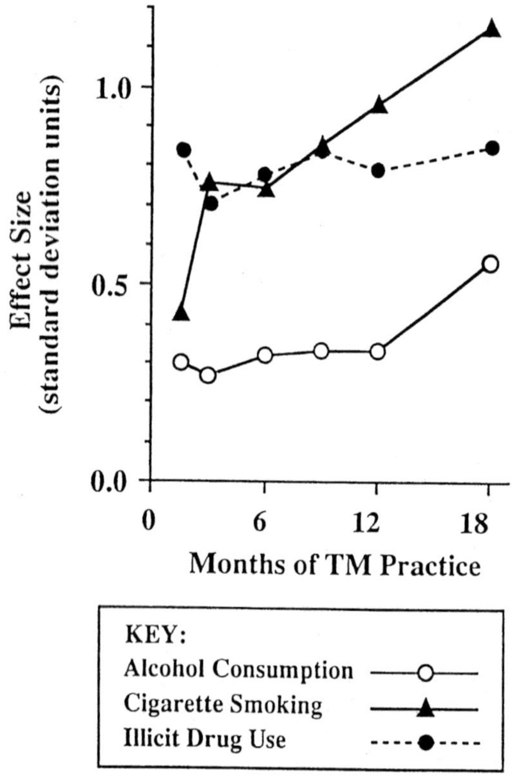

Contrary to rapid declines in abstinence for standard treatments seen in Hunt et al., the TM time course shows a gradual increase in effect sizes over time for alcohol and cigarettes, indicating increased abstinence and reduced use of these chemicals with TM practice over the long term. Steeper slopes for TM at the beginning of the graph for cigarettes and at the end for alcohol are probably due to incomplete compensation by the regression analysis for the few studies reporting either very short or very long study lengths relative to the other studies.

For the illicit drugs time course, the initial TM effect size was large and remained quite steady over time. The larger initial effect for illicit drugs (at 6 weeks) compared to the other chemicals is likely to be due largely to an initial 15-day abstinence from illicit drugs required of individuals prior to starting TM. The purpose of this voluntary requirement is not to prescribe lifestyle changes over the long term but to allow the clearest start of TM practice, since it has been found that illicit drug usage interferes with initial clarity of experience (Aron & Aron, 1983). However, once the individual starts TM, no prescription for abstaining from drug use is made since it is presumed that as a person spontaneously changes from "the inside," negative lifestyles will naturally fall off over time. In contrast to a precipitous drop in abstinence rates, followed by continuing declines for standard drug programs reported by Hunt et al., the stability of large TM effect sizes on illicit drugs indicates that subjects are successfully abstaining over the long term.

The overall time course for effect sizes depicted in Figure 6 is consistent with results of the strongest longitudinal studies on percentage abstinent for TM. For example, Royer (this volume) found the TM effect on smoking cessation increased linearly over time, to a 51% cessation rate (81% if reduction rates are also included) at 22 months for regular TM practitioners, compared to Hunt et al.'s rate of 25% at 12 months. Abstinence rate increased to 65% over an 18-month period in Taub et al.'s study (this volume) of skid-row-type alcoholics compared to Hunt et al.'s 35% alcohol abstinence rate. Finally, in a study of serious drug abusers (Geisler, 1978), abstinence increased to 89% at 18 months after TM instruction compared to Hunt et al.'s heroin abstinence rate of 25%. Given that abstinence rates for standard programs may continue to decline up to 2 years after treatment, the longer follow-up for TM studies should, if anything, have made it more difficult to sustain abstinence.

DISCUSSION

The use of quantitative statistical methods helps to clarify the issue raised in Klajner et al.'s (1984) narrative review regarding the efficacy of TM for substance abusers. Improved psychological functioning in known substance abusers (mainly prisoners) practicing TM was approximately twice as large as that produced by other forms of meditation and relaxation even for the general population. These psychological changes may, in turn, contribute to TM's distinctive effect on actual substance use. The current meta-analysis indicated the effect size of TM was substantially higher than for other treatments for each substance type: for alcohol, TM effects are 1.5 to 8 times larger than other treatments; for cigarettes, TM effects are from 2 to 5 times larger; and for illicit drugs, TM effects are 1.5 to 6 times larger. Also, TM appears different in its time course. Whereas with standard treatments success rates generally fall off over time, effects of TM appear to increase or at least remain stable over time.

Moreover, the impact of TM does not appear attributable to non-specific treatment effects, such as attention from trainer, expectancy, social support, or subjects' motivation to change. The magnitude of TM's effect compared with relaxation and standard treatments argues strongly against this. Relaxation methods tend to be similar to TM on most of these non-specific factors, yet their effects were substantially less than TM (.13 versus .55 for alcohol). If anything, sustained attention from trainers (and accompanying social support) should have been greater for the relaxation groups because initial training took place for a longer period (average 5 weeks) than TM (one week). The influence of such factors as initial motivation, attention from trainer, and social support also might be anticipated to be greater in some standard treatments (e.g., "face-to-face" counseling in smoking cessation clinics), yet these results were quite small compared to TM (in this case, .18 versus .90). Specifically, with regard to initial subject motivation to decrease substance use, it must be recalled that in contrast to these programs, TM is not explicitly introduced as a substance treatment program. Therefore, TM subjects are not selecting this program in order to reduce substance use. Moreover, these effects do not appear to be an artifact of TM subjects volunteering or choosing to participate. Although the majority of adolescents in Tobler's studies (1986) were assigned to their prevention class, and there were "incentives" for the DUI offenders to participate (Wells-Parker, personal communication, 1993), the results for the voluntary treatments reported in Kottke et al. (1988) and for the relaxation studies also were substantially smaller than for TM. Also, the time course of TM outcomes are in direct contrast to those of nonspecific treatment or placebo effects, which tend to be short-lived.

Several other potential alternative explanations for these results (other than the "distinctive" mechanics of the TM technique–see Conclusion) are briefly considered. While most of the published meta-analyses included only longitudinal and experimental studies, the TM meta-analysis included some retrospective surveys and cross-sectional studies to increase statistical power. However, TM's effects can not be attributed to inflated results due to inclusion of weaker studies because well-designed studies yielded equal or larger effect sizes than the weaker studies. The majority of TM studies drew from general populations rather than heavy abuser groups. Yet favorable results for TM also are not due to the overinclusion of casual users because TM effects for known abusing samples (or subsamples) were substantially larger than for the general population.

Eight of the 19 TM studies conducted secondary analyses on the effect of regularity of TM practice. They showed that when only the subset of regular TM practitioners (as opposed to all TM subjects) was compared with untreated controls, the average effect size was proportionally increased by 25% (from .74 to 1.00). The presence of such a "dose response" relation supports the hypothesis that it is the actual practice of TM (rather than other non-specific factors) that produces positive outcomes. The results for the current meta-analysis, however, cannot be attributed to inclusion of only regular meditators' results, because the effect size averages are based on the *total* sample of meditators (including irregular practitioners) available at posttest in each study. However, more effort in future primary studies and meta-analyses is needed to reliably estimate the impact of experimental attrition prior to posttest as well as the effect of regularity of treatment practice on substance use outcomes.

Another consideration is that TM follow-up times were generally longer than for standard treatments. However, the longer follow-up periods should have worked against producing larger TM results since the time course for standard treatments indicates a precipitous drop 3 months after completing treatment followed by a continuous gradual decline over the long term. Even for those meta-analyses with brief pre-posttest periods (e.g., Tobler, 1986), the magnitude of their effects still did not approach those of TM. It could be argued that because TM is self-directed, treatment is continuous and without end, and that this accounts for its success. Yet, other meditation and relaxation treatments which are also self-directed failed to produce psychological effects comparable to the psychological effects of TM on known substance abusers in the current meta-analysis, or on the general population in prior meta-analyses (e.g., Eppley et al., 1989). Moreover, TM's effect on actual substance use was substantially larger than that of relaxation, even though the pre-post intervals for TM (10.6 months) and relaxation (12.2 months) were comparable.

With a few exceptions, the studies of both TM and other treatment modalities relied primarily on self-report measures of substance abuse. Although there is evidence that self-report measures can provide a reliable estimate of actual substance use (as seen in Taub et al., this volume), future studies should augment "soft" self-report measures with "hard" indicators such as biochemical assays, incarcerations, or family/social validation procedures. In any event, for the present comparisons, use of self-report measures should have similarly affected outcomes for both TM and other treatments.

Thus, the results for TM do not appear attributable to the above potential alternative explanations. However, TM's results were compared to those for broad treatment types, on the basis of available meta-analyses, and *not* to specific programs. Even in the case of the relaxation studies, where we collected all primary published studies, there was not a sufficient number of cases to provide sufficient statistical power to allow meaningful comparisons with the specific relaxation treatments comprising this broader category. Thus, future meta-analyses on this topic should include an exhaustive search of both published and unpublished primary studies on promising treatments so that TM's effect can be compared with the effects of other *specific* programs or more narrowly defined treatment subtypes. Information on experimental attrition, treatment compliance, strength of experimental design, pre-posttest interval, treatment duration, and other factors that may potentially influence results should be uniformly coded and adjusted for statistically as necessary. Also, the time course of these primary studies should be quantified in a uniform and rigorous way so that their patterns over time can be statistically compared via appropriate dynamical methods.

Although meta-analysis provides a viable tool for statistically comparing results from many studies on different treatment types, it cannot substitute for (although it can valuably augment) rigorous experiments within which different treatments can be experimentally compared under identical conditions. It is recommended that future primary studies involve random assignment of heavy users to several promising treatment and usual-care control conditions as well as following consumption of various substances over a minimum two-year period using "hard" as well as "soft" measures of degree of substance abuse. It is also recommended that changes at the physiological, psychological, social, and spiritual levels be simultaneously monitored to assess their potential mediating role in treatment success.

CONCLUSION

Alcoholics Anonymous and other experts in the addiction field (e.g., Marlatt & Marques, 1977) have long acknowledged the critical role that meditation and relaxation may play in the recovery process. However, they do not provide clear criteria by which specific techniques should be chosen for practice. Statistical meta-analysis provides a useful tool for objectively determining the relative efficacy of different treatment programs.

Our review of prior meta-analyses on the general population (in Section II) showed that TM relative to other forms of meditation and relaxation significantly reverses physiological and psychological factors leading to substance abuse (thereby promoting primary prevention). As predicted, the current meta-analysis (in Section III) establishes that:

- these psychological improvements produced by TM generalize to known substance abusers (thereby promoting secondary prevention and addictions treatment);
- relative to control conditions, TM produces a significant effect on reducing use of alcohol, cigarettes, and illicit drugs in both the general population (further indicating secondary prevention) and in heavy users (demonstrating treatment efficacy);

- TM's effect on reducing use of these substances is also significantly larger than those produced by relaxation and other prevention and treatment programs;
- the time course for TM is distinctive with abstinence being maintained or increased over the long term (indicating effective relapse prevention).

The striking success of this natural technique thus holds important policy implications for both the treatment and prevention of substance abuse. TM appears to offer a highly cost-effective approach that can stand as a sole treatment for chemical dependency or serve as a useful adjunct to standard treatments (e.g., Bleick, this volume; Taub et al., this volume). As mentioned earlier, published statistical meta-analyses may not have featured or separately analyzed all promising individual treatment approaches. For example, it has been recently reported that a few largely residential programs (although losing about one-third of their clients during the first 6 weeks) show impressive reductions in relapse rate for those who stay the course for at least one year (Falco, 1992). However, such in-residence programs are highly expensive. For a private, non-profit treatment-center, the cost is approximately $10,000 for 4-6 weeks of treatment (Hazelden, 1991); when medicalized, treatment costs can soar up to $30,000 over the same period. The cost of TM is minuscule by comparison and includes life-long "check-ups" and knowledge sessions at any TM center world-wide at no additional cost (Denniston, 1986).

The total costs to the nation of alcohol, nicotine, and drug abuse are staggering. It is estimated that as much as $550 billion dollars is lost annually due to substance-related medical problems (such as cancer and heart disease), crime, decline in corporate productivity, chemical dependence treatment, and auto insurance losses paid (Orme-Johnson, this volume). The best controlled TM studies show abstinence rates for alcohol, cigarettes and illicit drugs of 51%-89% over an 18-22 month period (Geisler, 1978; Royer, this volume; Taub et al., this volume). Therefore, if the TM program could be taught on a large enough scale to drug users, and the above abstinence rates sustained over the long-term, literally hundreds of billions of dollars could be saved annually. Primary and secondary prevention through the societal effects of collective practice of the Transcendental Meditation and TM-Sidhi program could result in additional massive savings to the nation (Orme-Johnson, this volume).

What can account for this simple technique's apparently dramatic effects on reduced substance abuse? Multidimensional, interacting factors appear to underlie the emergence of addictive behavior. When one or more of these fundamental dimensions of life (spirit, mind, body, social behavior, and environment) are deficient or imbalanced, people become at risk for adopting addictive behavior as a means to fulfill unmet needs. While conventional treatments of substance dependence often employ several modalities, they may target more surface levels of functioning, such as attitudes and behavior, failing to root out the deeper causes of addiction. If deeper imbalances are not eliminated, initial effects may only be temporary, with addictive behaviors resurfacing again and again despite numerous attempts at abstinence. This may account for the rapid declines in abstinence following completion of most standard treatment programs (Hunt et al., 1971; Surgeon General, 1988).

In contrast, the dramatic effect of TM in reducing substance abuse may be due to its ability to address the "whole" of addiction rather than its "parts" from the deepest possible level. From the perspective of Maharishi's Vedic Psychology, TM brings the practitioner back "home to the Self," to a simple, self-referral experience of silent inner Being which has been lost to us amidst the frenetic activity of contemporary life. In recontacting this transcendental level of life, all the more manifest or active levels of functioning are said to be spontaneously nourished as well. Consistent with this view, research on TM documents this apparently holistic, positive effect at all levels–spiritual, psychological, physiological, social, and environmental. Therefore, repeated experiences of transcendence through TM should gradually culture a state of such inner fulfillment and balance that any need to seek fulfillment outside the self through substance use would be entirely eliminated. This would explain why, over the course of time, TM practice leads naturally to increasing drug abstinence.

Self-recovery through TM thus may provide the basis, not only for recovery from chemical dependency, but for unfolding one's full potential which is the natural birthright of all human beings.

NOTES

1. Hedge's correction factor for bias due to small sample sizes (Hunter & Schmidt, 1990) was applied to all effect size estimates by dividing by 1 + .75/(N – 3).

2. Weights were calculated as the logarithm of sample size times the study design code, following a scheme used by Kottke et al. (1988) in their analysis.

3. Levin and Lehman's (1991) meta-analysis on the effects of desipramine on cocaine addiction reported their results in combined p values which could not be converted into effect sizes.

4. There were two cases on smoking cessation where results were combined with larger categories. (1) In a meta-analysis on the effects o the drug clonidine on nicotine addiction (Covey & Glassman, 1991), results of the 5 primary studies with long-term follow-up, averaging 4.9 months, were combined with Kottke et al.'s (1988) category of nicotine replacement therapies (pharmacological treatments). (2) Only 6 published relaxation studies on smoking cessation were located which met our inclusion criteria (Brown & Lichtenstein, 1981; Griffith & Crossman, 1983; Patel & Carrughers, 1977; Ravensborg, 1976; Schneider et al., 1992; Schubert, 1983). These studies were combined with Kottke et al.'s nonconventional (nonpharmacological) treatment category.

5. Bangert-Drowns (1988) and Bruvold (1990) highly overlapped with the larger Tobler (1986) study, and their overall effect sizes were quite similar; Lam, Sze, Sacks, and Chalmers (1987) almost entirely overlapped with Kottke et al. (1988), and their overall effect sizes were again very similar.

6. Because standard deviations and number of intervention groups varied between treatment categories, Welch's modification of the planned comparison (Maxwell & Delaney, 1990, p. 146) was performed to avoid underestimating the level of Type I error.

7. In this analysis, the relationship between the number of degrees of freedom and the number of cases is mathematically complex because of the modified planned comparison which was used (see note 6).

8. The illicit drugs evaluated include not only "hard drugs" like heroin but also "soft" drugs like cannabis. However, given the similarity in relapse rates across diverse substances, the time course for this broader drug category would be anticipated to be similar to others reviewed by Hunt et al. (1971).

REFERENCES

Abrams, A. I. (1989). A follow-up study of the effects of the Transcendental Meditation program on inmates at Folsom prison. In R. Chalmers, G. Clements, H. Schenkluhn, & M. Weinless (Eds.), *Scientific research on Maharishi's Transcendental Meditation and TM-Sidhi program: Collected Papers* (Vol. 3) (pp. 2108-2112). Vlodrop, Netherlands: Maharishi Vedic University Press.

Abrams, A. I., & Siegel, L. M. (1978). The Transcendental Meditation program and rehabilitation at Folsom State Prison: A cross-validation study. *Criminal Justice and Behavior, 5*(1), 3-20.

Alcoholics Anonymous World Services, Inc. (1981). *Twelve steps and twelve traditions*. New York: Author.

Alexander, C. N. (1982). Ego development, personality and behavioral change in inmates practicing the Transcendental Meditation technique or participating in other programs: A cross-sectional and longitudinal study. *Dissertation Abstracts International, 43*(2), 539B.

Alexander, C. N. (1993). Transcendental Meditation. In R. J. Corsini (Ed.), *Encyclopedia of Psychology* (2nd ed.). New York: Wiley Interscience.

Alexander, C. N., Cranson, R., Boyer, R. W., & Orme-Johnson, D. W. (1987). Transcendental consciousness: A fourth state of consciousness beyond sleep, dreaming and waking. In J. Gackenbach (Ed.), *Sleep and dreams: A sourcebook* (pp. 282-312). New York: Garland.

Alexander, C. N., Gerace, D., Rainforth, M. V., & Beto, Z. (in press). Developing higher states of consciousness: Theory, subjective experiences, and research. In J. Gackenbach, C. N. Alexander, & H. Hunt (Eds.), *Higher states of consciousness: Theoretical and experimental perspectives*. New York: Plenum.

Alexander, C. N., Langer, E., Newman, R., Chandler, H., & Davies, J. L. (1989). Transcendental Meditation, mindfulness and longevity: An experimental study with the elderly. *Journal of Personality and Social Psychology, 57*, 950-964.

Alexander, C. N., Rainforth, M.V., & Gelderloos, P. (1991). Transcendental Meditation, self-actualization, and psychological health: A conceptual overview and statistical meta-analysis. *Journal of Social Behavior and Personality, 6*, 189-247.

Alexander, C. N., & Sands, D. (1993). Meditation and relaxation. In F. N. McGill (Ed.), *McGill's survey of the social sciences: Psychology*. Pasadena, CA: Salem Press.

Alexander, C. N., Swanson, G. C., Rainforth, M.V., Carlisle, T. W., & Todd, C. C. (1993). A prospective study on the Transcendental Meditation program in two occupational settings: Effects on stress-reduction, health, and employee development. *Anxiety, Stress and Coping: An International Journal, 6*, 245-262.

Alford, G. S., Koehler, R. A., & Leonard, J. (1991). Alcoholics Anonymous-Narcotics Anonymous model inpatient treatment of chemically dependent adolescents: 2-year outcome study. *Journal of Studies on Alcohol, 52*(2), 118-125.

Aron, E. N., & Aron, A. (1982). Transcendental Meditation program and marital adjustment. *Psychological Report, 51*, 887-890.

Aron, E. N., & Aron, A. (1983). The patterns of reduction of drug and alcohol use among Transcendental Meditation participants. *Bulletin of the Society of Psychologists in Addictive Behaviors, 3*(1), 28-33.

Aron, A., Orme-Johnson, D. W., & Brubaker, P. (1981). The Transcendental Meditation program in the college curriculum: A 4-year longitudinal study of effects on cognitive and affective functioning. *College Student Journal, 15*(2), 140-146.

Badawi, K., Wallace, R. K., Orme-Johnson, D. W., & Rouzere, A. M. (1984).

Electrophysiologic characteristics of respiratory suspension periods occurring during the practice of the Transcendental Meditation program. *Psychosomatic Medicine, 46*(3), 267-276.

Bangert-Drowns, R. L. (1988). The effects of school-based substance abuse education: A meta-analysis. *Journal of Drug Education, 18*(3), 243-264.

Beckman, L. J., & Bardsley, P. E. (1986). Individual characteristics, gender differences, and dropout from alcoholism treatment. *Alcohol and Alcoholism, 21*, 213-224.

Benson, H., & Wallace, R. K. (1972). Decreased drug abuse with Transcendental Meditation: A study of 1,862 subjects. In C. J. D. Zarafonetis (Ed.), *Drug abuse: Proceedings of the international conference*, Philadelphia: Lea and Febiger.

Bleick, C. R. (this volume). Case histories: Using the Transcendental Meditation program with alcoholics and addicts. *Alcoholism Treatment Quarterly.*

Bleick, C. R., & Abrams, A. I. (1987). The Transcendental Meditation program and criminal recidivism in California. *Journal of Criminal Justice, 15*, 211-230.

Brautigam, E. (1977). Effects of the Using the Transcendental Meditation program on drug abusers: A prospective study. In D. W. Orme-Johnson & J. T. Farrow (Eds.), *Scientific research on the Transcendental Meditation program: Collected papers* (Vol. 1) (pp. 506-514). West Germany: MERU Press.

Brickman, P., Rabinowitz V., Karuza, J., Coates, D., Cohn, E., & Kidder, L. (1982). Models of helping and coping. *American Psychologist, 37*, 368-384.

Brooks, J. S., & Scarano, T. (1985). Transcendental Meditation in the treatment of post-Vietnam adjustment. *Journal of Counseling and Development, 64*, 212-215.

Broome, V. J. (1989). *Relationship between participation in Transcendental Meditation and the functionality of marriage.* Doctoral dissertation. University of the Witerwatersrand, Johannesburg, South Africa.

Brown, H. P., & Peterson, J. H. (1990). Rationale and procedural suggestions for defining and actualizing spiritual values in the treatment of dependency. *Alcoholism Treatment Quarterly, 7*(3), 17-42.

Brown, R. A., & Lichtenstein, E. (1981). Effects of monitored nicotine fading and anxiety management training on smoking reduction. *Addictive Behaviors, 6*, 301-305.

Brownell, K. D. (1982). The addictive disorders. In C. M. Franks, P. C. Kendall, & K. D. Brownell (Eds.), *Annual review of behavior therapy: Theory and practice* (pp. 208-272). New York: Guilford Press.

Brownell, K. D., Marlatt, G. A., Lichtenstein, E., & Wilson, G. T. (1986). Understanding and preventing relapse. *American Psychologist, 41*, 765-782.

Bruvold, W. H. (1990). A meta-analysis of the California school-based risk reduction program. *Journal of Drug Education, 20*(2), 139-152.

Bujatti, M., &. Riederer, P. (1976). Serotonin, noradrenaline, dopamine metabolites in Transcendental Meditation technique. *Journal of Neural Transmitters, 39*, 257-267.

Catalano, R. F., Hawkins, J. D., Wells, E. A., & Miller, J. (1990-91). Evaluation of the effectiveness of adolescent drug abuse treatment, assessment of risks for relapse, and promising approaches for relapse prevention. *The International Journal of the Addictions, 25*(9A & 10A), 1085-1140.

Cattell, R. B. (1946). *The description and measurement of personality*. New York: World.

Cavanaugh, K. L., King, K. D., & Ertuna, C. (1989). *A multiple-input transfer function model of Okun's misery index: An empirical test of the Maharishi effect*. Paper presented at the Annual Meeting of the American Statistical Association. Washington, D. C., August 6-10, 1989. An abridged version of this paper appears in *Proceedings of the American Statistical Association, Business and Economics Statistics Section* (Alexandria, Virginia: American Statistical Association), 565-570.

Chandler, H. M. (1991). Transcendental Meditation and awakening wisdom: A ten-year longitudinal study of self-development. *Dissertation Abstracts International, 51*(106), 5048.

Chandler, H. M., & Alexander, C. N. (in review). Transcendental Meditation and advanced self-development in adulthood: A ten year longitudinal study. *Human Development*.

Chatlos, J. C. (1989). Adolescent dual-diagnosis: A 12-step transformational model. *Journal of Psychoactive Drugs: A Multidisciplinary Forum, 21*(2), 189-201.

Christopher, J. (1988). *How to stay sober: Recovery without religion*. Buffalo: Prometheus Books.

Clarke, J. C., & Saunders, J. B. (1988). *Alcoholism and problem drinking: Theories and treatment*. New York: Pergamon Press.

Cohen, J. (1977). *Statistical power analysis for behavioral sciences*. New York: Academic Press.

Cook-Greuter, S. R. (1990). Maps for living: Ego development stages from symbiosis to conscious universal embeddedness. In M. L. Commons, C. Armons, L. Kohlberg, F. A. Richards, T. A. Grotzer, & J. D. Sinnott (Eds.), *Adult development 2: Models and methods in the study of adolescent and adult thought*. New York: Praeger.

Covey, L. S., & Glassman, A. H. (1991). A meta-analysis of double-blind placed controlled trials of clonidine for smoking cessation. *British Journal of Addiction, 86*, 991-998.

Cranson, R. W., Orme-Johnson, D. W., Gackenbach, J., Dillbeck, M. C., Jones, C. H., & Alexander, C. N. (1991). Transcendental Meditation and improved performance on intelligence-related measures: A longitudinal study. *Personality and Individual Differences, 12*, 1105-1116.

Cronkite, R. C., & Moos, R. H. (1980). Determinants of the posttreatment functioning of alcoholic patients: A conceptual framework. *Journal of Consulting and Clinical Psychology, 48*(3), 305-316.

Cummings, C., Gordon, J., & Marlatt, G. (1980). Relapse: Strategies of prevention and prediction. In W. Miller (Ed.), *The addictive behaviors*. Oxford: Pergamon Press.

Denniston, D. (1986). *The Transcendental Meditation book: How to enjoy the rest of your life*. Fairfield, IA: Fairfield Press.

Denny, M. R., Baugh, J. L., & Hardt, H. D. (1991). Sobriety outcome after alcoholism treatment with biofeedback participation: A pilot inpatient study. *International Journal of the Addictions, 26*(3), 335-341.

Dillbeck, M. C. (1982). Meditation and flexibility of visual perception and verbal problem solving. *Memory and Cognition, 10*(3), 207-215.

Dillbeck, M. C. (1990). Test of a field theory of consciousness and social change: Time series analysis of participation in the TM-Sidhi program and reduction of violent death in the U.S. *Social Indicators Research, 22*, 399-418.

Dillbeck, M. C., & Abrams, A. I. (1987). The application of the Transcendental Meditation program in corrections. *International Journal of Comparative and Applied Criminal Justice, 11*, 111-132.

Dillbeck, M. C., Assimakis, P. D., Raimondi, D., Orme-Johnson, D. W., & Rowe, R. (1986). Longitudinal effects of the Transcendental Meditation and the TM-Sidhi program on cognitive ability and cognitive style. *Perceptual and Motor Skills, 62*, 731-738.

Dillbeck, M. C., & Orme-Johnson, D. W. (1987). Physiological differences between Transcendental Meditation and rest. *American Psychologist, 42*, 879-881.

Dillbeck, M. C., Orme-Johnson, D. W., & Wallace, R. K. (1981). Frontal EEG coherence, H-reflex recovery, concept learning, and the TM-Sidhi program. *International Journal of Neuroscience, 15*, 151-157.

Dongier, M., & Schwartz, G. (1989). Feasibility of effective psychopharmacological treatments for alcoholism. *British Journal of Addiction, 84*(2), 227-228.

Donovan, D. M. (1988). Assessment of addictive behaviors: Implications of an emerging biopsychosocial model. In D. M. Donovan, & G. A. Marlatt (Eds.), *Assessment of addictive behaviors*. New York: Guilford Press.

Donovan, D. M., Kivlahan, D. R., & Walker, R. D. (1986). Alcoholic subtypes based on multiple assessment domains: Validation against treatment outcome. In M. Galanter (Ed.), *Recent developments in alcoholism*. New York: Plenum Press.

Donovan, D. M., & Marlatt, G. A. (1988). *Assessment of addictive behaviors*. New York: Guilford Press.

Elliot, D. S., Huizinga, D., & Ageton, S. S. (1985). *Explaining delinquency and drug use*. Beverly Hills: Sage.

Ellis, G. A., & Corum, P. (this volume). Removing the motivator: A holistic solution to substance abuse. *Alcoholism Treatment Quarterly*.

Emrick, C. D. (1975). A review of psychologically oriented treatment of alcoholism II: The relative effectiveness of different treatment approaches and the effectiveness of treatment versus no-treatment. *Journal of the Study of Alcohol, 35*, 534-549.

Eppley, K. R., Abrams, A. I., & Shear, J. (1989). Differential effects of relaxation techniques on trait anxiety: A meta-analysis. *Journal of Clinical Psychology, 45*, 957-974.

Erikson, E. H. (1968). *Identity, youth and crises*. New York: Norton.

Falco, M. (1992). *The making of a drug-free America: Programs that work.* Alexandria, VA: Time Books.

Farinelli, L. (1989). Possibilita di applicazioni della tecnologia della coscienza in aspetti de medicccina preventiva: Una ricera pilota. In R. Chalmers, G. Clements, H. Schenkluhn, & M. Weinless (Eds.), *Scientific research on Maharishi's Transcendental Meditation and TM-Sidhi program: Collected papers* (Vol. 3) (pp. 1830-1845). Vlodrop, Netherlands: Maharishi Vedic University Press.

Farrow, J. T., & Hebert, J. R. (1982). Breath suspension during the Transcendental Meditation technique. *Psychosomatic Medicine, 44*(2), 133-153.

Frew, D. R. (1974). Transcendental Meditation and Productivity. *Academy of Management Journal, 17*, 362-368.

Friedman, A. S., & Glickman, N. W. (1986). Program characteristics for successful treatment of adolescent drug abuse. *Journal of Nervous and Mental Disease, 174*(11), 669-679.

Friend, K. E. (1975). *An experimental deception for the primary study and ancillary data relating Transcendental Meditation to decreases in alcohol and tobacco usage*. Unpublished manuscript. Graduate School of Business, University of Chicago, Chicago, IL.

Gay, L. R. (1981). *Educational research: Competencies for analysis and application*. Columbus, OH: Merrill.

Geisler, M. (1978). Therapeutische wirkungen der Transcendentalen meditation auf drogenkonsumenten (Therapeutic effects of Transcendental Meditation in drug abusers). *Zeitschrift fur Klinische Psychologie, 7*, 235-255.

Gelderloos, P. (1987). Psychological health and development of students at Maharishi International University: A controlled longitudinal study. *Modern Science and Vedic Science, 1*, 471-487.

Gelderloos, P., Goddard, P. H. III, & Ahlstrom, H. H., & Jacoby, R. (1987). Cognitive orientation towards positive values in advanced participants of the TM and TM-Sidhi program. *Perceptual and Motor Skills, 64*, 1003-1012.

Gelderloos, P., Hermans, H. J. M., Ahlstrom, H. H., & Jacoby, R. (1990). Transcendence and psychological health: Studies with long-term participants of the TM and TM-Sidhi program. *Journal of Psychology, 124, 177-197.*

Gelderloos, P., Walton, K. G., Orme-Johnson, D. W., & Alexander, C. N. (1991). Effectiveness of the Transcendental Meditation program in preventing and treating substance misuse: A review. *International Journal of the Addictions, 26*, 293-325.

Glaser, J. (this volume) Clinical applications of Maharishi Ayur-Veda in chemical dependency disorders. *Alcoholism Treatment Quarterly.*

Glass, G.V., McGaw, B., & Smith, M. L. (1981). *Meta-analysis in social research.* Beverly Kills, CA: Sage.

Goleman, D. J., & Schwartz, G. E. (1976). Meditation as an intervention in stress reactivity. *Journal of Consulting Clinical Psychology, 44*, 456-466.

Gorski, T. T., & Miller, M. (1986). *Staying sober.* Independence, MO: Independence Press.

Gorski, T. T. (1989). *Understanding the twelve-steps: An interpretation and guide for recovering people.* New York: Prentice Hall/Parkside.

Greaves, G. B. (1980). An existential theory of drug dependence. In D. Lettieri, M. Sayers, and H. Pearson (Eds.), *Theories of drug abuse.* Washington, DC: National Institute on Drug Abuse.

Griffith, E. E., & Crossman, E. (1983). Biofeedback: A possible substitute for smoking, experiment I. *Addictive Behaviors, 8,* 77-285.

Hawkins, J. D., Lishner, D., & Catalano, R. F. (1985). Childhood predictors and the prevention of adolescent substance abuse. In C. L. Jones & R. J. Battjes (Eds.), *Etiology of drug abuse: Implications for prevention* (pp. 75-126). National Institute on Drug Abuse Research Monograph.

Hazelden Foundation. (1991). *Hazelden News and Professional Update.* Minnesota: Hazelden.

Hedges, L. (1984). Estimation of effect size under nonrandom sampling: The effects of censoring studies yielding statistically insignificant mean differences. *Journal of Educational Statistics, 9,* 61-85.

Hedges, L. V., & Olkin, L. I. (1980). Vote counting methods in research synthesis. *Psychological Bulletin, 88,* 359-369.

Hester, R. K., & Miller, W. R. (1989). *Handbook of alcoholism treatment approaches: Effective alternatives.* Elmsford, NY: Pergamon Press.

Hjelle, L. A. (1974). Transcendental Meditation and psychological health. *Perceptual and Motor Skills, 39,* 623-628.

Hollister, L. E. (1990). Treatment outcome: A neglected area of drug abuse research. *Drug and Alcohol Dependence, 25,* 175-177.

Hunt, W. A., Barnett, L. W., & Branch, L. G. (1971). Relapse rates in addiction programs. *Journal of Clinical Psychology, 27,* 455-456.

Hunter, J. E., & Schmidt, F. L. (1990). *Methods of meta-analysis.* New York: Sage.

James, W. (1902/1958). *The varieties of religious experience.* New York: Mentor-NAL.

Jones, M. C. (1968). Personality correlates and antecedents of drinking patterns in adult males. *Journal of Consulting Clinical Psychology, 26,* 1-15.

Johnson, B. D., Goldstein, P. J., Preble, E., Schmeidler J., Lipton, D., Spunt, B., & Miller, T. (1985). *Taking care of business: The economics of crime by heroin abusers.* Lexington, MA: Lexington Books.

Jung, C. J. (1933). *Modern man in search of soul.* San Diego: Harcourt Brace Jovanovich.

Jurich, A., & Polson, C. C. (1984). Reasons for drug use: Comparison of drug users and abusers. *Psychological Reports, 55,* 371-378.

Katz, D. (1977). Decreased drug use and prevention of drug use through the Transcendental Meditation program. In D. W. Orme-Johnson & J. T. Farrow (Eds.), *Scientific research on Maharishi's Transcendental Meditation and TM-Sidhi program: Collected papers* (Vol. 1). West Germany: MERU Press.

Kember, P. (1985). The Transcendental Meditation technique and postgraduate academic performance. *British Journal of Educational Psychology, 55*, 164-166.

Klajner, F., Hartman, L. M., & Sobell, M. B. (1984). Treatment of substance abuse by relaxation training: A review of its rationale, efficacy and mechanisms. *Addictive Behavior, 9*, 41-55.

Klitzner, W. (1987). *Report to Congress on the nature and effectiveness of federal, state and local drug prevention/education programs, part II: An assessment of the research on school-based prevention programs.* In U.S. Department of Education, Office of Planning, Budget and Evaluation, Washington, DC: DHHS/U.S. Government Printing Office.

Kofoed, L. L., Tolson, R. L., Atkinson, R. M., Toth, R. L., & Turner, J. A. (1987). Treatment compliance of older alcoholics: An elder specific approach is superior to "mainstreaming." *Journal of Studies on Alcohol, 48*, 47-51.

Kottke, T. T., Battista, R. N., Defriese, G. H. & Brekke, M. L. (1988). Attributes of successful smoking cessation interventions in medical practice: A meta-analysis of 39 controlled trials. *Journal of the American Medical Association, 259*, 2883-2889.

Lam, W., Sze, P. C., Sacks, H. S., & Chalmers, T. C. (1987). Meta-analysis of randomized controlled trials of nicotine chewing-gum. *The Lancet,* July, 27-30.

Langer, E., Perlmutter, M., Chanowitz, B., & Rubin, R. (1988). Two new applications of mindfulness theory: Alcoholism and aging. *Journal of Aging Studies, 2* (3), 289-299.

Lazar, Z., Farwell, L., & Farrow, J. T. (1977). The effects of the Transcendental Meditation program on anxiety, drug abuse, cigarette smoking, and alcohol consumption. In D. W. Orme-Johnson & J. T. Farrow (Eds.), *Scientific research on Maharishi's Transcendental Meditation and TM-Sidhi program: Collected papers* (Vol. 1) (pp. 524-535). West Germany: MERU Press.

Levin, J. D. (1987). *Treatment of alcoholism and other addictions.* New Jersey: Aronson.

Levin, F. R., & Lehman, A. F. (1991). Meta-analysis of desipramine as an adjunct in the treatment of cocaine addiction. *Journal of Clinical Psychopharmacology, 11*(6), 374-378.

Long, J. V. F., & Scherl, D. J. (1984). Developmental antecedents of compulsive drug use: A report on the literature. *Journal of Psychoactive Drugs, 16*, 169-182.

Loevinger, J. (1976). *Ego development: Conceptions and theories.* San Francisco: Jossey-Bass.

Loevinger, J., Cohn, L. D., Bonneville, L. P., Redmore, C. D., Surcich, D. D., & Sargent, M. (1985). Ego development in college. *Journal of Personality and Social Psychology, 48*, 947-962.

MacClean, C. R. K., Walton, K. G., Wenneberg, S. R., Levitsky, D. K., Mandarino, J. V., Waziri, R., & Schneider, R. H. (1992). Altered cortisol response to stress after four months practice of the Transcendental Meditation program. *Society of Neuroscience Abstracts, 18*, 1541.

Maharishi Mahesh Yogi (1966). *The science of being and art of living*. Livingston Manor, NY: Maharishi International University Press.

Maharishi Mahesh Yogi (1969). *On the Bhagavad Gita: A translation and commentary, Chapters 1-6*. Baltimore, MD: Penguin.

Maharishi Mahesh Yogi (1986). *Life supported by natural law*. Washington, DC: Age of Enlightenment Press.

Maharishi Mahesh Yogi (1972). *Science of creative intelligence: Knowledge and experience* (Videotaped course syllabus). Los Angeles: MIU Press.

Marlatt, G. A. (1988). Matching clients to treatment: Treatment models and stages of change. In D. M. Donovan, & G. A. Marlatt (Eds.), *Assessment of addictive behavior* (pp. 474-483). New York: Guilford Press.

Marlatt, G. A., & George, W. H. (1984). Relapse prevention: Introduction and overview of the model. *British Journal of Addictions, 79*, 261-272.

Marlatt, G. A., & Marques, J. K. (1977). Meditation, self-control, and alcohol use. In R.B. Stuart (Ed.), *Behavioral self-management: Strategies, techniques, and outcomes* (pp. 117-153). New York: Brunner/Mazel.

Martin, S. E., Sechrest, L. B., & Redner, R. (Eds.). (1981). *New directions in the rehabilitation of criminal offenders*. Washington, DC: The National Research Council, National Academy of Sciences.

Maslow, A. H. (1964). *Religion, values and peak-experiences*. Columbus, OH: Ohio State University Press.

Maslow, A. H. (1968). *Toward a psychology of being* (2nd ed.). New York: Harper & Row.

Maxwell, S. E., & Delaney, H. D. (1990). Designing experiments and analyzing data: A model comparison perspective. Belmont, CA: Wadsworth.

McLellan, A. T., Alterman, A. I., Cacciola, J., Metzger, D., & O'Brien, C. P. (1992). A new measure of substance abuse treatment: Initial studies of the treatment services review. *The Journal of Nervous and Mental Disease, 180*(2), 101-110.

Miller, W. R., & Taylor, C. T. (1980). Relative effectiveness of bibliotherapy, individual and group self-control training in the treatment of problem drinkers. *Addictive Behavior, 5*, 13-24.

Monahan, R. J. (1977). Secondary prevention of drug dependence through the Transcendental Meditation program in metropolitan Philadelphia. *International Journal of the Addictions, 12*, 729-754.

Moore, T. (1992). *Care of the soul*. New York: Harper Collins.

Murphy, M. (1992). *The future of the body: Exploration into the further evolution of human nature*. New York: G.P. Putnam's Sons.

Murphy, T. J., Pagano, R. R., & Marlatt, A. (1986). Lifestyle modification with heavy alcohol drinkers: Effects of aerobic exercise and meditation. *Addictive Behaviors, 11*, 175-186.

Myers, T. I., & Eisner, E. J. (1974). *An experimental evaluation of the effects of karate and meditation*. Final report for the U.S. Army Institute for the Behavioral and Social Sciences, Social Processes Technical Area. American Institutes for Research, Washington, D.C.

Nidich, S. I. (1989). The Science of Creative Intelligence and the Transcendental Meditation program: Reduction of drug and alcohol consumption. In R. Chalmers, G. Clements, H. Schenkluhn & M. Weinless (Eds.), *Scientific research on Maharishi's Transcendental Meditation and TM-Sidhi program: Collected papers* (Vol. 3) (pp. 2115-2123). Vlodrop, Netherlands: Maharishi Vedic University Press.

Nystul, M. S., & Garde, M. (1977). Comparison of self-concepts of Transcendental Meditators and nonmeditators. *Psychology Report, 41*, 303-306.

O'Connell, D. F. (1991). The use of Transcendental Meditation in relapse prevention counseling. *Alcoholism Treatment Quarterly, 8* (1), 53-68.

O'Connell, D. F. (this volume). Possessing the self. *Alcoholism Treatment Quarterly.*

Oetting, R. R., & Beauvais, F. (1987). Peer cluster theory, socialization characteristics and adolescent drug use: A path analysis. *Journal of Counseling Psychology, 43*, 205-213.

Olson, R. P., Ganley, R., Devine, V. T., & Dorsey, G. C. (1981). Long-term effects of behavioral versus insight-oriented therapy with in-patient alcoholics. *Journal of Consulting and Clinical Psychology, 49*(6), 866-877.

Orford, J. (1985). *Excessive appetites: A psychological view of addictions.* New York: John Wiley & Sons.

Orme-Johnson, D. W. (1973). Autonomic stability and Transcendental Meditation. *Psychosomatic Medicine, 35*, 341-349.

Orme-Johnson, D. W. (1988). The cosmic psyche, an introduction to Maharishi's Vedic psychology: The fulfillment of modern psychology. *Modern Science and Vedic Science*. 2(2), 113-163.

Orme-Johnson, D. W. (this volume). Transcendental Meditation as an epidemiological approach to drug and alcohol abuse: Theory, research and Financial Impact Evaluation. *Alcoholism Treatment Quarterly.*

Orme-Johnson, D. W., Alexander, C. N., Davies, J. L., Chandler, H. M., & Larimore, W. E. (1988). International peace project in the Middle East: The effect of the Maharishi Technology of the Unified Field. *Journal of Conflict Resolution, 32*, 776-812.

Orme-Johnson, D. W., & Haynes, C. T. (1981). EGG phase coherence, pure consciousness, and TM-Sidhi experiences. *International Journal of Neuroscience, 13*, 211-217.

Ormrod, J. & Budd, R. (1991). A comparison of two treatment interventions aimed at lowering anxiety levels and alcohol consumption amongst alcohol abusers. *Drug and Alcohol Dependence, 27*, 233-243.

Ottens, A. J. (1975). The effect of Transcendental Meditation upon modifying the cigarette smoking habit. *Journal of the School of Health, 45*(10), 577-583.

Overbeck, K. D. (1982). Auswirkungen der Transzendentalen Meditation (TM) auf die psychische und psychosomatische Befindlichkeit. *Psychotherapie-Psychosomatik Medizinische Psychologie, 32*(6), 188-192.

Padelford, B. (1974). Relationship between drug involvement and purpose in life. *Journal of Clinical Psychology, 30*, 303-305.

Patel, C., & Carruthers, M. (1977). Coronary risk factor reduction through biofeedback-aided relaxation and meditation. *Journal of the Royal College of General Practitioners, 27*, 401-405.

Penner, W. J., Zingle, H. W., Dyck R., & Truch, S. (1974). Does an in-depth Transcendental Meditation course effect change in personalities of the participants? *Western Psychologist, 4*, 104-111.

Pelletier, K. R. (1974). Influence of Transcendental Meditation upon autokinetic perception. *Perceptual and Motor Skills, 39*, 1031-1034.

Rodin, J., Maloff, D., & Becker, H. S. (1984). Self-control: The role of environment and self-generated cues. In P. K. Levison (Ed.), *Substance abuse, habitual behavior and self-control* (pp. 9-47). Boulder, CO: Westview Press.

Ravensborg, M. R. (1976). Relaxation as therapy for addictive smoking. *Psychological Reports, 39*, 894.

Rokeach, M. (1981). A value approach to the prevention and reduction of drug abuse. In T. J. Glunn, C. G. Lukefield, & J. P. Ludford (Eds.), *Preventing Adolescent Drug Abuse* (WIDA Research Monograph No. 47.). Rockville, MD: National Institute on Drug Abuse.

Rohsenow, D. J., Smith, R. E., & Johnson, S. (1985). Stress management training as a prevention program for heavy social drinkers: Cognitions, affect, drinking, and individual differences. *Addictive Behaviors, 10*, 44-54.

Royer, A. (this volume). The role of the Transcendental Meditation technique in promoting smoking cessation: A longitudinal study. *Alcoholism Treatment Quarterly.*

Rush, T. V. (1979). Predicting treatment outcomes for juvenile and young adult clients in the Pennsylvania substance-abuse system. In G. M. Beschner (Ed.), *Youth.* Massachusetts: Lexington Books.

Sands, D. (this volume) Introducing Maharishi Ayur-Veda into clinical practice. *Alcoholism Treatment Quarterly.*

Saunders, J. B. (1988). Medical aspects of management therapy. In J. C. Clarke & J. B. Saunders (Eds.), *Alcoholism and problem drinking: Theories and treatment* (pp. 122-123). Oxford: Pergamon Press.

Schenkluhn, H., & Geisler, M. (1977). A longitudinal study of the influence of the Transcendental Meditation program on drug abuse. In D. W. Orme-Johnson and J. T. Farrow (Eds.), *Scientific research on the Transcendental Meditation program: Collected papers* (Vol. 1) (pp. 544-555). West Germany: MERU Press.

Schneider, R. H., Alexander, C. N., & Wallace, R. K. (1992). In search of an optimal behavioral treatment for hypertension: A review and focus on Transcendental Meditation. In E. H. Johnson, W. D. Gentry, & S. Julius (Eds.), *Personality, elevated blood pressure, and essential hypertension.* Washington, DC: Hemisphere Publishing Corp.

Schroeder, E. D. (1991). Family therapy and twelve-step programs: Complementary process. *Journal of Chemical Dependency Treatment, 4*(1), 87-109.

Schubert, D. K. (1983). Comparison of hypnotherapy with systematic relaxation in the treatment of cigarette habituation. *Journal of Clinical Psychology, 39*(2), 198-202.

Schwartz, G. E. (1982). Testing the biopsychosocial model: The ultimate challenge facing behavioral medicine. *Journal of Consulting and Clinical Psychology, 50*, 1040-1053.

Shafii, M., Lavely, R. A., & Jaffe, R. D. (1974). Meditation and marijuana. *American Journal of Psychiatry, 131*, 60-63.

Shafii, M., Lavely, R. A., & Jaffe, R. D. (1975). Meditation and the prevention of alcohol abuse. *American Journal of Psychiatry, 132*, 942-945.

Shiffman, S. (1979). The tobacco withdrawal syndrome. In N. M. Krasnegor (Ed.), *Cigarette smoking as a dependence process* (NIDA) Research Monograph No. 23, (pp. 158-184). Washington DC: U.S. Government Printing Office.

Shoemaker, R. H., & Sherry, P. (1991). Posttreatment factors influencing outcome of adolescent chemical dependency treatment. *Journal of Adolescent Chemical Dependency, 21*(1), 89-106.

Skinner, H. A. (1981). Assessment of alcohol problems: Basic principles, critical issues, and future trends. In Y. Israel, F. B. Glaser, H. Kalant, R. E. Popham, W. Schmidt, & R. G. Smart (Eds.), *Research advances in alcohol and drug problems* (Vol. 6) (pp. 319-369). New York: Plenum Press.

Solomon, R. L. (1977). An opponent-process theory of acquired motivation: The affective dynamics of addiction. In J. R. Maser & M. E. P. Seligman (Eds.), *Psychopathology: Experimental models* (pp. 66-103). San Francisco: W. H. Freeman.

Spotts, J. V., & Shontz, F. C. (1991). Drugs and personality: Comparison of drug users, nonusers, and other clinical groups on the 16PF. *The International Journal of the Addictions, 26*(10), 1019-1054.

Stanton, M. D., & Todd, T. C. (1979). Structural family therapy with drug addicts. In E. Kaufman & P. K. Kaufman (Eds.), *The family therapy of drug and alcohol abuse*. New York: Gardner Press.

Stark, M. J. (1992). Dropping out of substance abuse treatment: A clinically oriented review. *Clinical Psychology Review, 12*, 93-116.

Steffenhagen, R. (1980). Self-esteem theory of drug abuse. In D. Lettieri, M. Sayers, & H. Pearson (Eds.), *Theories of drug abuse*. Washington, DC: National Institute on Drug Abuse.

Subrahmanyam, S., & Porkodi, K. (1980). Neurohormonal correlates of Transcendental Meditation. *Journal of Biomedicine, 1*, 73-88.

Surgeon General (1988). *The health consequences of smoking & nicotine addiction*. A report of the Surgeon General, U.S. Department of Health and Human Services. Centers for Disease Control. Center for Health, Promotion and Education.

Taub, E., Steiner, S. S., Smith, R. B., Weingarten, E., & Walton, K. G. (this volume). Effectiveness of broad spectrum approaches to relapse prevention: A long-term, randomized, controlled trial comparing Transcendental Meditation, muscle relaxation and electronic neurotherapy in severe alcoholism. *Alcoholism Treatment Quarterly.*

Tennant, F. S. (1985). *Primer on neurochemistry of drug dependence.* West Covina, CA: Veract.

Throll, D. A. (1989). The effect of the Transcendental Meditation technique upon adolescent personality. In R. Chalmers, G. Clements, H. Schenkluhn, & M. Weinless (Eds.), *Scientific research on Maharishi's Transcendental Meditation and TM-Sidhi program: Collected papers* (Vol. 2) (pp. 1057-1065). Vlodrop, Netherlands: Maharishi Vedic University Press.

Tobler, N. S. (1986). Meta-analysis of 143 adolescent drug prevention programs: Quantitative outcome results of program participants compared to a control or comparison group. *Journal of Drug Issues, 16*, 537-568.

Travis, F. (1979). The Transcendental Meditation technique and creativity: A longitudinal study of Cornell University undergraduates. *Journal of Creative Behaviors, 13*(3), 169-180.

Turnbull, M. J., & Norris, H. (1982). Effects of Transcendental Meditation on self-identity indices and personality. *British Journal of Psychology, 73*, 57-68.

United States Department of Health and Human Services. (1986). *Toward a national plan to combat alcohol abuse and alcoholism: A report to the US Congress by the Secretary of Health and Human Services* Rockville, MD: Author.

United States Department of Health and Human Services. (1991). *Drug abuse and drug abuse research: The third triennial report to Congress from the Secretary. Department of Health and Human Services.* Rockville, MD: Author.

United States Department of Health and Human Services. (1992). *Drug abuse and drug abuse research (an update). The third triennial report to Congress from the Secretary, Department of Health and Human Services.* Rockville, MD: Author.

V., Rachel. (1992). The formless form: Buddhism and the twelve-step program. *Tricycle: The Buddhist Review, 1*(4), 32-36.

Van Den Berg, W. P., & Mulder, B. (1976). Psychological research on the effects of the Transcendental Meditation technique on a number of personality variables. *Gedrag: Tijdschrift voor Psychologie, 4*, 206-218.

Wallace, R. K. (1993). *The physiology of consciousness.* Fairfield, IA: Maharishi International University Press.

Walton, K. G., & Levitsky, D. (this volume). Role of Transcendental Meditation in reducing drug use and addictions: Neurochemical evidence and a theory. *Alcoholism Treatment Quarterly.*

Weiss, C. (1990). The immediate effect of the Transcendental Meditation technique and theoretical reflections upon the psychology and physiology of subjective well-being. In R. Chalmers, G. Clements, H. Schenkluhn, & M. Weinless (Eds.), *Scientific research on Maharishi's Transcendental Meditation and TM-Sidhi program: Collected papers* (Vol. 2) (1044-1046). Vlodrop, Netherlands: Maharishi Vedic University Press.

Wells-Parker, E. & Bangert-Drowns, R. (1990). Meta-analysis of research on DUI remedial interventions. *Alcohol, Drugs and Driving, 6*, 147-160.

Whitehead, A. N. (1978). (Corrected edition). D. Griffin & D. Sherburne (Eds.), *Process and reality.* New York: Free Press.

Whitfield, C. L. (1985). *Alcoholism and spirituality.* New York: Simon & Schuster.

Wills, T. A., & Shiffman, S. (1985). Coping and substance use: A conceptual framework. In S. Shiffman & T. A. Wills (Eds.), *Coping and substance abuse.* Orlando: Academic Press.

Yoder, B. (1990). *The recovery resource book.* New York: Simon & Schuster.

A Neuroendocrine Mechanism for the Reduction of Drug Use and Addictions by Transcendental Meditation

Kenneth G. Walton, PhD
Debra Levitsky, MS

INTRODUCTION

Chronic stress causes long-lasting neurochemical and endocrine imbalances which prolong psychological distress and impair coping abilities. Studies indicate these factors contribute to drug abuse. The Transcendental Meditation (TM) program appears to reverse these effects, providing a natural route to the experiences abusers are looking for–relief from distress and enhancement of well-being. Centered around stress, this article builds a neuroendocrine theory of addiction and of how the mental technology of TM counters addictive behaviors. The article first outlines the theory in general terms (Part I), then examines evidence for its various components

---

Kenneth G. Walton and Debra Levitsky are affiliated with the Department of Chemistry and Physiology at Maharishi International University in Fairfield, IA 52557.

Address correspondence to Ken Walton, Neurochemistry Laboratory, Faculty Box 1005, Maharishi International University, 1000 N. 4th St., Fairfield, IA 52557-1005.

[Haworth co-indexing entry note]: "A Neuroendocrine Mechanism for the Reduction of Drug Use and Addictions by Transcendental Meditation." Walton, Kenneth G. and Debra Levitsky. Co-published simultaneously in the *Alcoholism Treatment Quarterly* (The Haworth Press, Inc.) Vol. 11, No. 1/2, 1994, pp. 89-117; and: *Self-Recovery: Treating Addictions Using Transcendental Meditation and Maharishi Ayur-Veda* (ed: David F. O'Connell and Charles N. Alexander) The Haworth Press, Inc., 1994, pp. 89-117. Multiple copies of this article/chapter may be purchased from The Haworth Document Delivery Center [1-800-3-HAWORTH; 9:00 a.m. - 5:00 p.m. (EST)].

(Parts II and III), and finally provides a concise summary and conclusions (Part IV).

PART I: GENERAL THEORY OF EFFECTS OF TM ON DRUG USE AND ADDICTION

Although evidence indicates that the Transcendental Meditation program is an effective aid in both treating and preventing drug use (Alexander, Robinson & Rainforth, this volume; Gelderloos, Walton, Orme-Johnson & Alexander, 1991; Aron & Aron, 1980), a serious question remains, namely, what mechanisms of human physiology and of the TM program are responsible for its effectiveness? A framework for answering this question has been provided by the founder of the Transcendental Meditation program, Maharishi Mahesh Yogi. This theory for understanding how drug use arises, and how TM counters it, can be summarized as follows:

1. Stress-related experiences can disrupt or prevent optimal psychophysiological function and balance.
2. Substance abuse is an attempt to gain or regain optimal psychophysiological function and balance, but because either the types or quantities of the abused substances are unnatural, in the long run they give rise to further dysfunction and imbalance.
3. TM is a simple and natural way to optimize psychophysiological function and balance, thus removing the impetus for artificial attempts to do so through drugs.

Maharishi brought to light both the TM program and his understanding of its effects from the ancient Vedic tradition, including its central component, *Rik Veda*, which describes the mechanics of development of the full potential of mind and body. In his lectures and writings he has long held that stress can produce physiological imbalances that impair optimal function of the mind-body system (Maharishi Mahesh Yogi, 1963; 1969). Such imbalances he refers to as "residues" or "abnormalities" which are due to an overload of physical or psychological demands on the individual. These demands might also be called "stressors," and include daily hassles and the frustrations that result from lack of ability to satisfy desires. Such impairments or imbalances are held to adversely affect all aspects of life, including the ability to cope with subsequent stressors.

Physiological imbalances arising from the response to frequent or extreme stressors appear to set the stage for drug use and addiction. Such imbalances generally give rise to mental distress (Burchfield, 1979) which, in turn, may enhance the urge to take substances promising instant mood elevation or tension relief. However, although temporary relief may be provided, such relief soon wears off and leaves in its place additional physiological imbalances and/or further impairment of coping ability. The result is still more distress. In this way, the vicious cycle of addiction–increasing imbalance, distress, and drug use, producing more imbalances and distress–is created.

In addition to this theory of drug use and addiction, Maharishi has provided an explanation for the ability of TM to prevent or reverse this pattern. Direct experience as well as objective evidence indicates that a major effect of the TM technique is to establish optimal psychophysiological function (Alexander, Davies, Dixon, Dillbeck, Druker, Oetzel et al., 1990; Alexander, Rainforth & Gelderloos, 1991). This establishment of optimal balance in the mind and body appears to occur progressively with length of time practicing the technique (Dillbeck & Orme-Johnson, 1987; Eppley, Abrams & Shear, 1989; Walton, Pugh, Gelderloos, & Macrae, submitted), and apparently results from the repeated experience of "transcendental consciousness," a unique, completely natural state of consciousness systematically promoted by TM which is described further below (Alexander et al., 1990; 1991).

This brief explanation of the reduction of drug use through TM is stated in simple terms but can easily be elaborated in terminology familiar to physiologists. In particular, it can be argued that the optimal psychophysiological state is represented by the maintenance of an ideal state of *homeostasis* within an organism. Homeostasis refers to a state of relative balance and coordination among the various components and processes of the body's internal environment, especially the liquid environment of cells and tissues (Cannon, 1929). It reflects the body's ability to regulate itself for optimal function. The ideal state of homeostasis can be viewed as the most stable state of the physiology, one conferring the greatest resistance to disruptive influences or the most appropriate adaptive responses to the changing environment.

It is significant that maintenance of homeostasis, including attainment of the ideal state, appears to be a natural tendency of living organisms or of life itself. The famous nineteenth-century physiologist Claude Bernard was first to note this tendency. He proposed that this "fixity of the *milieu interieur*" was the very "condition of a free and independent life." This relative fixity of the internal medium was later given the name homeostasis by physiologist Walter Cannon (1929). It refers to the self-defined and self-regulated limits of such things as salt balance, acidity and nutrient level of the blood, in which the organism functions best. Many mechanisms exist to prevent the trespass of these limits.

Since ideal homeostasis is the most natural and balanced physiological state, it is not unreasonable to expect a state of psychological well-being–a high degree of contentment and confidence in meeting the challenges of daily life–to be associated with it. Accordingly, when physiological homeostasis is not ideal or not well maintained, an individual tends to experience psychological distress (Burchfield, 1979). Such a loss of balance or disruption of homeostasis appears due most often to stress.

Although stress has been defined in many ways, the following observations will suffice for understanding its role in the present discussion. It is recognized in stress physiology that when an organism is subjected to stressors, homeostasis can be disrupted or made less ideal. Such stressors may be provided by a limitless variety of common, everyday experiences, such as frustration, anger, fear, humiliation, strenuous exertion, and even apparently neutral or positive experiences, such as change of residence, marriage, promotion, or outstanding personal achievements (Goldberger & Breznitz, 1982). Subjection of a person to stressors sets into motion a concert of physiological responses which, taken as a whole, is termed the *stress response*. The stress response appears designed (1) to conserve and redirect energy stores to most effectively deal with the stressor at hand, and (2) to restore homeostasis when the emergency has passed.

Though the stress response was initially believed to be adaptive in every way, later research has demonstrated this is not always the case (Sapolsky, 1992; Sapolsky, Krey & McEwen, 1986). It seems to function best when of limited duration. When an organism is subjected to frequent or sustained stressors (chronic stress), especially when such stressors are unpredictable, the stress response may become ineffectual or even damaging, producing homeostatic imbalance and disease (Sapolsky, 1992; Sapolsky et al., 1986). Therefore, for individuals subjected to chronic stress, ideal homeostasis, and thus the optimal psychophysiological state, may remain far from attainment most of the time.

Viewed in this context, substance use is an attempt to optimize one's psychophysiological state with exogenous chemicals. If this view is correct, then suboptimal mechanisms for maintaining homeostasis–and the resulting suboptimal psychophysiological state–are partly responsible for the temptation to rely on tension-relieving or mood-altering substances. Such a condition of imbalance is envisioned to arise mainly from chronic stress (Walton et al., submitted). Evidence further suggests that ingestion of foreign substances provides only temporary or illusory relief from distress. This is partly because foreign substances are themselves stressors and therefore can lead to more imbalance and distress (Antelman, Caggiula, Knopf, Kocan & Edwards, 1992).

Evidence also appears to support the possibility that certain types of addictions can be caused by genetic defects. The view presented here does not exclude the possibility of genetic predisposition to addiction. For example, due to a genetic difference, one or more mechanisms involved in the maintenance of homeostasis may be weaker in certain individuals, inclining these individuals toward substance abuse. One of the strongest studies purporting to show a genetic predisposition to drug abuse supports this contention (see Part IV). However, evidence for chronic stress as the most prevalent influence weakening homeostatic mechanisms is more elaborate, and will be examined as a primary cause of drug abuse in this review.

The Role of TM

How does the TM program reverse the addictive cycle? Transcendental Meditation is a mental technique which allows the mind to settle down effortlessly to a wakeful but deeply restful state called "transcendental consciousness." Subjectively, this state is experienced as a conscious state without thought. This experience provides deep rest both physically and mentally (Alexander, Davies et al., 1990; Alexander, Rainforth & Gelderloos, 1991; Dillbeck & Orme-Johnson, 1987). Furthermore, Maharishi has proposed that repeated experience of this state promotes a progressive increase of psychophysiological integration outside of the practice (Maharishi Mahesh Yogi, 1969). Support for this view is found in studies showing lower levels of autonomic arousal (see Dillbeck & Orme-Johnson, 1987), reduced levels of the stress-related hormone cortisol (Jevning, Wallace & Beidebach, 1992; Walton et al., submitted), enhanced EEG coherence (Dillbeck & Bronson, 1981), improved health (e.g., Alexander, Langer, Newman, Chandler & Davies, 1989; Alexander et al., 1991; Schneider, Alexander & Wallace, 1992) and more effective activity (e.g., Frew, 1974; Kember, 1985) as a result of TM practice.

Evidence indicates there are several ways this enhanced psychophysiological balance removes the motivation for substance abuse. Firstly, enhanced balance of the neuroendocrine system gives rise to increased behavioral efficacy and inner contentment, and thus to a reduced urge for instant mood elevation or tension relief (see for reviews Alexander et al., this volume; Gelderloos et al., 1991). Secondly, enhanced neuroendocrine balance reawakens the body's natural healing mechanisms (Walton et al., submitted), ability to cope with stressors (Sapolsky, 1992) and ability to fulfill desires (Frew, 1974; Kember, 1985), thus preventing the future build-up of distress and frustration. Thirdly, enhanced psychophysiological balance and inner contentment appear to increase one's sensitivity to, and desire to avoid, the damaging side-effects of substances of abuse (Gelderloos et al., 1991).

Therefore, because TM restores homeostatic balance and optimizes the psychophysiological state naturally and holistically, it appears to eliminate the vicious cycle of substance abuse, replacing it with a "virtuous cycle" of ever-increasing balance, integration and resistance to disruptive influences. While this explanation is both internally consistent and supported by behavioral data, the question remains whether it is also supported by neurochemical and endocrine evidence. The next two sections explore this question.

PART II: EVIDENCE FOR CHRONIC STRESS AS A CAUSE OF DRUG USE AND ADDICTION

Establishment and maintenance of homeostasis in the physiology involves the coordinated function of several systems, most conspicuously the nervous and endocrine systems. Among the crucial components of the central nervous system responsible for maintaining homeostasis are the hypothalamus, the hippocampus, the locus coeruleus and the raphe nuclei. These areas, shown diagrammatically in Figure 1, interface with the endocrine system principally through the hypothalamic-pituitary-adrenocortical (HPA) axis, the sympatho-adrenomedullary axis, and the parasympathetic nervous system. This latter system, with the relevant central and peripheral serotonergic components, may form another major axis. Each of these neuronal components of the machinery maintaining homeostasis is introduced below. Among brain structures, the locus coeruleus has been identified as a key site for biochemical changes associated with tolerance and addictions (Nestler, 1992). Therefore, this brain area and its possible connection to substance abuse are reviewed first.

The Locus Coeruleus

The locus coeruleus (LC), or "blue spot," in the brain stem is the largest nucleus of norepinephrine-containing neurons in the brain (Dahlstrom & Fuxe, 1964). LC neurons project prominently to the brain's fear-anxiety-defense centers in the limbic system (e.g., Blanchard & Blanchard, 1979; LeDoux, Cicchetti, Xagoraris & Romanski, 1990). There they release the neurotransmitter norepinephrine (NE) in response to real or apparent threats to survival (Amaral & Sinnamon, 1977; Aston-Jones & Bloom, 1981; Jacobs, 1986). The LC has been believed responsible for one or more of a variety of functions, including the regulation of: (1) arousal (Jouvet, 1972), (2) vigilance (Aston-Jones, 1985), (3) reward-extinction

(Mason & Fibiger, 1978), (4) fear-anxiety (Redmond & Huang, 1979), (5) memory-learning (Amaral & Foss, 1975), or (6) the cardiovascular system (Scriabine, Clineschmidt & Sweet, 1976). A more holistic perspective views the LC as an alarm-aversion system which functions in concert with reward systems to promote surviv-al-maximizing behavior in vertebrates (Morton, B.E., personal communication; Redmond & Huang, 1979).

Extensive evidence indicates that the LC is involved in the adaptive changes underlying drug tolerance and dependence. For example, the *acute* effects of opiate drugs include inhibiting the firing rate of LC neurons (Aghajanian & Wang, 1986). Under *chronic* opiate treatment, on the other hand, LC neurons recover their pre-treatment firing rates, thus developing "tolerance" to the acute inhibitory actions of opiates (Aghajanian, 1978). This is significant for the theory examined here because agents that inhibit LC output, such as opiate drugs, are known to reduce anxiety, fear and anger, while those that excite LC output tend to increase these emotions.

When the neurotransmitter, serotonin, is secreted in the LC, the sensitivity of the LC to excitatory input is lowered (Aston-Jones, Akoka, Charlety & Chouvet, 1991). Therefore, increased serotonergic activity in the LC would appear to be a natural means of reducing anxiety, fear and anger. Serotonin also exercises important roles in regulation of the hypothalamic-pituitary-adrenocortical axis, another key player in homeostatic maintenance. These and other important influences of serotonin will be further discussed below.

The HPA Axis

A second major system responsible for the maintenance of homeostasis is the HPA axis. Traditionally, the HPA axis has been thought to involve three principal components: the hypothalamus, the pituitary gland, and the adrenal cortex. In this long-accepted scheme, stressors excite the HPA axis by causing nerve impulses to be transmitted from the periphery of the body through unknown "higher centers" of the brain to terminate in the hypothalamus. The hypothalamus then secretes corticotropin releasing factor (CRF), which travels through the bloodstream to the pituitary. CRF stimulates pituitary secretion of adrenocorticotropic hormone (ACTH),

FIGURE 1. Major brain areas and endocrine glands involved in adaptive mechanisms which regulate homeostasis. Minus signs signify inhibitory influences of serotonin (top arrow) and cortisol (three arrows right of center).

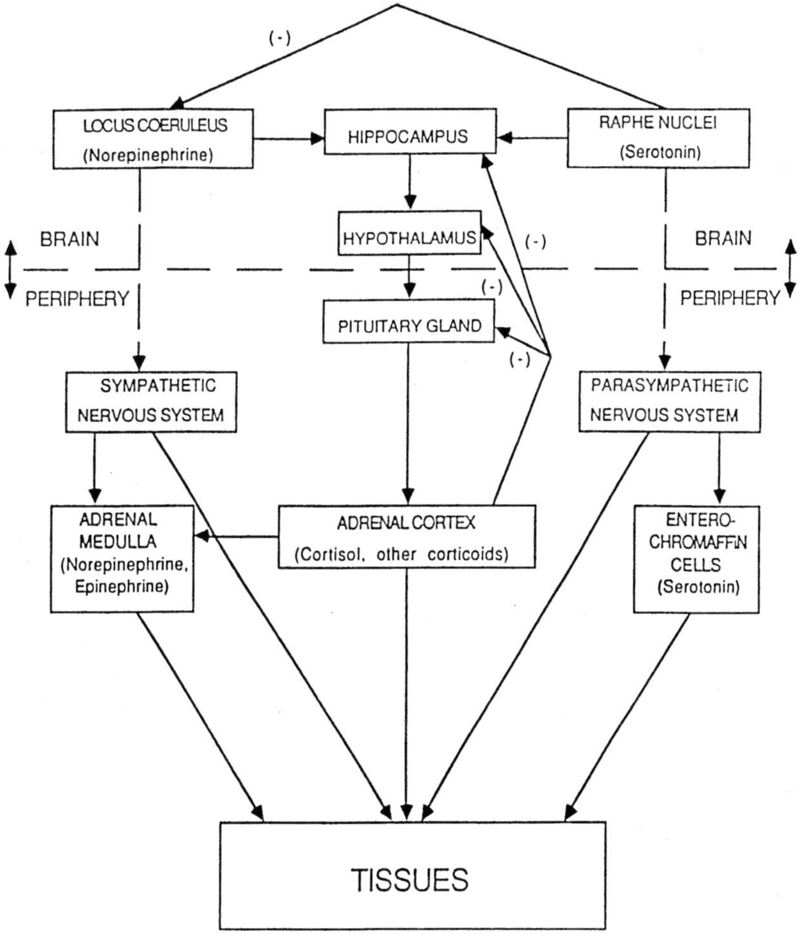

which then travels to the adrenal cortex, causing the secretion of the steroid hormone, cortisol. Cortisol affects a wide variety of target tissues throughout the body, including the nervous system. The adrenal cortex also secretes other steroids important in maintaining homeostasis, including mineralocorticoids, which are involved in maintaining salt balance, and dehydroepiandrosterone (DHEA), the major precursor of anabolic steroids, whose effects often counter those of cortisol. Although these other steroids also appear adversely affected by chronic stress (see Walton et al., submitted), the mechanisms for their regulation are less well known than those of cortisol and will not be discussed here.

The best known effects of cortisol are to mobilize energy stores for immediate energy needs, to enhance sensitivity of tissues to other stress-related neurohormones, and to inhibit immune and inflammatory responses. Together, these effects enhance the organism's ability to respond to acute stressors, as well as to restore homeostasis. After the stressor is removed and the initial steps in restoration of homeostasis have been completed, negative feedback mechanisms turn off the heightened secretion of cortisol, thus returning cortisol to its prior level (see Figure 1).

Recent evidence supports inclusion of an additional brain component, the hippocampus, as part of the HPA system. This evidence suggests that the hippocampus, a portion of the limbic system, may mediate one of the key negative feedback mechanisms regulating secretion of adrenal steroids. Due to its greater density of cortisol receptors (intracellular proteins that bind cortisol and help carry out its effects) the hippocampus has a much greater sensitivity to cortisol than do other parts of the brain (Sapolsky, 1992). Neuron pathways project from the hippocampus through other brain centers to the hypothalamus, where CRF secretion is effected. Further evidence has shown that the hippocampus affects three aspects of HPA activity: initial cortisol response to stress, circadian rhythm of cortisol, and feedback inhibition of cortisol (Sapolsky, 1992).

The Raphe Nuclei

A third major system involved in adaptation to stress centers around serotonin. The principal brain sources of serotonergic neuron terminals are the bilateral raphe nuclei of the midbrain. Like the LC, the raphe contain a small number of neurons that branch out to innervate virtually all other areas of the brain. Although the signaling roles of serotonin in the brain are many, attempts have been made to conceptually unify these roles in relation to the organism as a whole. A theory advanced over 30 years ago (Brodie, Spector & Shore, 1959) has been generally supported by subsequent studies.

Based on the seminal work of Hess, Brodie et al. (1959) reviewed extensive pharmacological studies suggesting that brain serotonin integrates function of the somatomotor nervous system (governing voluntary bodily actions) with function of the parasympathetic branch of the autonomic nervous system (governing involuntary functions of visceral organs). Thus, serotonin may in fact be the major mediator of Hess's "trophotropic" division of the nervous system, i.e., those centers oriented to the economy, restitution and protection of cells and tissues. Observable signs of trophotropic dominance are drowsiness and sleep, increased parasympathetic activity, decreased skeletal muscle tone and decreased motor activity.

Hess's "ergotropic" system, on the other hand, is composed of those subcortical mechanisms integrating function of the sympathetic branch of the autonomic nervous system with somatomotor activities preparing the body for assertive responses to the environment, especially in cases of perceived threat. Observable signs of ergotropic dominance are arousal, increased sympathetic activity, enhanced skeletal muscle activity and tone, and an activated psychic state. Brodie et al. (1959) proposed that norepinephrine is the primary mediator of this system.

Figure 1 uses dotted lines to depict the relationship between the LC and the sympatho-adrenomedullary system, as well as that between the raphe nuclei and the parasympathetic nervous system. This is because Brodie's proposals, though generally supported by later work, are still considered speculative. Parallel to the sympatho-adrenomedullary system there is a less-well-studied parasympatho-enterochromaffin cell system, with the vagus nerve (primarily parasympathetic) controlling release of serotonin from the enterochromaffin cells selectively into the lumen of the intestine (Ahlman, DeMagistris, Zinner & Jaffe, 1981), where it affects digestion, or into the bloodstream (Meirieu, Pairet, Sutra & Ruckebusch, 1986) where it may influence all bodily tissues, much as sympathetic stimuli induce adrenal medullary release of epinephrine and norepinephrine into the circulation. Unlike the adrenal hormones, however, a possible hormonal role of serotonin continues to be debated.

Regardless of the exact relationship of their influences, there is ample evidence that the monoamine neurotransmitters (serotonin, epinephrine, norepinephrine and dopamine) play vital roles in the maintenance of homeostasis under stress, as illustrated by the following primitive but graphic example. Using reserpine to deplete neuronal stores of monoamine transmitters, Rosecrans and DeFeo (1965) showed that stressing rats by daily exposure to 30 minutes of forced restraint caused half the animals to lose their lives within 32 days. None of the untreated control animals (receiving an injection of saline alone) died, and only 4% of the reserpine controls (receiving reserpine in saline but no stress) died. This shows that adaptation to this physically mild (mainly "psychological") stressor is greatly hampered by the reduced supply of monoamines. The three systems and the neurotransmitters or hormones discussed here appear to be the principal components responsible for maintaining homeostasis in a changing environment. Thus, a background has now been provided for examining the theory of drug abuse described in Part I above.

Chronic Stress and Drug Use

Having reviewed these adaptive mechanisms, what specific role or roles might they play in connecting chronic stress to drug use? The peripheral circle of the diagram in Figure 2 shows an expanded version of the theory of drug abuse delineated in Part I. The additional components included in this illustration provide the focus for a more detailed discussion of the neurochemistry involved. At the top, as described before, is the experience of chronic stress, including not only the negative emotions such as anger, frustration and fear, but also overwhelming positive emotions–in short, any experience that temporarily taxes the ability of adaptive mechanisms to maintain homeostasis. Some of the mechanisms taxed by chronic stress are now known, and the hippocampally-mediated feedback inhibition of the HPA axis appears to be one of these.

Studies of the feedback inhibition of cortisol, partly responsible for the rapid drop of cortisol after a stressor has passed, indicate that chronic stress reduces the sensitivity of the hippocampus to cortisol by reducing the number of cortisol receptors present (Sapolsky, 1992; Sapolsky, Krey & McEwen, 1984a). This reduced sensitivity is associated with an impaired ability of the hippocampus to signal

FIGURE 2. Proposed vicious cycle relating chronic stress to drug use.

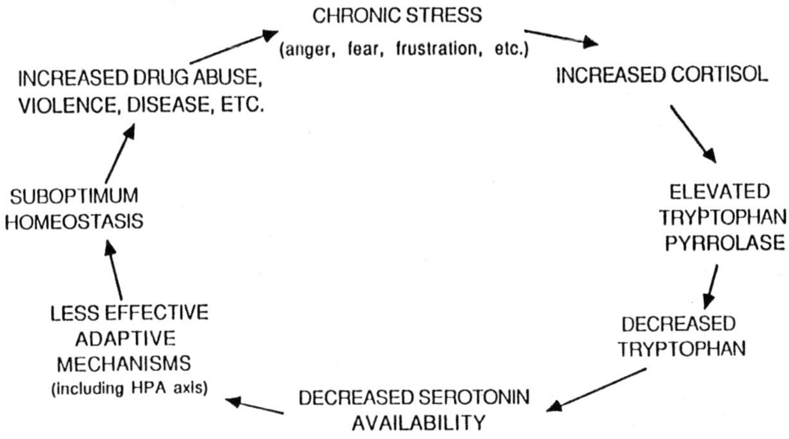

the HPA axis to turn down cortisol secretion, consequently producing cortisol hypersecretion (Sapolsky, 1992; Sapolsky, Krey & McEwen, 1984b).

Cortisol hypersecretion can have many damaging effects. One such effect is to induce synthesis of enzymes in the liver that break down the amino acids which are precursors for the monoamines (Knox, Piras & Tokuyama, 1966). For simplicity, only one of these enzymes, tryptophan pyrrolase, which breaks down the serotonin precursor, L-tryptophan, is shown in Figure 2. However, the enzyme breaking down tyrosine, precursor of epinephrine, norepinephrine and dopamine (the other three monoamines discussed above), is also induced.

Though this ability of cortisol to reduce monoamine precursors has long been known in animals, its significance for humans has only recently been considered. Studies in humans now show that cortisol (actually dexamethasone, its synthetic analog) lowers availability of these precursors in the plasma (Maes, Jacobs, Suy, Minner, Leclerccq, Christiaens & Raus, 1990). Since the level of these precursors is an important component in the regulation of synthesis of the respective monoamines, this likely results in decreased availability of the monoamine neurotransmitters themselves (reviewed in Walton et al., submitted). A case in point is the decreased availability of serotonin, which apparently leads to lowered effectiveness of adaptive mechanisms regulating cortisol.

Serotonin appears involved in both (1) the initial secretion of glucocorticoids such as cortisol, and (2) the subsequent negative feedback which returns the cortisol to its basal level. Some of the supportive evidence for these involvements includes the observations that serotonin levels in rat brains vary in parallel with the diurnal rhythm of plasma corticosterone (the cortisol analog in rats) (Scapagnini, Moberg, Van Loon, de Groot & Ganong, 1971), and that a variety of serotonin agonists (drugs capable of initiating serotonin-like actions in the body) activate the HPA axis (Bagdy, Cologero, Murphy & Szemeredi, 1989). Moreover, destruction of brain serotonin neurons, which effectively reduces serotonin levels in the hippocampus, significantly decreases the hippocampal receptors for cortisol, resulting in a lower efficacy of feedback regulation of cortisol levels (Seckl, Dickson & Fink, 1990). Furthermore, agents which enhance serotonin cause an increase in these receptors (Seckl & Fink, 1992) and presumably enhance feedback regulation. Thus, the end effect of decreased serotonin availability, at least in the rat, is expected to be chronic hypersecretion of cortisol (Sapolsky et al., 1984a; 1984b). If the same mechanisms are at work in humans, as suggested by a wide variety of studies, then the cycle shown in Figure 2 continues. This suboptimum homeostasis appears to lead to other imbalances which would encourage use of substances to alleviate the associated unpleasant emotions.

Although several of these steps have been studied directly only in rodents, a variety of findings support the same role for serotonin in HPA-axis regulation in humans. For example, when the serotonin precursor is administered for two weeks or more, the average cortisol level is reduced (Brodie, Sack & Siever, 1973), suggesting that the normal subjects studied were in fact experiencing a substantial level of chronic stress which had impaired normal negative feedback and raised their cortisol levels (see Walton et al., submitted). Furthermore, more stressful states, such as hostility and depression, have been correlated with elevated cortisol levels. For example, men with high levels of hostility show a three-fold larger rise in cortisol levels during daytime activities than men with low levels of hostility (Pope & Smith, 1991). Similarly, many depressed patients show a generalized impairment of HPA function, including increased ACTH and cortisol secretion (Sachar, Puig-Antich, Ryan, Asnis, Rabinovich, Davies & Halpern, 1985; Seckl et al., 1990). Other evidence indicates that depressives, while ill, secrete substantially more cortisol, have more secretory episodes, more minutes of active secretion, marked elevations of cortisol throughout day and night, both at the beginning and at the end of secretory episodes, and active secretion of cortisol during late evening and early morning hours when secretion is normally minimal (Sachar, Hellman, Roffward, Halpern, Fukushima & Gallagher, 1973). These alterations in cortisol regulation and levels in depression may be particularly significant, since many cases of depression are relieved by serotonin-enhancing drugs. After effective treatment, the patients' patterns of cortisol secretion normalize. Impairments of HPA function similar to those found in depression have been reported in other mental and behavioral disorders as well, including psychosis, panic disorder, alcoholism and anorexia nervosa (e.g., Chrousos & Gold, 1992; Seckl et al., 1990). Suggestions of serotonin deficiencies also are present in all these disorders, and both these types of adaptive deficiencies have been discussed as a basis of increased disease incidence (Walton et al., submitted). Thus, a lowered serotonin availability, such as that which arises from chronic stress, may be responsible for some of the deranged activities of the HPA axis that are found in many disorders and diseases.

At this point on the vicious cycle linking chronic stress with drug use, it is clear that neurochemical mechanisms exist which could account for the connection between chronic stress, loss of effectiveness of adaptive mechanisms, and suboptimal homeostasis. The last step is the use of foreign substances in an attempt to correct this suboptimal psychophysiological state.

The ability of serotonin to inhibit activity of the LC (Aston-Jones et al., 1991) was mentioned above. When serotonin availability is substantially reduced by chronic stress, through the steps just described, could this cause LC activity to become chronically elevated? And could this explain increased feelings of anxiety, anger, fear and frustration that contribute to the negative cycle of chronic stress and drug use? The answer to both questions appears to be yes.

Evidence indicates that LC activity is increased by both chronic and acute stress. [See for example Nisenbaum, Zigmond, Sved & Abercrombie (1991).] Evidence also suggests this could be due, at least in part, to the reduction of serotonin by chronic stress, thus removing a tonic inhibitory influence on LC activity (Kuriyama, Kanmori & Yoneda, 1983; Walton et al., submitted). Since increased LC activity can activate fear, anger and aggression centers (see above), the logic of the cycle in Figure 2 appears complete. Moreover, there is evidence that drug use is an attempt to block this excessive LC activity. All classes of drugs of abuse (including: sedative-hypnotics such as the barbiturates, the benzodiazepines, alcohol and marijuana; opiate narcotics; stimulants such as the amphetamines and cocaine; and nicotine) transiently inhibit LC activity while simultaneously relieving anxiety and fear (Holdefer & Jensen, 1987; Pitts & Marwah, 1988; Sanna, Concas, Serra & Biggio, 1990; Schwartz, Suzdak & Paul, 1987; Seitin, Franchimont, Massotte & Dresse, 1990; Shirae & Morton, 1991; Tallman, Paul, Skolnick & Gallager, 1980). Thus, drugs of abuse can help reduce the experience of acute stress, but because these drugs are themselves stressors (Antelman et al., 1992), in the long run they only cause further depletion of serotonin (Kuriyama et al., 1983; Walton et al., submitted).

PART III: NEUROCHEMICALLY, HOW MIGHT TM PREVENT OR COUNTER EFFECTS OF CHRONIC STRESS?

Findings discussed in the preceding section indicate that chronic stress can cause malfunction of adaptive mechanisms, or at least can cause these mechanisms to function at far-from-optimal levels. This section examines some neurochemical changes resulting from the practice of TM that may prevent or reverse such altered functions, along with a preliminary verification in normal subjects.

Central in the evidence presented above is support for a specific example, a smaller vicious cycle of effects of stress on regulation of the HPA axis. In this cycle, chronically elevated cortisol is responsible for chronically reduced availability of serotonin, and reduced serotonin, in turn, appears responsible for lowered efficacy of the hippocampal "brake" on cortisol secretion into the bloodstream (Figures 1, 2). Either side of this cycle, the reduction of serotonin caused by high cortisol or the increase of cortisol caused by low serotonin, could be important for the beneficial effects of TM. Results to date are consistent with effects on both sides, and these will be summarized here.

Figure 3 shows five sites in the proposed cycle of drug abuse at which TM might produce primary effects (see numbered arrows). Arrow 2 points to the decreased availability of serotonin in the drug abuse cycle. Evidence that practice of TM increases serotonin first appeared in 1976 (Bujatti & Riederer, 1976). An increased rate of excretion of 5-HIAA, the principal metabolite of serotonin, was found in meditators immediately prior to a 30-minute TM session in the afternoon, compared to non-meditator control subjects who merely rested for the same length of time. This was followed by a further 5-HIAA rise in TM practitioners during the session itself. When dietary intake of serotonin is precluded, as in this study, urinary excretion of 5-HIAA gives a reasonable indication of serotonin metabolism or turnover throughout the body. This observation suggests that practice of TM causes (1) an increase in serotonin

FIGURE 3. Proposed "virtuous" cycle by which the Transcendental Meditation program appears to reduce or prevent drug use and addictions.

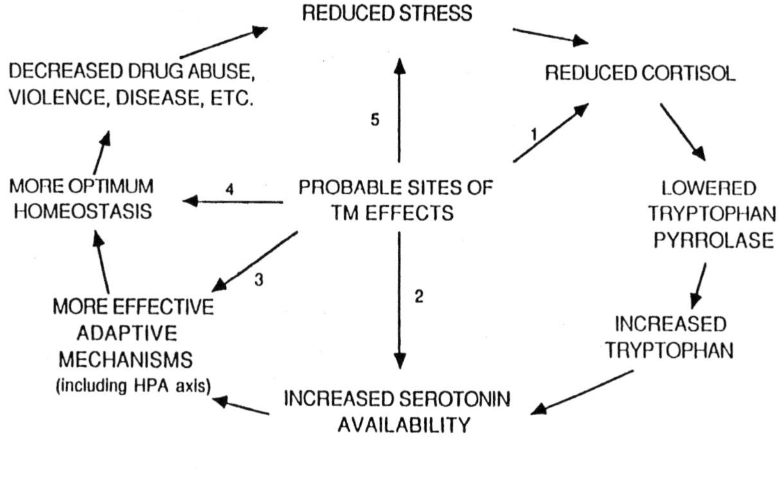

during individual TM sessions, and (2) higher average serotonin availability with regular practice of TM over long periods. A variety of studies in our laboratory support this interpretation (Pugh, & Walton, unpublished data; Walton et al., submitted). However, direct effects of TM on cortisol, for example through reduction of HPA "drive," might explain the longitudinal increase in serotonin.

The effect of TM on cortisol levels (Figure 3, arrow 1) is remarkably similar to its effect on serotonin, except in the reverse direction. The bulk of evidence indicates that cortisol drops acutely during individual TM sessions and averages lower over long periods of time in regular meditators (Jevning et al., 1992). Both effects appear cumulative, i.e., long-term practitioners show a greater reduction during a session, as well as lower baseline levels, compared to short-term practitioners (Jevning, Wilson & Davidson, 1978; Jevning et al., 1992). Because adequate serotonin is necessary to maintain the optimal braking effect of the hippocampus on the HPA axis, long-term reduction of plasma cortisol is the expected result of greater serotonin availability. Therefore, the longer-term changes in cortisol could be caused by increased serotonin availability, the exact reverse of the situation described above, where changes in serotonin could be caused by changes in cortisol levels. Both the serotonin changes and the cortisol changes arising from TM practice may reflect improved adaptive mechanisms (Figure 3, arrow 3) and more optimal homeostasis (Figure 3, arrow 4), as explained below.

According to the scheme in Part II, decreased baseline cortisol and increased serotonin availability reflect a more adaptive, healthier neuroendocrine profile than the opposite. Work with animals in the wild, for example, indicates that low baseline cortisol, with a robust rise under acute stress, is associated with the dominant members of social groups, who are also generally healthier and less violent or aggressive than their subordinate counterparts (Sapolsky, 1990). Sapolsky (1990) interpreted this profile to mean that dominant animals normally experience less stress, but that when they do encounter challenges, the cortisol rises appropriately and robustly to meet the challenge. Practicing the TM technique, therefore, might be predicted to cause the cortisol profile of a person who had been experiencing chronic stress (that is, most anyone in the current social environment) to become more like that of the dominant animals.

In apparent confirmation, a recent study in our laboratory indicated that practice of the TM technique for only four months can produce such changes. Young men were randomly assigned to TM or to a cognitive approach to reducing stress. After four months, the TM group had assumed a more optimal cortisol profile, i.e., lower baseline with higher response to acute challenge (MacLean, Walton, Wenneberg, Levitsky, Mandarino et al., 1992). This is precisely what would be expected if serotonin also were functioning more normally. Serotonin is not only involved in the maintenance of effective negative feedback of cortisol via the hippocampus, thus helping to maintain low baseline cortisol values, but also is necessary for the most robust CRF response in the hypothalamus in the face of acute stressors (see Walton et al., submitted). Thus, in the normal subjects used in this study, some of whom were occasional drinkers and a few of whom were smokers, four months of regular practice of the TM technique produced changes in the direction of optimal function of the HPA axis. This finding provides prospective evidence that TM improves adaptive mechanisms and homeostasis (arrows 3 and 4, Figure 3).

There is also evidence of a cross-sectional nature which supports improvement of adaptive mechanisms by TM. In a recent study in our laboratory, long-term practitioners compared to age- and occupation-matched controls showed indications of more optimal adaptive mechanisms and more ideal homeostasis in seven measures of neuroendocrine activity (Walton et al., submitted). Other cross-sectional studies have also supported such effects of TM (e.g., Dillbeck & Orme-Johnson, 1987; Goleman & Schwartz, 1976).

Relating such changes in adaptive mechanisms more directly to the question of drug use, it is proposed that both (1) a reduction in the LC stimulant CRF (such reduction being a required step in lowering average cortisol level), and (2) an increase in the LC inhibitor serotonin, would minimize excessive LC activity. Thus, these effects of TM would reduce chronic stimulation of the anger and fear centers and disinhibit reward centers. This neuroendocrine mechanism could underlie the feeling of well-being that results from the TM program, and might, through the combination of these effects, account for the decreased desire for drugs of abuse. The fact that decrease of drug and alcohol use due to TM tends to be gradual and spontaneous rather than the result of a sudden, rational decision (e.g., Alexander et al., this volume; Royer, this volume) may provide further evidence for progressive optimization of adaptive mechanisms as the underlying mechanism of reduced substance use in TM meditators.

Thus, evidence appears to support the conclusion that, through changes in adaptive mechanisms, a more ideal state of homeostasis is restored and more steadfastly maintained through TM practice. With such improved physiological function, it is likely that an individual would also become more competent to deal with challenges that might previously have evoked psychological distress, and therefore would be less likely to suffer the build-up of chronic stress.

There may be, however, an alternative explanation. If the practice of TM were to reduce chronic psychological stress directly (Figure 3, arrow 5), then from the scheme pictured in Figure 3, all the neurochemical and endocrine changes might be simply the natural consequences of reduction of psychological stress. If this is the case, then the unusual effectiveness of the TM program (see Alexander et al., this volume) may reside in its ability to more effectively eliminate psychological stress than other meditation and stress-reduction techniques. In comparisons with other techniques, such a difference in stress reduction has, in fact, been found (Alexander et al., 1991; Eppley et al., 1989). Thus, due to the interconnectedness of physical and psychological stress, it may be impossible to identify where in Figure 3 the benefits of TM begin or might be most important. Moreover, the optimization of one site, such as serotonin availability, may not mean the end of improvements at other sites due to TM. Such a multifaceted improvement of adaptive mechanisms might well continue until states far beyond the current notion of normal are attained, as the Vedic tradition has long held (Alexander et al., 1990; 1991).

PART IV: A THEORY OF ADDICTION AND THE NEUROENDOCRINE EFFECTS OF TM: SUMMARY AND CONCLUSIONS

This description of key neurochemical components of addiction and of the role of TM in preventing or reversing addiction relies on research in rodents, non-human primates and humans. The extent and clarity of the research appear to make the model realistic. The deleterious effects of chronic stress on the hypothalamic-pituitary-adrenal axis and on serotonin levels form the centerpieces of the theory.

Corresponding to the vicious cycle of chemical dependence, in which physiological imbalance and psychological distress lead to use of drugs that only produce more imbalance and distress, is a vicious cycle of loss of neural control of the HPA axis and reduction in availability of serotonin. The starting place in the cycle is probably the increased frequency of stressful experiences which transiently raise cortisol (Figure 2). At some point along the continuum, stressful experiences become frequent enough to cause substantial, long-lasting reductions in serotonin availability. These serotonin reductions appear to result from a cortisol-induced increase of the liver enzyme which metabolizes the serotonin precursor, tryptophan, so that plasma levels of tryptophan are reduced. This, in turn, reduces serotonin synthesis and thus also the availability of an adequate supply of serotonin for optimal modulation of various mechanisms maintaining homeostasis.

Two of the homeostatic mechanisms involving serotonin are crucial for optimal function of the HPA axis. Inadequate function of the first mechanism results in deficient serotonergic input to the hippocampus and as a consequence reduces the number of adrenocorticoid receptors needed by the hippocampus for its negative feedback (braking) role in cortisol regulation. Due to this loss of efficient feedback, the average level of cortisol rises, inducing more breakdown of tryptophan, further reducing serotonin in a vicious cycle that severely limits the functional range of these adaptive mechanisms. In the second serotonin-requiring mechanism, serotonin is involved in the release of CRF which drives the positive cortisol response to acute stressors. When this serotonergic function is inadequate, the CRF/cortisol response to acute challenge is weakened. This could contribute to the subjective experience of inability to cope with challenging situations (often reflected in high trait anxiety) and, once again, to the desire for relief through some outside source, such as drugs of abuse.

The subjective effects probably also are connected with changes in activity of the locus coeruleus. Serotonin exercises an inhibitory influence on activity of the locus coeruleus, thus reducing LC activation of brain centers for fear, anxiety and anger. Reduction of LC activity also disinhibits the brain centers for reward. Thus, when serotonin availability is low, allowing LC activity to rise, an increase of environmental demands would increase the likelihood that a person would experience negative emotions, such as fear, anxiety and anger, along with an increase in the feeling of inability to cope. Since feelings such as these are what tend to drive a person to seek external sources of relief (see Staggers, Alexander & Walton, this volume; Taub, Steiner, Smith, Weingarten & Walton, this volume), evidence that most or all drugs of abuse either directly inhibit LC activity (e.g., opiates, nicotine), or have at least a short-lived ability to raise serotonin, comes as no surprise.

Thus, because of serotonin's roles at multiple brain sites involved in successful interaction with the environment, its decreased availability may be one of the most important neurochemical components in the production of tendencies toward addiction. The apparent importance of this conclusion appears to warrant mention of some further supportive evidence.

In the rat, artificial enhancement of serotonergic activity reduces alcohol consumption in both an alcohol-preferring strain and a non-preferring strain (McBride, Murphy, Lumeng & Li, 1988). On the other hand, animals with reduced brain serotonin (produced by chemical lesion with the neurotoxin, 5,7-dihydroxytryptamine) increase their self-administration of cocaine (Loh & Roberts, 1990). These are isolated examples from a large body of fairly consistent findings in animals, all pointing to a preventive role of serotonin in drug craving or drug use.

Other recent evidence comes from studies in humans. A genetic disorder known as Tourette's syndrome is accompanied by lowered plasma tryptophan (the serotonin precursor) and signs of reduced serotonin in the brain as well as the periphery (Comings, 1990). The frequency of alcoholism and drug abuse associated with Tourette's is substantially increased (Comings & Comings, 1990). This is true not only in those who exhibit the symptoms of Tourette's but in relatives who are asymptomatic, recessive carriers of the genetic trait. The genetic locus for the disease appears to be the same as that of the liver enzyme that metabolizes tryptophan (Comings, Muhleman, Dietz & Donlon, 1991). The authors suggest that the defect in Tourette's syndrome results in greater breakdown of tryptophan in the liver. Thus, although produced by genetic predisposition instead of increased cortisol, a reduction of tryptophan similar to that proposed in the present theory appears both to reduce serotonin and to increase the incidence of alcoholism and drug abuse.

Consistent with this interpretation, reductions in the discomfort during withdrawal and in relapse to addiction have been obtained when the patient's diet is supplemented with a mixture containing tryptophan (Blum & Trachtenberg, 1988; Brown, Blum & Trachtenberg, 1990). However, the other ingredients in this mixture, i.e., *d*- and *l*-phenylalanine, *1*-glutamine and pyridoxal phosphate (vitamin B_6), may also contribute to these effects.

The findings with Tourette's and with amino acid supplementation appear to provide direct support for the theory discussed here, which posits chronic stress as a widespread source of serotonergic deficits predisposing to drug use. Tourette's syndrome also may provide an example of a genetic predisposition towards drug use that fits the general theory described in this paper, i.e., any genetic defect that impairs mechanisms maintaining homeostasis would be predicted to increase the incidence of drug abuse, as appears to be the case in Tourette's. In the chronic stress model, serotonergic deficits appear widespread in the body (Walton et al., submitted). This is apparently the case in Tourette's as well, and the frequency of other behaviors and disorders associated with serotonergic deficits is also increased (see Comings et al., 1991).

Thus, the evidence that practice of the Transcendental Meditation technique increases serotonin availability and decreases cortisol levels, as well as evidence that it reduces psychological stress and improves adaptive mechanisms, gives strong support to its ability to interrupt the cycle of drug abuse. Which of these effects might be primary cannot be deduced on the basis of the present data. However, evidence indicates that during each session of the practice, adaptive mechanisms tend to normalize, bringing the whole psychophysiological system to a more ideal state of homeostasis. This process appears progressive, so that each session of meditation builds on the balance fostered by previous sessions. At some point on this continuum of increasing psychophysiological integration, the system is no longer driven to seek artificial means of increasing serotonin or of otherwise decreasing activation of anxiety, fear and anger centers. The reduced activity of these centers, along with disinhibition of the reward centers, uphold the return of subjective well-being. The system appears now to be set on a "virtuous" cycle of ever-increasing balance and integration (Figure 3), enhancing both health and fulfillment in life.

REFERENCES

Aghajanian, G. K. (1978). Tolerance of locus coeruleus neurons to morphine and suppression of withdrawal response by clonidine. *Nature, 267*, 186-188.

Aghajanian, G. K. & Wang, Y. Y. (1986). Pertussis toxin blocks the outward currents evoked by opiate and alpha2-agonists in locus coeruleus neurons. *Brain Research, 371*, 390-394.

Ahlman, H., DeMagistris, L., Zinner, M., & Jaffe, B. M. (1981). Release of immunoreactive serotonin into the lumen of the feline gut in response to vagal nerve stimulation. *Science, 213*, 1254-1255.

Alexander, C. N., Davies, J. L., Dixon, C. A., Dillbeck, M. C., Druker, S. M., Oetzel, R. M., Muehlman, J. M., & Orme-Johnson, D. W. (1990). Growth of higher states of consciousness: The Vedic psychology of human development. In C. N. Alexander & E. J. Langer (Eds.), *Higher stages of human development: Perspectives on adult growth* (pp. 286-340). New York: Oxford University Press.

Alexander, C. N., Langer, E. J., Newman, R. I., Chandler, H. M., & Davies, J. L. (1989). Transcendental Meditation, mindfulness, and longevity: An experimental study with the elderly. *Journal of Personality and Social Psychology, 57*, 950-964.

Alexander, C. N., Rainforth, M. V., & Gelderloos, P. (1991). Transcendental Meditation, self-actualization and psychological health: A conceptual overview and statistical meta-analysis. *Journal of Social Behavior and Personality, 6*, 189-247.

Alexander, C. N., Robinson, P., & Rainforth, M. (this volume). Treating and preventing alcohol, nicotine, and drug abuse through Transcendental Meditation: A review and statistical meta-analysis. *Alcoholism Treatment Quarterly.*

Aron, A., & Aron, E. N. (1980). The Transcendental Meditation program's effect on addictive behavior. *Addictive Behaviors, 5*, 3-12.

Amaral, D. G., & Foss, J. A. (1975). Locus coeruleus lesions and learning. *Science, 188*, 377-379.

Amaral, D. G., & Sinnamon, H. M. (1977). The locus coeruleus: Neurobiology of a central noradrenergic nucleus. *Progress in Neurobiology, 9*, 147-196.

Antelman, S. M., Caggiula, A. R., Knopf, S., Kocan, D. J., & Edwards, D. J.

(1992). Amphetamine or haloperidol 2 weeks earlier antagonized the plasma corticosterone response to amphetamine: Evidence for the stressful/foreign nature of drugs. *Psychopharmacology, 107*, 331-336.

Aston-Jones, G. (1985). Behavioral functions of the locus coeruleus derived from cellular attributes. *Physiological Psychology, 13*, 118-126.

Aston-Jones, G., Akaoka, H., Charlety, P., & Chouvet, G. (1991). Serotonin selectively attenuates glutamate-evoked activation of noradrenergic locus coeruleus neurons. *Journal of Neuroscience, 11*, 760-769.

Aston-Jones, G., & Bloom, F. E. (1981). Norepinephrine-containing locus coeruleus neurons in behaving rats exhibit pronounced responses to non-noxious environmental stimuli. *Journal of Neuroscience, 1*, 887-900.

Bagdy, G., Cologero, A., Murphy, D., & Szemeredi., K. (1989). Serotonin agonists cause parallel activation of the sympathoadrenomedullary system and the hypothalomo-pituitary-adrenal axis in conscious rats. *Endocrinology, 125*, 2664-2669.

Blanchard, D. C., & Blanchard, R. J. (1979). Defensive behaviors in rats following septal and septal-amygdala lesions. *Journal of Comparative Physiology and Psychology, 93*, 378-380.

Blum, K., & Trachtenberg, M. C. (1988). Neurogenetic deficits caused by alcoholism: Restoration by SAAVE™, a neuronutrient intervention adjunct. *Journal of Psychoactive Drugs, 20*, 297-313.

Brodie, B. B., Spector, S., & Shore, P. A. (1959). Interaction of drugs with norepinephrine in the brain. *Pharmacological Reviews, 11*, 548-564.

Brodie, H. K. H., Sack, R., & Siever, L. (1973). Clinical studies of L-5-hydroxtryptophan in depression. In J. Barchas & E. Usdin (Eds.), *Serotonin and behavior* (pp. 549-559). New York: Academic Press.

Brown, R. J., Blum, K. & Trachtenberg, M. C. (1990). Neurodynamics of relapse prevention: A neuronutrient approach to outpatient DUI offenders. *Journal of Psychoactive Drugs, 22*, 173-187.

Bujatti, M., & Riederer, P. (1976). Serotonin, noradrenaline, dopamine metabolites in Transcendental Meditation technique. *Journal of Neural Transmission, 39*, 257-267.

Burchfield, S. R. (1979). The stress response: A new perspective. *Psychosomatic Medicine, 41*, 661-672.

Cannon, W. B. (1929). Organization for physiological homeostasis. *Physiological Reviews, 19*, 399-431.

Chrousos, G. P., & Gold, P. W. (1992). The concepts of stress and stress system disorders. *Journal of the American Medical Association, 267*, 1244-1252.

Comings, D. E. (1990). Blood serotonin and tryptophan in Tourette syndrome. *American Journal of Medical Genetics, 36*, 418-430.

Comings, D. E., & Comings, B. G. (1990). A controlled family history study of Tourette's syndrome, II: Alcoholism, drug abuse, and obesity. *Journal of Clinical Psychiatry, 51*, 281-287.

Comings, D. E., Muhleman, D., Dietz, Jr., G. W., & Donlon, T. (1991). Human tryptophan oxygenase locked to 4q31: Possible implications for alcoholism and other behavioral disorders. *Genomics, 9*, 301-308.

Dahlstrom, A., & Fuxe, K. (1964). Evidence for the existence of dopamine-containing neurons in the central nervous system I: Demonstration of monoamines in the cell bodies of brainstem neurons. *Acta Physiologica Scandinavica Supplement, 222*, 1-55.

Dillbeck, M. C., & Bronson, E. C. (1981). Short-term longitudinal effects of the Transcendental Meditation technique on EEG power and coherence. *International Journal of Neuroscience, 14*, 147-151.

Dillbeck, M. C., & Orme-Johnson, D. W. (1987). Physiological differences between Transcendental Meditation and rest. *American Psychologist, 42*, 879-881.

Eppley, K., Abrams, A., & Shear, J. (1989). The differential effects of relaxation techniques on trait anxiety: A meta-analysis. *Journal of Clinical Psychology, 45*, 957-974.

Frew, D. R. (1974). Transcendental Meditation and productivity. *Academy of Management Journal, 17*, 362-368.

Gelderloos, P., Walton, K. G., Orme-Johnson, D. W., & Alexander, C. N. (1991). Effectiveness of the Transcendental Meditation program in preventing and treating substance misuse: A review. *International Journal of the Addictions, 26*, 293-325.

Goldberger, L., & Breznitz, S. (1982). *Handbook of stress: Theoretical and clinical aspects*. New York: The Free Press.

Goleman, D. J., & Schwartz, G. E. (1976). Meditation as an intervention in stress reactivity. *Journal of Consulting and Clinical Psychology, 44*, 456-466.

Holdefer, R. N., & Jensen, R. A. (1987). The effects of peripheral D-amphetamine, and epinephrine on maintained discharge in the locus coeruleus with reference to the modulation of learning and memory by these substances. *Brain Research, 417*, 108-117.

Jacobs, B. L. (1986). Single unit activity of locus coeruleus neurons in behaving animals. *Progress in Neurobiology, 27*, 183-194.

Jevning, R., Wallace, R., & Beidebach, M. (1992). The physiology of meditation: A review. A wakeful hypometabolic integrated response. *Neuroscience and Biobehavioral Reviews, 16*, 415-424.

Jevning, R., Wilson, A. F., & Davidson, J. M. (1978). Adrenocortical activity during meditation. *Hormones and Behavior, 10*, 54-60.

Jouvet, M. (1972). The role of monoamines and acetylcholine neurons in the regulation of the sleep waking cycle. *Ergebnisse der Physiologie, Biologischen Chemie und Experimentellen Pharmakologie, 64*, 166-307.

Kember, P. (1985). The Transcendental Meditation technique and academic performance: A short report on a controlled, longitudinal pilot study. *British Journal of Educational Psychology, 55*, 164-166.

Knox, W. E., Piras, M. M., & Tokuyama, K. (1966). Induction of tryptophan pyrrolase in rat liver by physiological amounts of hydrocortisone and secreted glucocorticoids. *Enzymologia Biologica et Clinica, 7*, 1-10.

Kuriyama, K., Kanmori, K., & Yoneda, Y. (1983). Preventive effect of alcohol on stress-induced alterations in metabolism and function of biogenic amines and gamma-aminobutyric acid (GABA) in neuroendocrine system. In L. A. Pohorecky, & J. Brick (Eds.), *Stress and alcohol use* (pp. 404-420). New York: Elsevier.

LeDoux, J. E., Cicchetti, P., Xagoraris, A., & Romanski, L. M. (1990). The lateral amygdaloid nucleus: Sensory interface of the amygdaloid in fear conditioning. *Journal of Neuroscience, 10*, 1062-1069.

Loh, E. A., & Roberts, D. C. S. (1990). Break-points on a progressive ratio schedule reinforced by intravenous cocaine increase following depletion of forebrain serotonin. *Psychopharmacology, 101*, 262-266.

Maclean, C. R. K., Walton, K. G., Wenneberg, S. R., Levitsky, D. K., Mandarino, J. V., Waziri, R., & Schneider, R. H. (1992). Altered cortisol response to stress after four months' practice of the Transcendental Meditation program. *Society of Neuroscience Abstracts, 18*, 1541.

Maes, M., Jacobs, M-P., Suy, E., Minner, B., Leclerccq, C., Christiaens, F., & Raus, J. (1990). Suppressant effects of dexamethasone on the availability of L-tryptophan and tyrosine in healthy controls and in depressed patients. *Acta Psychiatrica Scandinavica, 81*, 19-23.

Maharishi Mahesh Yogi (1963). *Science of being and art of living: Transcendental Meditation*. New York: Signet.

Maharishi Mahesh Yogi (1969). *On the Bhagavad-Gita: A translation and commentary, Chapters 1-6*. Harmondsworth, Middlesex, England: Arkana (Penguin).

Mason, S. T., & Fibiger, H. C. (1978). 6-OHDA lesion of the dorsal noradrenergic bundle alters extinction of passive avoidance. *Brain Research, 152*, 209-214.

McBride, W. J., Murphy, J. M., Lumeng, L., & Li, T. (1988). Effects of Ro 15-4513, fluoxetine and desipramine on the intake of ethanol, water and food by the alcohol-preferring (P) and non-preferring (NP) lines of rats. *Pharmacology. Biochemistry and Behavior, 30*, 1045-1050.

Meirieu, O., Pairet, M., Sutra, J. F., & Ruckebusch, M. (1986). Local release of monoamines in the gastrointestinal tract: An in vivo study in rabbits. *Life Sciences, 38*, 827-834.

Nestler, E. J. (1992). Molecular mechanisms of drug addiction. *Journal of Neurosciences, 12*, 2439-2450.

Nisenbaum, L. K., Zigmond, M. J., Sved, A. F., & Abercrombie, E. D. (1991). Prior exposure to chronic stress results in enhanced synthesis and release of hippocampal norepinephrine in response to a novel stressor. *Journal of Neuroscience, 11*, 1478-1484.

Pitts, D. K,, & Marwah, J. (1988). Cocaine and central monaminergic neurotransmission: A review of electrophysiological studies and comparison to amphetamines and antidepressants. *Life Sciences, 42*, 949-968.

Pope, M. K., & Smith, T. W. (1991). Cortisol excretion in high and low cynically hostile men. *Psychosomatic Medicine, 53*, 386-392.

Redmond, D. E., & Huang, Y. H. (1979). Current concepts II: New evidence for a locus coeruleus-norepinephrine connection with anxiety. *Life Sciences, 25*, 2149-2162.

Rosecrans, J. A., & DeFeo, J. J. (1965). The interrelationships between chronic restraint stress and reserpine sedation. *Archives Internationales de Pharmacodynamie et de Therapie, 157*, 487-498.

Sachar, E. J., Hellman, L., Roffward, H. P., Halpern, F. S., Fukushima, D. K., & Gallagher, T. F. (1973). Disrupted 24-hour patterns of cortisol secretion in psychotic depression. *Archives of General Psychiatry, 28*, 19-24.

Sachar, E. J., Puig-Antich, J., Ryan, N. D., Asnis, G. M., Rabinovich, H., Davies, M., & Halpern, F. S. (1985). Three tests of cortisol secretion in adult endogenous depressives. *Acta Psychiatrica Scandinavica, 71*, 1-8.

Sanna, E., Concas, A., Serra, M., & Biggio, G. (1990). In vivo administration of ethanol enhances the function of the GABA-dependent chloride channel in the rat cerebral cortex. *Journal of Neurochemistry, 54*, 696-698.

Sapolsky, R. M. (1990). Adrenocortical function, social rank, and personality among wild baboons. *Biological Psychiatry, 28*, 862-878.

Sapolsky, R. M. (1992). *Stress, the aging brain, and the mechanisms of neuron death*. Cambridge, Massachusetts: The MIT Press.

Sapolsky, R. M., Krey, L. C., & McEwen, B. S. (1984a). Stress down-regulates corticosterone receptors in a site-specific manner in the brain. *Endocrinology, 114*, 287-292.

Sapolsky, R. M., Krey, L. C., & McEwen, B. S. (1984b). Glucocorticoid-sensitive hippocampal neurons are involved in terminating the adrenocortical stress response. *Proceedings of the National Academy of Sciences USA, 81*, 6174-6177.

Sapolsky, R. M., Krey, L. C., & McEwen, B. S. (1986). The neuroendocrinology of stressed aging: The glucocorticoid cascade hypothesis. *Endocrine Review, 7*, 284-301.

Scapagnini, U., Moberg, G., Van Loon, G., de Groot, J., & Ganong, W. (1971). Relation of brain 5-hydroxytryptamine content to the diurnal variation in plasma corticosterone in the rat. *Neuroendocrinology, 7*, 90-96.

Schneider, R. H., Alexander, C. N., & Wallace, R. K. (1992). In search of an optimal behavioral treatment for hypertension: A review and focus on Transcendental Meditation. In E. H. Johnson, W. D. Gentry, & S. Julius (Eds.), *Personality, elevated blood pressure and essential hypertension*. Washington, DC: Hemisphere Publishing Corporation.

Schwartz, R. D., Suzdak, P. D., & Paul, S. M. (1987). GABA and barbiturate-mediated 36C1 ion uptake in rat brain synaptoneurosomes: Evidence for rapid desensitization of the GABA receptor-coupled chloride channel. *Molecular Pharmacology, 30*, 419-426.

Scriabine, A., Clineschmidt, B. U., & Sweet, C. S. (1976). Central noradrenergic control of blood pressure. In H. W. Elliot (Ed.), *Annual reviews of pharmacology and toxicology, Vol 16*. Palo Alto: Annual Reviews.

Seckl, J. R., Dickson, K. L., & Fink, G. (1990). Central 5, 7-dihydroxytryptamine lesions decrease hippocampal glucocorticoid and mineralocorticoid receptor messenger ribonucleic acid expression. *Journal of Neuroendocrinology, 2*, 911-916.

Seckl, J. R., & Fink, G. (1992). Antidepressants increase glucocorticoid and mineralocorticoid receptor mRNA expression in rat hippocampus in vivo. *Neuroendocrinology, 55*, 621-626.

Seitin, V., Franchimont, M., Massotte, L., & Dresse, A. (1990) Comparison of the effect of morphine on locus coeruleus noradrenergic and ventral tegmental area dopaminergic neurons in vitro. *Life Sciences, 46*, 1879-1885.

Shirae, D. T., Morton, B. E. (1991). Tetrahydrocannibinol raises basal and GABA-mediated synaptoneurosome 36-chloride ion influx. *Society of Neuroscience Abstracts, 17*, 1521.

Staggers, Jr., F., Alexander, C. N., & Walton, K. G. (this volume). Importance of reducing stress and strengthening the host in drug detoxification: The potential offered by Transcendental Meditation. *Alcoholism Treatment Quarterly.*

Tallman, J. F., Paul, S. M., Skolnick, P., & Gallager, D. S. (1980). Receptors for the age of anxiety: Pharmacology of the benzodiazepines. *Science, 207*, 274-281.

Taub, E., Steiner, S. S., Smith, R. B., Weingarten, E. & Walton, K. G. (this volume). Effectiveness of broad spectrum approaches to relapse prevention in severe alcoholism: A long-term, randomized, controlled trial of Transcendental Meditation, EMG biofeedback and electronic neurotherapy. *Alcoholism Treatment Quarterly.*

Walton, K., Pugh, N., Gelderloos, P., & Macrae, P. (submitted). Mechanisms of prevention through stress reduction: Suggestive results on corticosteriods, salt excretion and negative emotions. *Journal of Hypertension.*

Transcendental Meditation as an Epidemiological Approach to Drug and Alcohol Abuse: Theory, Research, and Financial Impact Evaluation

David Orme-Johnson, PhD

We dance round in a ring and suppose,
But the Secret sits in the middle and knows.

–Robert Frost

INTRODUCTION

The epidemic of drug and alcohol abuse is part of a larger complex of problems that arise from stress in collective consciousness. Collective consciousness is held to be a field that permeates society, with the individual as its basic unit. Stress in individuals means dysfunction of physiological and cognitive adaptive systems, which results in inability to fulfill desires and, consequently, a lack of

---

David Orme-Johnson is Chairman of the Department of Psychology at Maharishi International University, 1000 N. Fourth Street, Fairfield, IA 52557-1034.

[Haworth co-indexing entry note]: "Transcendental Meditation as an Epidemiological Approach to Drug and Alcohol Abuse: Theory, Research, and Financial Impact Evaluation." Orme-Johnson, David. Co-published simultaneously in the *Alcoholism Treatment Quarterly* (The Haworth Press, Inc.) Vol. 11, No. 1/2, 1994, pp. 119-168; and: *Self-Recovery: Treating Addictions Using Transcendental Meditation and Maharishi Ayur-Veda* (ed: David F. O'Connell and Charles N. Alexander) The Haworth Press, Inc., 1994, pp. 119-168. Multiple copies of this article/chapter may be purchased from The Haworth Document Delivery Center [1-800-3-HAWORTH; 9:00 a.m. - 5:00 p.m. (EST)].

fulfillment. Stressed individuals create stress in collective consciousness, which is experienced throughout society as tension, anxiety, and lethargy. Stress in collective consciousness, in turn, causes people to take alcohol and drugs as an attempt to reestablish balance and gain an illusion of optimal state of functioning and fulfillment. However, alcohol, tobacco, and drugs instead invariably throw the system out of balance, leading to a vicious cycle of escalating stress in both the individual and society.

This paper presents the theory of Maharishi Mahesh Yogi, which suggests that experience of the silent basis of the mind, transcendental consciousness, is the direct experience of the unified field of nature's intelligence. This experience, which can be systematically gained through Maharishi's Transcendental Meditation and TM-Sidhi program, can break the vicious cycle of growing individual and collective stress, reestablish balance, and cultivate optimal psychophysiological functioning, thus reducing the urge to further consume alcohol and drugs. Extensive research, reviewed in this paper, shows that when 1% of the population practices the Transcendental Meditation program or the square root of 1% practices the TM and TM-Sidhi program in a group an influence of coherence is created in collective consciousness, reducing all the various stress-related social problems.

The financial savings of widespread application of this program to reduce stress in collective consciousness are estimated to be hundreds of billions of dollars per year. The research indicates that this program is a highly effective and inexpensive public health measure to "immunize" the entire population against stress and its symptoms, drug and alcohol abuse.

THEORY

A Multidimensional Epidemic: Drug and alcohol abuse are part of a multidimensional international epidemic that involves virtually every area of society, including the criminal justice system, health, education, social welfare, and the economy (Bureau of Justice Statistics [BJS] Bulletin, 1993, p. 8). An estimated 38 million Americans (15% of the population) are chemically addicted to alcohol or drugs (Yoder in Hazelden Foundation, 1991). Moreover, if each addict affects three family members, then 60% of the population is directly or indirectly affected by use of these substances (Yoder, 1990, p. v).

The problem of crime is so closely interrelated with drug and alcohol abuse that they must be considered part of the same epidemic. Alcohol and drug use is a contributing factor in 54% of all violent crimes, 40% of property crimes, and 64% of public order crimes in the U.S. (Yoder in Hazelden Foundation, 1991, p. 52). Heroin addicts commit an average of 178 criminal offenses per year (Johnson et al., 1985). In 1991, drug related offenses were the largest single cause of federal imprisonment, accounting for 14,738 new sentences (BJS Bulletin, 1993, p. 8).

If tobacco use is included in the picture, which it should be, since nicotine is an addictive drug, then the public health implications of this epidemic become even more staggering. Twenty percent of the industrialized world's current population–at least 250 million people, more than the population of the United States–will die of smoking-related diseases (Peto, Lopez, Boreham, Thum, & Heath, 1992). In the U.S. almost 400,000 people will die of smoking related diseases, and 18 million will experience alcohol-related health problems (U.S. Dept. of Health and Human Services, 1990a).

The epidemic of drugs, alcohol, and crime also seriously affects the economy. For example, alcohol and drugs account for 52% of all traffic fatalities (in Hazelden Foundation, 1991). Because it raises insurance premiums, and lowers productivity, drug and alcohol abuse costs corporations $93 billion a year (Harwood et al., 1984; Rice et al., 1990). These addictions also increase the tax burden due to costs for treatment, incarceration, and social welfare to care for the afflicted individuals and their families.

Our educational system is heavily implicated in this multidimensional epidemic. One in four high school students has a drinking problem (Horton, 1985), and one-third of all school children in the U.S. have used an illicit drug (U.S. Dept. of Health and Human Services, 1991). More than 135,000 students carry a gun to school, and in 1990 over half a million violent crimes occurred around American schools, a majority of which were drug or alcohol related (Children's Defense Fund, 1991). Education should be our front line defense against this epidemic, but instead our schools are a breeding ground for drug abuse and violence. Clearly a fresh perspective on education is needed, as one component of a strategy for curbing the epidemic.

Social Stress as the Cause of the Epidemic: Linsky, Colby, and Straus (1986) have pioneered in the concept of social stress as the underlying cause of crime, disease, and maladaptive behavior such as drug and alcohol abuse. In their analysis, social stress is a component process of the social system as a whole that may not be predictable from knowledge about individuals. They operationalize social stress in three categories: economic stressors (e.g., business failures, unemployment, workers on strike, personal bankruptcies, and mortgage foreclosures); family stressors (e.g., divorces, abortions, illegitimate births, infant deaths); and other stressors (new welfare cases, high school dropouts, state residence less than 5 years). In two studies, Linsky and Straus use these parameters to measure the stress level of the 50 states in a "State Stress Index" (SSI). They found that the SSI was predictive of maladaptive behavior as indicated by the level of crime, disease, accidents of all kinds, and suicides. They found that the SSI was significantly correlated with cirrhosis and lung cancer, indirect measures of alcohol and cigarette related behavior. In another study, Linsky, Straus, and Colby (1985) found that social stress as variously defined (e.g., the SSI, barriers to upward mobility, structurally induced role conflict) was a significant predictor of death rate from alcoholism, alcohol psychosis, and per capita alcohol consumption, once other variables were controlled. They also found that social stress is correlated with smoking, and that smoking in turn is correlated with death from respiratory cancer (Linsky, Colby, & Straus, 1986). Drug use is indirectly related to social stress because social stress is a good predictor of crime, particularly violent crime (Yoder in Hazelden Foundation, 1991, p. 52), and half of violent crime is attributed to drug and alcohol use. Thus *there is strong evidence that alcohol, tobacco, and drug use are all elevated by social stress.*

These studies indicate that drug and alcohol abuse are not just individual aberrations but are manifestations of underlying imbalances in society. Just as a systemic disease gives rise to localized symptoms, so too does stress in society give rise to drug and alcohol abuse. Without knowledge of the systemic aspect of the disease process, one would be inclined to treat each symptom topically, which would be extremely difficult, and ineffective because it would miss the cause of the problem. Similarly, it is simplistic and reductionist to treat drug and alcohol abuse as individual and independent processes, because they are enmeshed in a wider complex of problems related to economy, the family, poor health, poor nutrition, crime, poverty, racism, lack of fulfillment, and lack of purpose, direction, and something for which to live.

Limitations of the Social Stress Model: The social stress model has a number of shortcomings. For one thing, it is difficult to separate cause and effect in the model. Family problems, such as divorce, may cause alcohol abuse, but then drinking may also cause family problems. In Linsky and Straus's model *social stress variables* such as business failures, unemployment, strikes, personal bankruptcies, divorces, abortions, infant deaths, and high school dropouts are hypothesized to be the *cause* of *maladaptive behavior variables* such as alcohol and drug problems, crime, disease, accidents of all kinds, and suicides. But the opposite may also be true. The maladaptive behavior variables such as alcohol and drug problems, crime, disease, accidents, and suicides may cause change in the social stress variables: business failures, unemployment, strikes, personal bankruptcies, divorces, abortions, infant deaths, high school dropouts, etc. The correlation between the two sets of variables only indicates that they are part of a single interacting system.

In our view, both social stress variables and maladaptive behavior variables are *symptoms of the same epidemic*, not causes. There is no real causal level specified by current social stress models that points to a way of treating this epidemic. How do we reduce social stress? We cannot tell people not to have business failures or not to go on strike or get divorced any more than we can effectively tell them not to drink, smoke, or take drugs.

Concepts of Collective Consciousness in the Social Sciences: All the main streams of contemporary sociological theory–conflict theory, structural-functional theory, and symbolic interaction theory–view society in terms of direct *behavioral* and symbolic interactions between individuals and groups. In this view individuals and society are completely localized entities which interact with each other in very complex ways but which are in their essence separate. Such a "collective consciousness," if it exists, might well be the unambiguous causal level missing from the social stress model.

However, several of the founding theorists of modern psychology and sociology have proposed the concept of consciousness as a field through which individuals may be fundamentally connected. One of the founding fathers of modern psychology, Gustav Fechner, for example, described a unity or continuity of "general consciousness" underlying the discontinuities of consciousness associated with each individual, accessible in principle simply through lowering the threshold of conscious experience (in James, 1898/1977). William James, the founder of psychology as an academic discipline in America, suggested that the brain may serve to reflect or transmit, rather than produce, consciousness, which in turn may be conceived as a transcendental, infinite continuity underlying the phenomenal world (ibid). Emile Durkheim, considered one of the founders of modern sociology, proposed that a *conscience collective* was the essence of the underlying social fabric unifying individuals in society. This "collective consciousness" was described by Durkheim as the mind of society, created when "the consciousness of the individuals, instead of remaining isolated, becomes grouped and combined" (1951, pp. 310, 312, 313). Carl Jung also talks of a *collective unconscious* as the repository of humanity's collective experience that embodies archetypal patterns that are actualized by individuals and society as specific individual personalities and social roles (Campbell, 1949).

None of these theories of collective consciousness, however, were operationalized and therefore they did not engender any scientific research or practical programs for the betterment of society. Consequently, they never became major components of mainstream social science theory or research (McDougall, 1920/1973).

Maharishi's Principles of Collective Consciousness: In sharp contrast to the early theories of psychology, Maharishi Mahesh Yogi's (e.g., 1977) theory of collective consciousness has testable consequences which have been extensively researched, and it has practical applications which promise to dramatically reduce and eventually eliminate the drug-alcohol-crime epidemic. Maharishi's theory of collective consciousness has its roots in the Vedic[1] tradition of India. In the Vedic literature, the Yoga Sutras of Patanjali, one of the "six systems of Indian philosophy" (Prasada, 1978), states *tat sannidhau vairatyagah* which means "in the vicinity of coherence [yoga], hostile tendencies are eliminated." In this view, meditation produces coherence in the field of collective consciousness, which then penetrates throughout society and influences everyone, reducing stress in the whole system, thus eliminating the manifestations of stress, such as hostility and drug and alcohol abuse.

"Consciousness" is defined as the ground of awareness on which all thought processes and behaviors depend (Maharishi, 1966). For example, when we are drowsy and dull, our thoughts and behavior are full of mistakes and create suffering. Collective consciousness is the wholeness of consciousness of an entire group. Just as an individual consciousness can be drowsy and stressed or wide awake and happy, so too can collective consciousness. For example, each family has a characteristic collective consciousness. When we go into a home of a happy family, we feel a harmonious influence and our behavior becomes more relaxed and open. Similarly, each city, state, and country has a characteristic collective consciousness (Maharishi Mahesh Yogi, 1977). When we enter a city with a high crime rate, we sense it and feel tense and uneasy.

In Maharishi's theory of collective consciousness, the quality of collective consciousness at each subordinate level contributes to the quality of collective consciousness at a higher level. For example, stressed individuals create stress in the family consciousness. Stressed family consciousnesses create stress in the city consciousness, urban stress influences the state's collective consciousness, and so on, ultimately to the collective consciousness of the entire globe (Maharishi Mahesh Yogi, 1977, p. 122). We propose that the epidemic of drugs and alcohol abuse arises from stress in all levels of collective consciousness, from family consciousness to world consciousness, and therefore, must ultimately be treated on the world level.

Maharishi's theory of collective consciousness holds that there is a reciprocal relationship between individual consciousness and collective consciousness (Maharishi Mahesh Yogi, 1977, p. 124). That is, each individual influences the collective consciousness of the society, and, at the same time, each individual is influenced by the collective consciousness. The stress of everyone else in the world is influencing us, just as our stress is influencing everyone else in the world, through the field of collective consciousness (Maharishi Mahesh Yogi, 1977, pp. 122-124).

Biochemistry of Stress: Since the individual is the basic unit of collective consciousness, the source of stress in collective consciousness is stress in the individual. To understand stress in the individual and collective consciousness and how it relates to drug and alcohol abuse, we will review some of the recent stress research. In recent years a great deal has been discovered about stress (Chrousos & Gold, 1992; Sapolsky, 1992). Stress is conceptualized as a generalized response of the system that occurs when the pressure of experience exceeds a threshold. Overload of the system breaks it down. The components of the stress system are the corticotropin-releasing hormone and the norepinephrine/autonomic system, the pituitary-adrenal axis, and the limbs of the autonomic system. The stress response mobilizes bodily resources to support an adaptive response to environmental challenges while maintaining homeostatic balance. Basically, the purpose of the stress response is to fulfill desires. The problem comes when the system malfunctions due to chronic overstimulation. The system may become depleted and lose the ability to cope with challenges. Or the set points of the system may become reset so that the system may fail to return to optimal baseline levels, as in hypertension.

Stress has a wide range of effects on psychiatric, endocrine, and inflammatory disorders as well as susceptibility to these disorders. The stress system is strongly influenced by cognitive and emotional factors. The exigencies of modern life increase the risk of action of the stress system and raise the prevalence of stress-related diseases (Elliot & Eisendorfer, 1982).

Thus, stress in the individual involves an imbalance in the delicate and complex neurochemical systems that regulate adaptive responses. These imbalances get transmitted from individual to individual in society both behaviorally and via collective consciousness.

TM has been found to have the opposite biochemical effects of stress, which is reviewed below in the section on research.

Stress in Collective Consciousness: In Maharishi's view, all problems in society are expressions of stress throughout the system as a whole, i.e., in its collective consciousness. Maharishi states:

"All occurrences of violence, negativity and conflict, crises, of problems in any society are just the expression of growth of stress in collective consciousness. When the level of stress becomes sufficiently great, it bursts out into large-scale violence, war, and civil uprising necessitating military action" (1979, p. 38).

When stress in collective consciousness builds up to an extreme degree, then it will inevitably burst out in violence and conflict, such as a race riot or drug war. Just as any spark can kindle a fire in dry grass, any unfortunate event can have catastrophic results when there is great stress in collective consciousness (Maharishi Mahesh Yogi, 1986a, pp. 83-84). Stress, originating in the individual, is thus held to be the basis of all problems in society, including alcohol and drug abuse, negativity, violence, terrorism, and national and international conflicts (Maharishi Mahesh Yogi, 1986a, pp. 80-85). They are all aspects of the same epidemic.

The Theoretical Model: Figure 1 illustrates how drug abuse and crime are just two of the many symptoms of the multidimensional epidemic caused by stress in collective consciousness. Behavioral symptoms and the underlying field of stress in collective consciousness are shown to reciprocally interact within the circle of society. Underlying and outside society is the unified field of natural law, the source of order in nature.

In order to reduce stress in the individual and in collective consciousness, one must step out of the vicious cycle of stress in social behavior and collective consciousness, and go to a deeper underlying level of natural law, the unified field of natural law (to be discussed below). In Maharishi's theory, the unified field is a field of pure consciousness that is the source of order and coherence not only in society, but in nature.

According to Maharishi, the unified field of natural law can easily and effortlessly be experienced as transcendental consciousness through the Transcendental Meditation technique.

> The Transcendental Meditation technique is an effortless procedure for allowing the excitations of the mind to settle down until the least excited state of mind is reached. This is a state of inner wakefulness with no object of thought or perception, just pure consciousness aware of its own unbounded nature. It is

> wholeness, aware of itself, devoid of differences, beyond the division of subject and object–transcendental consciousness. It is a field of all possibilities, where all creative potentialities exist together, infinitely correlated yet unexpressed. It is a state of perfect order, the matrix from where all the laws of nature emerge. (1977, p. 123)

How many meditators are theoretically needed to produce a measurable increase in coherence in an entire society? A large body of

FIGURE 1. This illustration shows drug and alcohol abuse as part of a multidimensional complex of behavioral symptoms (Level 1) that arise from stress in an underlying abstract field of collective consciousness (Level 2). The circle represents the usual system of reciprocal interaction of stress in collective consciousness and its behavioral symptoms. Underlying the circle is the unified field of natural law, the source of nature's infinite organizing power, which governs the universe in perfect orderliness (Level 3). When the unified field of natural law is outside the circle of the behavioral/collective consciousness system of society, incoherence and conflict predominate in society.

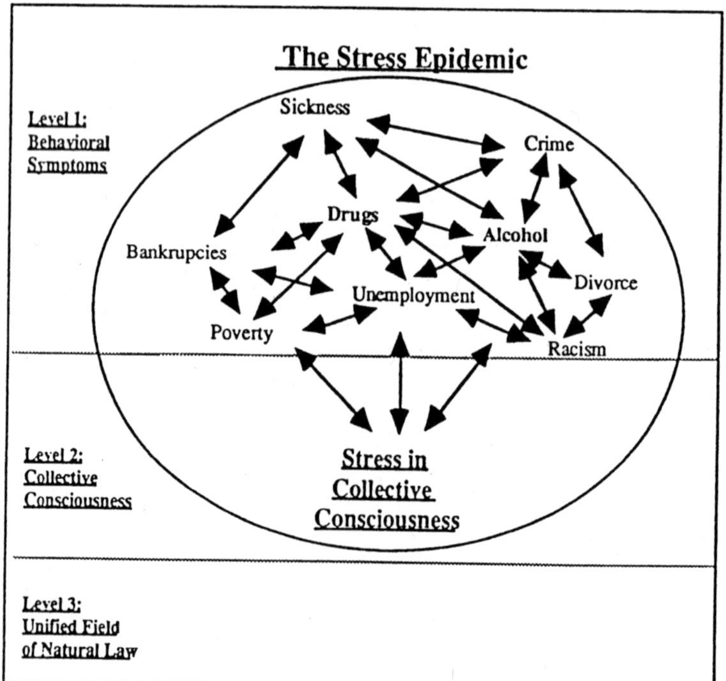

scientific research reviewed below has found that as little as one percent of a population practicing the TM program or an even smaller number, on the order of the square root of 1% of a population, collectively practicing the TM-Sidhi program is sufficient to produce a measurable and holistic influence of harmony and integration in the entire population (c.f. Maharishi Mahesh Yogi, 1986a, p. 76).

To understand how such a remarkably small group could influence an entire population we can consider analogous phenomena in physical systems. In systems governed by wavelike interactions, the strength of elements that are interacting coherently is proportional to the square of their number, while the influence of elements that are interacting incoherently is only proportional to their number. As a result, when a number proportional to the square root of the total elements are interacting coherently, then the coherent influence outweighs the incoherent influence of all the other elements in the system. An example of this principle is laser light. Through the coherent emission of a number of photons that is proportional to the square root of the total, the entire system undergoes a phase transition in which all the photons begin to interact coherently, generating the laser light.

In a similar manner, Maharishi's theory predicts that the coherent influence generated by the square root of 1% of the population experiencing the field of pure consciousness will combine to create a powerful influence of coherence in the entire society. Maharishi comments on this point in referring to pure consciousness as the transcendental level of nature's functioning:

> This transcendental level of nature's functioning is the level of infinite correlation. When the group awareness is brought in attunement with that level, then a very intensified influence of coherence radiates and a great richness is created. Infinite correlation is a quality of the transcendental level of nature's functioning from where orderliness governs the universe. (1986a, p. 75)

Figure 2 illustrates this idea. When there is a sufficient number of meditators in society, they enliven the unified field of nature's intelligence, the "Constitution of the Universe" said to govern all of nature in perfect orderliness. These individuals neutralize stress and radiate coherence in collective consciousness, which fosters ideal social relationships on the behavioral level.

If stress in the collective consciousness creates the drug problem, then neutralizing the stress in the whole society in one stroke would solve it. The difficulty dealing with the drug problem by any other means (unaided by creating coherence in collective consciousness) is that the solution *must* be systemic. Alcohol and drug abuse have

FIGURE 2. This figure illustrates the transformation of society that comes about when 1% of the population practices the Transcendental Meditation technique, or the square root of 1% practices the TM-Sidhi program. The sphere of society is expanded to include the unified field of natural law, whose infinite organizing power creates coherence in society, resulting in ideal social behavior in which the individual and society are always fully mutually supportive.

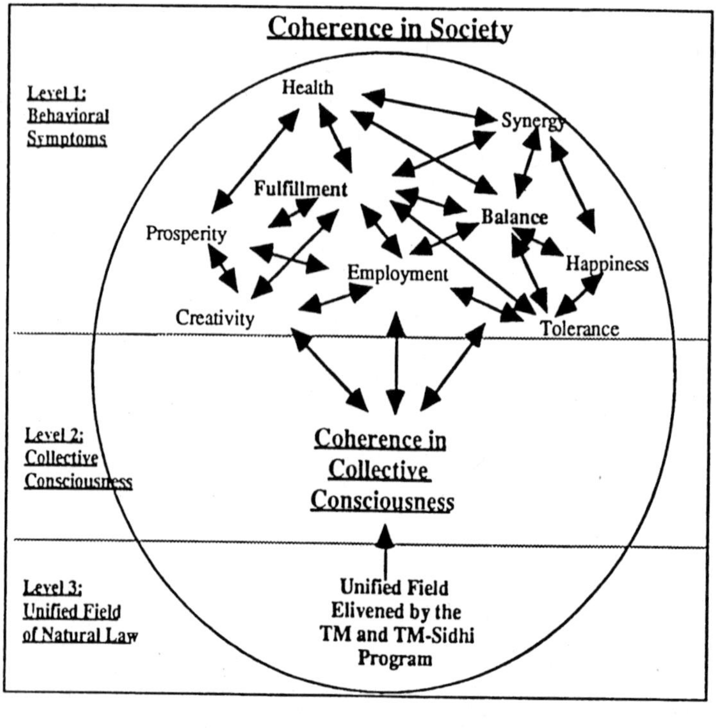

many complex determinants–economic, political, historical, individual, ethnic–that must all be addressed simultaneously if a drug free society is to become a stable reality. The beauty of Maharishi's approach to drug abuse is that it deals with the whole system at once through its collective consciousness, which is possible because collective consciousness touches every level of life in society.

Corroborating Insights from Modern Scientists: In Maharishi's (1966, 1977, 1986a) analysis, the unified field of natural law that has recently been glimpsed by modern physics is the same reality that India's ancient Vedic Science, Plato, and virtually all of the world's philosophical traditions have identified as the source of order in nature (Hagelin, 1987, 1989). Maharishi's assertion that the source of order in nature is a field of consciousness is supported by the statements of many of the leading scientists of our time. For example, Sir Arthur Eddington, who provided empirical confirmation of Einstein's General Theory of Relativity, wrote: "The idea of a universal Mind or Logos would be, I think, a fairly plausible inference from the present state of scientific theory; at least it is in harmony with it" (1984, p. 206; c.f. Dossey, 1989, p. 125).

The eminent astronomer, mathematician, and author Sir James Jeans wrote:

> When we view ourselves in space and time, our consciousness are obviously the separate individuals of a particle-picture, but when we pass beyond space and time, they may perhaps form ingredients of a single continuous stream of life. As it is with light and electricity, so may it be with life; the phenomena may be individuals carrying on separate existences in space and time, while in the deeper reality beyond space and time we may all be members of one body. (1981, p. 204; c.f. Dossey, 1989, p. 125)

Thus we see that Jeans intuited that the most basic level of consciousness is a continuum that interconnects everyone and everything. It has been argued that quantum field theory gives consciousness an ontologically fundamental position. As the French physicist Bernard D'Espagnat (1979) commented in a *Scientific American* article: "The doctrine that the world is made up of objects whose existence is independent of human consciousness turns out to be in conflict with quantum mechanics and with the facts established by experiment." Max Planck, the father of quantum theory, more directly said, "I regard consciousness as fundamental. I regard matter as derivative from consciousness" (quoted in Klein, 1984).

Thus, both ancient and modern seers have apprehended that the basis of natural law underlying human society is an unbounded field of consciousness. But it has remained for Maharishi's revival of Vedic knowledge to bring to the world the practical significance of this theoretical framework. Through the widespread availability of a simple technology for experiencing the unified field of natural law–Maharishi's Transcendental Meditation program–research on collective consciousness has taken a foothold and has demonstrated its ability to solve the otherwise recalcitrant worldwide epidemic of stress-related disorders. The research indicates that the Transcendental Meditation and TM-Sidhi program is a practical technology to "immunize" the entire population against the stress epidemic, which can substantially reduce and eventually eliminate alcohol and drug abuse.

RESEARCH

Research on the Individual: The individual is the unit of collective consciousness. Therefore, in order to reduce stress and create coherence in society, it is necessary to reduce stress and create coherence in the individual. Hans Selye, who was the foremost pioneer of stress research, summarized the research on Maharishi's Transcendental Meditation technique as follows:

> Research already conducted shows that the physiological effects of Transcendental Meditation are exactly the opposite of those identified by medicine as being characteristic of the body's effort to meet the demand of stress. The TM technique is a method which so relaxes the human central nervous system that . . . it doesn't suffer from stress . . . And I think that if you can relax the nervous system so that it can really relax, really be at its best in responding non-specifically to any demand, that is an ideal solution. (cited in Oates, 1976, pp. 214-217)

Since Selye made that statement, there have been three major meta-analyses which corroborate it. A meta-analysis conducted on the 32 physiological studies of the Transcendental Meditation technique compared with simple rest while sitting quietly with eyes closed found that TM produced significantly greater reduction in somatic arousal than simply resting quietly, as measured by basal skin resistance, respiration rate, and plasma lactate (Dillbeck & Orme-Johnson, 1987; also, see the review paper on the physiological effects of TM by Jevning, Wallace, & Beidebach, 1992). In addition, Walton, Pugh, Gelderloos, & Macrae (submitted) have recently shown that TM normalizes the biochemistry, an extremely important finding in explaining its effects on substance abuse.

A second meta-analysis by Eppley, Abrams, and Shear (1989) considered all the research on the effects of meditation and relaxation on anxiety (146 independent outcomes), and found that TM produces significantly greater reduction in trait anxiety (i.e., chronic stress) than is provided by any other meditation or relaxation technique. Studies with the strongest experimental design (random assignment to groups and low attrition) showed the largest effects for TM and the greatest contrast between TM and other meditation and relaxation techniques.

A third exhaustive meta-analysis of 42 independent outcomes found that the effect produced by TM on overall self-actualization as indicated primarily by the Personality Orientation Inventory (POI) was significantly larger than that produced by other forms of meditation and relaxation, controlling for duration of intervention and strength of experimental design (Alexander, Rainforth, & Gelderloos, 1991). This meta-analysis shows that practice of TM develops realization of the individual's unique potential, and increases capacity for warm interpersonal relationships, thus satisfying some of the motivation for alcohol and drug abuse.

Reviews of some 24 studies show that the Transcendental Meditation technique is highly effective for treating drug abuse in the individual (Alexander, Robinson, & Rainforth, this volume; Gelderloos, Cavanaugh, & Davies, 1991). Moreover, there are eight studies showing its effectiveness for prison rehabilitation (Bleick & Abrams, 1987; Dillbeck & Abrams, 1987).

These meta-analyses and reviews are only a small fraction of the research on the Transcendental Meditation technique. Over 500 studies have been conducted at more than 200 universities and research institutions in 30 countries, all supporting the conclusion that TM reduces stress and increases coherence in the individual.

The First Research on Collective Consciousness: Research on collective consciousness began in 1974, when researcher Garland Landrith of Maharishi International University (MIU) tested Maharishi's prediction on crime rate in 4 Midwestern cities where 1% of the population had learned the TM technique. He reported that crime rate decreased significantly the year after each became 1% cities, compared with other cities of similar size and geographic location. In the tradition of naming findings after the scientists who discovered them (e.g., the Doppler Effect, the Meissner Effect) this finding has been named the Maharishi Effect in honor of Maharishi who predicted it and provided the technology to implement it (Borland & Landrith, 1977). Because at least half of crime is alcohol and drug related, it can be inferred from the reduction in crime that alcohol and drug abuse must have decreased also.

Extension of the Original Crime Study: Using FBI data, the original study of 4 cities was expanded to include 11 cities that had over 25,000 population (Borland & Landrith, 1977), and by using data from local police for cities with 10,000 population, it was expanded again to include all 24 cities that had reached 1% of their population practicing the TM technique in 1972 (Dillbeck, Landrith, & Orme-Johnson, 1981). The finding of significant reduction in crime rate was replicated both times. In the second replication, not only did crime rate decrease the year after 1% was reached, but the crime rate trend was lower for those cities over the following six years, controlling for total population, geographic region, college population, unemployment rate, median education level, stability of residence, percentage of persons 15-29 years old in the population, and a number of other variables (see Figure 3).

Causal Analysis of Crime Reduction in 160 Cities: The most comprehensive studies of the Maharishi Effect on the city level employed causal analyses of crime trends over a period of seven

FIGURE 3. Twenty-four cities in which 1% of the population had been instructed in the Transcendental Meditation program by 1972 displayed significant decreases in crime rate during the next year (1973) and a decreased crime rate trend during the subsequent five years (1972-1977 in comparison to 1967-1972). This finding was in contrast to an overall increase in crime in 24 control cities matched for geographic region, population, college population, and crime rate, statistically controlling for a number of other demographic variables.

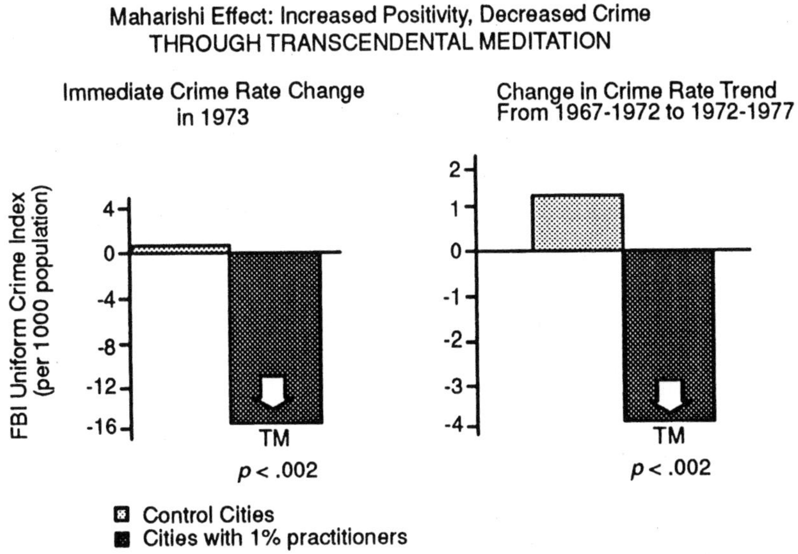

years in random samples of 160 U.S. cities and 50 Standard Statistical Metropolitan Areas (SSMA's), the latter sample representing approximately half the urban population of the U.S. (Dillbeck, Banus, Polanzi, & Landrith, 1988). These studies, which were published in *The Journal of Mind and Behavior*, found that cities and metropolitan areas with higher proportions of meditators in 1973 had reduced crime trends for the next six years. In neither study did the level of crime predict the number of meditators in the population in future years. Thus, TM practice apparently influenced the crime rate but crime rate did not influence TM practice, suggesting that TM practice was the causal element in the correlation between the two. Both studies statistically controlled for virtually all demographic variables known to influence crime, and a significant and stable causal structure was found for both samples, the 160 cities and the 50 SSMA's. These studies provide powerful evidence that the Transcendental Meditation and TM-Sidhi program can significantly reduce the drug-alcohol-crime epidemic.

The TM-Sidhi Program and Reduced Stress in Collective Consciousness: A major breakthrough in the Maharishi Effect research came in 1976 with the development of the more powerful TM-Sidhi program. The incredible power of the TM-Sidhi program on impacting collective consciousness was discovered in 1978 during Maharishi's Ideal Society Campaign, which was conducted in selected provinces in 20 countries. Maharishi sent teams of teachers of the Transcendental Meditation technique to these countries in order to try to inspire 1% of the local populations to learn the technique in order to create an ideal society. As it happened, these teachers practiced the TM-Sidhi program together in groups, particularly the powerful Yogic Flying technique (Orme-Johnson & Gelderloos, 1988; Travis & Orme-Johnson, 1990). It was discovered that groups of the order of the square root of 1% of a population collectively practicing the TM-Sidhi program were sufficient to produce a measurable and holistic influence of harmony and integration in the entire population (Dillbeck, Cavanaugh, Glenn, Orme-Johnson, & Mittlefehldt, 1987; c.f. Maharishi Mahesh Yogi, 1986a, p. 76).

For example, the first study of TM and TM-Sidhi groups was conducted on the state level in Rhode Island, and was published in *The Journal of Mind and Behavior.* It found improvements on a quality of life index that included crime, deaths, unemployment, *alcohol consumption, cigarette consumption*, pollution, motor vehicle fatalities, and accidents (Dillbeck et al., 1987). Thus, this study showed the direct influence of the Maharishi Effect on reducing alcohol and cigarette consumption, as well as indirectly through reduced crime, as well as motor vehicle accidents and fatalities, since over 50% of accidents are alcohol related. These results suggest that the meditator groups reduced the stress and tension in collective consciousness, so that the population felt more balanced and therefore less impelled to drink and smoke.

Decreased Urban Crime in Metro Manila, New Delhi, and Washington D.C.: Other research conducted in a variety of urban settings around the world has also shown that the TM and TM-Sidhi program can reduce the stress epidemic as seen in reduced crime. Studies published in *The Journal of Mind and Behavior* found that in Metro Manila, Philippines during a period when a TM and TM-Sidhi group was established there from August 1984 to January 1985 there was an 12.1% reduction in weekly crime totals. Similarly, there was an 11% reduction in daily crime totals from November 1980 to March 1981 attributed to a TM and TM-Sidhi group in that city (Dillbeck et al., 1987). A study of weekly violent crime in Washington, D.C. found an 11.8% decrease from October 1981 to October 1983 attributed to a group established in Washington at that time. Detailed analysis of other possible causes of the decreases in these cities found that they could not be attributed to changes in police policies or procedures, or to trends and cycles in the data. During the entire time the group of TM and TM-Sidhi participants was in Washington from 1981 to 1986, violent crime decreased almost 40%, but returned to a trend of increasing crime after the group left (see Figure 4).

Establishing a U.S. National TM and TM-Sidhi Group: The square root of 1% of a population is a relatively small number, making controlled studies even on the national and world level possible. For example, the square root of 1% of the U.S population is currently approximately 1,600, and the square root of 1% of the world population is approximately 7,000. Since 1979, a group of Transcendental Meditation and TM-Sidhi participants ranging in size from a few hundred to over 8,000 has gathered twice a day at Maharishi International University in Fairfield, Iowa (pop. 9,648) for the purpose of creating coherence in the U.S. and world. The effects of this group have been studied on the town of Fairfield, the state of Iowa, the U.S., and the whole world.

Fairfield: A study of violent crime in Fairfield found that it has 1/3 the rate of violent crime of other non-suburban towns of 5,000 to 10,000 population in Iowa and 1/7 the rate of violent crime of U.S. towns under 10,000 (see Figure 5, Orme-Johnson & Chandler, 1993). Because of the high association of violent crime and drug and alcohol abuse (Yoder in Hazelden Foundation, 1991, p. 52), this finding suggests that the Fairfield community has been relatively protected from the drug-alcohol-crime epidemic (see Figure 5).

FIGURE 4. From October 1981 to mid-1986, a group of 250 to 400 experts in the Transcendental Meditation and TM-Sidhi program was located in Washington, D.C. During this period, violent crime decreased from 15,045 to 9,423 per year, a reduction of almost 40%. Two research studies conducted during this period found that other variables were unable to explain this effect, and that the reduction in crime occurred at those precise times when the group of TM-Sidhi participants was largest.

Reduced Violent Crime in Washington, D.C., 1981-86 through the Transcendental Meditation and TM-Sidhi-Program

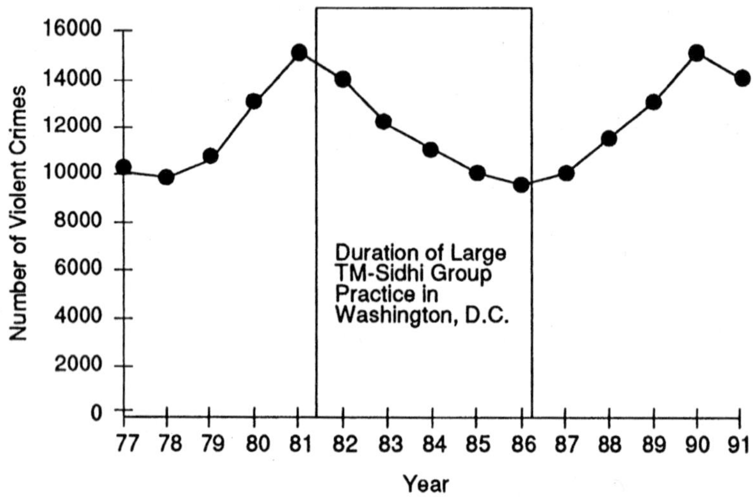

Iowa: The research on social stress by Straus, Linsky, and Bachman-Prehn (1989) found that Iowa had moved from the second lowest state on social stress in 1976 to the lowest state (along with South Dakota) in 1982, three years after MIU established its TM-Sidhi group (MIU moved to Iowa in 1974). They attribute low levels of social stress to stability in the social structure and low population density. These are undoubtedly strong contributive factors to reduced crime in the state. However, the research by Reeks (1990) shows that the meditators also had an influence. Conducting a careful time series analysis that controlled for cycles and trends in the data, she found that the group of TM and TM-Sidhi participants at MIU had significant effects on reducing three major indices of social stress in Iowa: crime, unemployment, and traffic

FIGURE 5. Fairfield, Iowa (pop. 9,648) is the home of Maharishi International University (MIU), where a large group of students, faculty, staff, and community members regularly practice the Transcendental Meditation and TM-Sidhi program twice daily. The average rate of violent crime per year in Fairfield from 1976 to 1991 (the period in which MIU has been in Fairfield for which data is available) was less than 1/3 the average rate of violent crime in other non-suburban towns in Iowa of 5,000 to 10,000 population ($p < .0001$). In addition, the rate of violent crime in Fairfield was approximately 1/7 that of non-suburban towns under 10,000 in the U.S. as a whole ($p < .0001$). The average rate of violent crime of Iowa towns was 1/2 the average rate of all U.S. towns ($p < .0001$). The error bars are standard errors of the mean of yearly crime change from 1976 to 1991. (Source: *Iowa Uniform Crime Report, 1990.* Iowa Department of Public Safety, Plans, Training, and Research Bureau. Wallace State Office Building, Des Moines, Iowa, 50319; and *FBI Uniform Crime Report 1990: Crime in the United States.* U.S. Department of Justice, Federal Bureau of Investigation. U.S. Government Printing Office, Washington, D.C., 20402.)

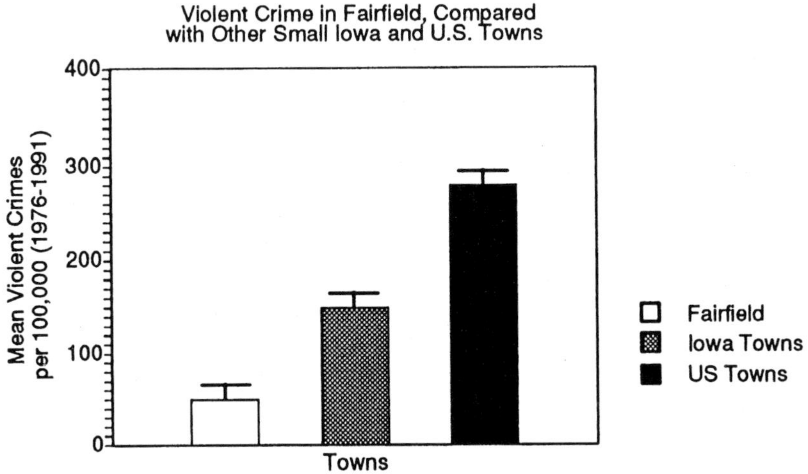

fatalities. Using monthly data from 1979 to 1986 she found that increases in the size of the coherence creating group resulted in decreases in social stress the same month or one month later that could not be explained by seasonal changes, business cycles, or holidays. A group of 1,600 TM and TM-Sidhi participants at MIU accounted for 548 fewer crimes per month (-5.4%), 5,792 fewer people unemployed (-5.8%) and 13 fewer traffic fatalities (-24.6%) in Iowa.

The United States: More than half of the violent deaths in America due to traffic accidents, suicides, and homicides are drug and alcohol related. A study published in *Social Indicators Research* found a significant effect of the MIU group on U.S. violent deaths per week (homicides, suicides and traffic fatalities) from 1979 to 1985. The square root of 1% of the U.S. population in 1985 was approximately 1,550, and the study found that an increase in TM and TM-Sidhi group size at MIU from zero to 1,550 corresponded to a decrease of 106 fatalities per week (see Figure 6). The study used time series analysis that controlled for seasonal fluctuations, trends, and drifts in the data (Dillbeck, 1990). A similar time

FIGURE 6. Two studies using time series impact assessment analysis found a significant reduction in weekly fatalities due to motor vehicle accidents, homicides, and suicides in the United States (1982-1985) and Canada (1983-1985) during periods in which the size of the group practicing the Transcendental Meditation and TM-Sidhi program at Maharishi International University in Fairfield, Iowa, exceeded the square root of 1% of the U.S. population, or of the U.S. and Canadian population together for an effect seen in Canada. During periods when the size of the group was smaller than the square root of 1% of the U.S. and Canadian populations, fatality rates were higher.

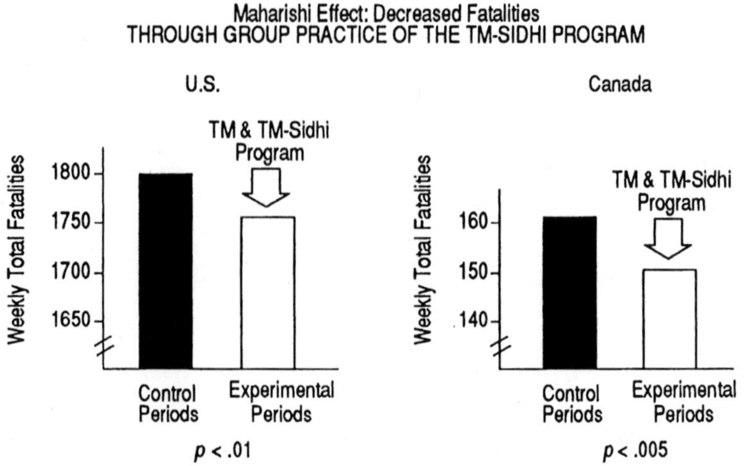

series analysis found a reduction in violent deaths in Canada when the threshold of 1,600 for North America was reached (Assimakis, in press).

Economic factors, such as unemployment and inflation, are closely linked to drug and alcohol abuse. Using state-of-the-art time series analyses, research presented at the Business and Economics Statistics Section of the American Statistical Association by Cavanaugh and his collaborators found strong evidence that the MIU TM and TM-Sidhi group significantly reduced the misery index of inflation and unemployment for both the U.S. and Canada, controlling for a number of economic factors (Cavanaugh, 1987; Cavanaugh & King, 1988; Cavanaugh, King, & Ertuna, 1989, see Figure 7 and Savings section below).

Another study of the effects of the group practice of the TM and

FIGURE 7. This study used time series impact assessment analysis to investigate the relationship between the economic "misery index"–defined as the sum of the monthly inflation rate and unemployment rate–and the number of participants in the group practice of the Transcendental Meditation technique and TM-Sidhi program at Maharishi International University in Fairfield, Iowa. During the period April 1979 to January, 1987, the misery index substantially decreased in the U.S. and Canada and during following months when more than 1,500 people practiced daily in this group program. When the group was over 1,700, the effect was even bigger.

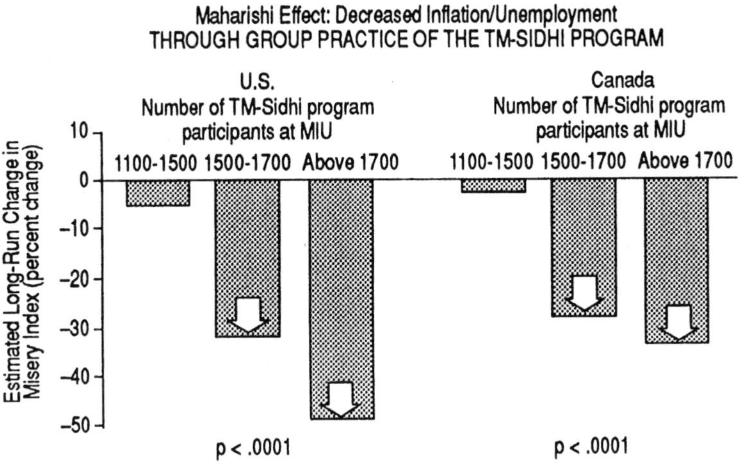

TM-Sidhi program at MIU on quality of life in the United States used an equally weighted composite index of 12 social indicators from the fields of crime, justice, health, education, economic welfare, creativity, marital stability, and safety (including alcohol consumption per capita and cigarette consumption per capita) for the 25-year period from 1960 through 1984 (Orme-Johnson, Gelderloos, & Dillbeck, 1988). The magnitude of the Maharishi Effect was estimated by the "Maharishi Effect Index" that took into account the percentage of TM participants distributed throughout the United States as well as the square of the number of TM and TM-Sidhi participants in the group practice at MIU.

Analysis of the quality-of-life index showed a virtually continuous downward trend in the overall quality of life in the United States from 1960 to 1975. This negative trend began to level off starting in 1975. During the years 1982-1984, when the group of Transcendental Meditation and TM-Sidhi program participants at MIU was large enough to have a predicted effect on national consciousness, there was a dramatic increase in U.S. quality of life. The total improvement of 7.17% on the quality-of-life index over this three-year period was 5.2 times greater than any three-year improvement in the prior 22 years. Clearly, an unprecedented change in recent U.S. history had occurred.

A further analysis of the different quality-of-life variables in this study used a multivariate method of analysis of covariance structures (e.g., Jöreskog & Sörbom, 1979; Long, 1983) implemented by the LISREL VI program (Jöreskog & Sörbom, 1986). The covariance structure model combines the approaches of factor analysis and structural equation causal modeling to assess the impact of independent variables on a set of latent variables underlying a group of observed variables. Two quality-of-life factors were found, a general factor and a second factor, and the MIU TM and TM-Sidhi group had a significant effect on both factors, accounting for 80.4% of the variance of the general factor and 60.3% of the secondary factor.

These studies provide strong evidence that the MIU TM and TM-Sidhi group has significantly reduced the drug-alcohol-crime epidemic in the United States, as seen in a reduction of many alcohol and drug related variables, including those cited above in research involving deaths due to suicides, homicides, and traffic fatalities, a reduction in inflation and unemployment, and an improvement in the general quality of life, including reduced alcohol and cigarette consumption.

The International Peace Project in the Middle East: One of the major symptoms of the stress epidemic is international conflict. An experimental test of the application of the Maharishi Effect on international conflict in Lebanon and national quality of life in Israel was published in the *Journal of Conflict Resolution* (Orme-Johnson, Alexander et al., 1988). This study took place in 1983 in Israel during the war in Lebanon for a two-month period (August and September). The project was funded in part through a grant in honor of William Ellinghaus, then president of American Telephone and Telegraph Company, from the Fund for Higher Education. Predictions were lodged in advance with scientists in the U.S. and in Israel. The variables, such as traffic accidents, crime rate, and fires, all of which are major problems in Israel, were selected because they had been used in previous experiments. As a measure of the war in Lebanon, two war variables, war deaths and war intensity, were derived by content analysis of a major newspaper and other media sources using a scaling method modeled after Azar's (1982). Other variables included the Israeli national stock market and the national mood from content analysis of a major newspaper. All variables were derived from publicly available data sources. All are highly relevant to the stress epidemic of which drug and alcohol misuse are a part.

Figure 8 shows that the overall composite index composed of all the variables mentioned above and the size of the coherence creating group closely track one another. Statistical analysis using the Box-Jenkins (1976) ARIMA (auto-regressive, integrated, moving averages) time series methods of transfer functions showed that change in the size of the coherence creating group significantly led change in the composite index by one day, controlling for any seasonal fluctuations in the data, as well as controlling for changes in the weather and holidays. This means that the up and down variations in the size of the coherence creating group were followed by a corresponding variation in the overall quality of life in the region, supporting a casual interpretation.

FIGURE 8. Based on previous research, scientists predicted that the collective practice of the Transcendental Meditation and TM-Sidhi program by a group in Jerusalem would increase positive trends and decrease negativity in the Middle East. The sociological parameters measured were lodged in advance with an independent review board of scientists in the U.S. and Israel. This study indicated that increasing the numbers of participants engaged in Maharishi's Transcendental Meditation and TM-Sidhi program improved the quality of life in Israel as measured by an index comprised of decreases in crime rate, traffic accidents, fires, and the number of war deaths in Lebanon, and by increases in the national stock market and improvements in national mood.

Maharishi Effect: Improved Quality of Life
and Reduced Conflict
THROUGH GROUP PRACTICE OF THE TM-SIDHI PROGRAM

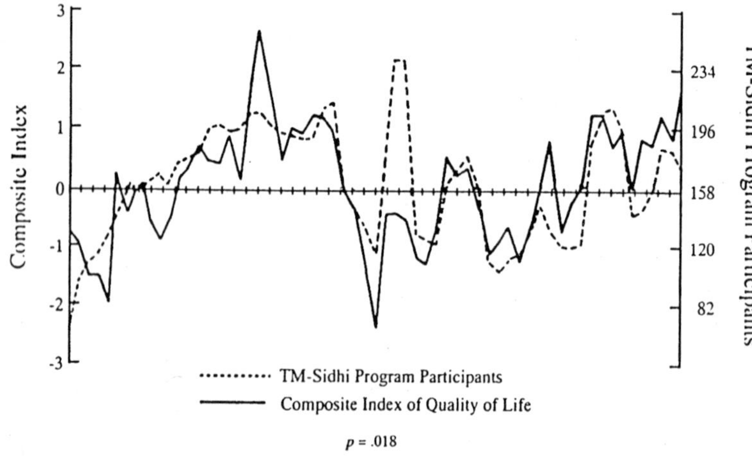

Another very interesting finding in this study was that when the individual variables were combined into a composite variable, the results were the clearest, as seen in Figure 8, which shows the clear covariance between the composite of all the raw data and the coherence creating group. Adding the individual variables together is a type of signal averaging that enhances the common variance. As a result, the composite of all the variables most clearly shows their common variance. The finding that changes in the composite variable correspond most clearly to changes in the coherence creating group is strong empirical evidence that the common variance underlying these diverse social processes was in fact generated by the coherence creating group functioning at a fundamental level of natural law (Orme-Johnson, Alexander et al., 1988, p. 806). This study demonstrates that the TM and TM-Sidhi program addresses the complex of stress in society at the basis of the drug and alcohol epidemic.

Replication of Reduced War in Lebanon: Experimental replication is the most powerful test of the reliability of a new discovery. These dramatic results on the Lebanon war have now been replicated seven times with a statistical probability of less that 10^{-19}, or one in ten million trillion, that the results were due to chance (Davies & Alexander, 1989). This study, which was presented at the annual conference of the American Political Science Association in 1989, found that during the seven coherence creating assemblies large enough to have a predicted impact on the war in Lebanon, war fatalities decreased by an average of 71%, war injuries decreased by 68%, and cooperation among antagonists increased by 66%. The degree of statistical certitude of this finding is unheard of even in the physical sciences, lending strong support to the reliability and legitimacy of the theory and empirical evidence of the Maharishi Effect.

The Global Maharishi Effect: Drug abuse is a global phenomenon, with drug trade being a major international problem. For this reason the Maharishi Effect must be established on a global level to eliminate the stress epidemic completely. The global Maharishi Effect was first demonstrated in late 1983.

After seeing the results of the first study in the Middle East, even before the evidence of extensive replication was amassed, Maharishi inspired an assembly of 7,000 practitioners of the Transcendental Meditation and TM-Sidhi program, the square root of 1% of the world's population, in order to give the world a "Taste of Utopia." In addition, he created a tradition of holding large assemblies every quarter of the year, with the intention of raising world consciousness and demonstrating effects that would inspire the world leadership to establish permanent coherence creating groups as sustained peace keeping forces in every country.

A study of the effects of these assemblies on worldwide international conflicts, terrorism, and economic confidence was presented at the American Political Science Association and American Psychological Association in 1989 and 1990, respectively (Orme-Johnson, Dillbeck, Alexander, Chandler, & Cranson, 1989; Orme-Johnson, Cavanaugh et al., 1989). This study found that on the three occasions when the world assemblies approached the 7,000 threshold needed for global coherence, international conflicts decreased by more than 30%, according to a content analysis of the *New York Times* and *London Times*, and that international terrorism decreased by more than 70%, using data compiled by the Rand Corporation. In addition, the World Index of international stock prices in the 19 major industrial countries increased significantly, indicating increased economic confidence. As in other studies, time series analysis ruled out the possibility that the results were spuriously due to cycles, trends, or drifts in the measures used. The study also showed that the results were not due to changes that usually occur during the year-end holiday seasons when two of the assemblies were held.

This study provides evidence of the application of the TM and TM-Sidhi program to reduce global stress as a possible means to treat the global epidemic of drug and alcohol abuse.

Improved U.S./Soviet Relations: Drugs are often an international problem. The evidence that the Maharishi Effect improves international relations is important to finding a lasting solution to the drug abuse problem.

International tensions are the apex of the stress epidemic. The most dramatic political change of the twentieth century is the warming of relations between the superpowers with its enormous worldwide implications. In some of the studies reviewed above, the Maharishi Effect had a calming effect in trouble-spot areas in which the Americans and Soviets were involved on opposite sides, indicating indirectly and sometimes directly that the coherence creating groups soothed the relations between the superpowers. This evidence is further strengthened by studies of the statements of heads of state. For example, one study analyzed statements by the President of the United States (President Reagan) published by the U.S. government's Office of the Federal Register of National Archives and Records Administration in the *Weekly Compilation of Presidential Documents* from April 1985 to September 1987. The study found that increased coherence in U.S. national consciousness through the Maharishi Effect was reflected in the increased positivity of the President's statements about the USSR.

Another study on the effects of the MIU TM and TM-Sidhi group on U.S.-Soviet relations used the data base from the Zurich Project on East-West Relations, which has tracked U.S.-Soviet relations by content analysis of news events from 1979 to 1986. When the group reached the threshold of the square root of 1% of the U.S. population (1500-1700), U.S. actions towards the Soviets began to become significantly more positive. U.S. behavior towards the Soviets became even more positive when the MIU group was over 1,700, and moreover, Soviet behavior towards the U.S. also became significantly more positive when the group was largest (Gelderloos, Cavanaugh, & Davies, 1990). This data is the first empirical demonstration of why East-West relations have suddenly improved (see Figure 9).

Research on the Mechanism of the Maharishi Effect in Relation to Substance Abuse: Preliminary studies have found evidence of physiological effects of coherence creating groups. One study found that at the time when the MIU group was practicing the TM-Sidhi program, the EEGs of three subjects in a distant laboratory became significantly more coherent with each other in the alpha and beta frequencies (Orme-Johnson, Dillbeck, Wallace, & Landrith, 1982).

In another experiment, the relationship between the EEGs of pairs of subjects in different rooms in the laboratory were studied. One subject was meditating while the other was working on a task on a computer. Both subjects were blind to the purpose of the experiment. It was found that increased EEG coherence in the meditating subject was significantly correlated with increased EEG coherence in the other subject doing the computer task (Travis & Orme-Johnson, 1989).

A third experiment that has direct bearing on the problem of drug and alcohol addiction studied serotonin turnover as a function of the size of the TM and TM-Sidhi group (Pugh, Walton, & Cavanaugh, 1988). Serotonin is a neurotransmitter that, along with other neurotransmitters, appears to play a vital role in regulation of homeostasis

FIGURE 9. This study investigated the contribution of a large coherence creating group at Maharishi International University in the U.S. towards improvement in relations between the U.S. and the Soviet Union from 1979 to 1986. The study was of monthly ratings of cooperation and conflict, obtained from independent investigators (the Zurich Project on East-West Relations) of all interactions of the U.S. towards the Soviet Union and of the Soviet Union towards the U.S. Time series analysis showed that during the months following periods when the size of the coherence creating group was above the predicted thresholds (i.e., above 1,500 and 1,700), there was a significant improvement in U.S. actions towards the USSR. In months after the group size was above 1,700, Soviet actions towards the U.S. also significantly improved. The overall impact of the coherence creating group on the U.S.-Soviet interaction was highly significant ($p < .00001$).

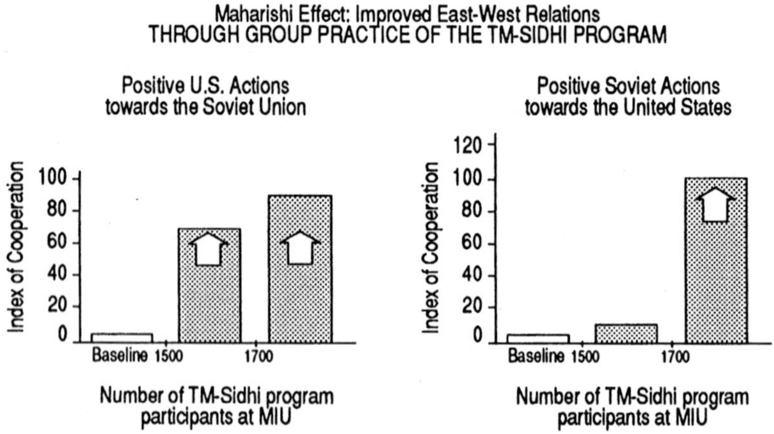

(see Walton & Levitsky, this volume, on a neurochemical theory of TM's effects on drug abuse). In four studies that used time series analysis of daily levels of serotonin metabolite 5-HIAA in the urine, Pugh et al. (1988) found that increasing the group size of TM and TM-Sidhi participants increased serotonin, both in meditators in the group and in non-meditators who were not in the group and who had no direct contact with the meditators. The experiments showed that daily variations in ambient temperature could not account for the results.

These experiments suggest that the people who practice the TM and TM-Sidhi program have a direct effect on increasing neurochemical balance in the larger population essential to reducing stress and thus preventing drug and alcohol addiction.

In conclusion, the research on the Maharishi Effect shows that it reduces stress and increases coherence throughout all levels of society–individual, city, state, nation, and international, treating the stress epidemic systematically. The following section reviews the financial implications of utilizing this technology.

FINANCIAL IMPACT OF THE TRANSCENDENTAL MEDITATION PROGRAM

Expenses Due to Drug and Alcohol Abuse: The economic implications of this technology to "vaccinate" the population against stress are enormous. Just as the stress epidemic degrades the quality of life in every sphere of individual and collective existence, so too does it deplete personal and national resources in every area. Drug and alcohol abuse, two of the major symptoms of the epidemic, cost the nation an estimated $562 billion per year, almost 10% of the GNP. Table 1 shows some of the major sources of expenditures that can be attributed to drug and alcohol abuse.

The national health bill in 1993 is likely to exceed $900 billion. In the U.S., cigarette smoking accounts for 400,000 deaths per year (McGinnis & Foege, 1993), including 21% of all coronary heart disease, and 87% of lung cancer, two of the leading causes of death. In addition, smoking contributes substantially to chronic bronchitis, emphysema, and lung cancer, which are major causes of disability (U.S. Department of Health and Human Services, 1990a, p. 136). In 1990, 25.5% of the U.S. population smoked, which although down from a high of 42% in 1955, still means that 64 million people have the addiction. From one-third to one-half of these people will die from smoking, many in the prime of life, resulting in a mean loss of 23 years of life (Peto et al., 1992).

An exhaustive survey conducted by the U.S. Department of Health and Human Services (1990b) found that a small proportion of the population, which for the most part consists of users of tobacco and drugs, and abusers of alcohol, accounts for 40%-70% of all premature deaths, a third of all cases of acute disability, and two-thirds of all cases of chronic disability. Another study found

TABLE 1. US Expenditures per Year Due to Drug and Alcohol Abuse.

Source of Expenditure	Total Expense per Year ($ Billions)	% Due to Drugs and Alcohol	Expense Due to Drugs and Alcohol ($Billions)
Health	$900.0	23%*	$207.0
Crime	$200.0	50%	$100.0
Corporations	----	----	$93.0
Loss of 1% or workforce due to imprisonment	$140.0	50%	$70.0
Treatment Cost	----	100%	$38.0
Auto Insurance Losses Paid[1]	$107.9	50%	$53.9
Total	----	----	**$561.9**

Source: Extrapolated from 1987 figures from The National Underwriter Co., Cincinnati. Found in *Statistical Abstract.*
* This number includes the effects of smoking on health.

that simply removing smoking and drinking could reduce health utilization by 25% (Scheffler & Pringer, 1980). Studies have shown that 10% of the population accounts for 75% of the nation's health care costs (Garfinkle, Riley, & Iannacchione, 1988) and the high-cost people tend to be smokers and drinkers (Zook & Moore, 1980). On the basis of these studies, it is conservatively estimated that smoking, alcohol and drug use account for 33% of the medical care expenditures, or $300 billion per year.

The cost of crime in the U.S. in 1990 was $200 billion–$80 billion in federal, state and local government expenditures for the criminal justice system, police, and corrections (BJS, 1993; Congressional Budget Office [CBO], 1990), and another $120 billion in victim expenses for medical and lost property (Cohen, 1990). If drugs and alcohol account for half of crime, then they induce a financial burden to society of over $100 billion per year for their effects on crime alone.

An additional expenditure from drug and alcohol related crimes is for lost productivity of those who are in prison. There are currently 1.2 million inmates in prisons and other correctional institutions (BJS, 1992, pp. 2, 3), which is approximately 1% of the workforce. If half of crime is attributed to drugs and alcohol (Yoder, 1990, p. 52), then so too is half of the prison population. The loss of .5% of the workforce translates into a 1.25% loss in the GDP, which is $70 billion (CBO Report, 1990).

If 15% of the population suffers from drug and alcohol addiction, with a mean treatment expense of $10,000 per person, this accounts for another $38 billion. The expense of alcohol and drugs to corporations is estimated to be $93 billion (Harwood et al., 1984; Rice et al., 1990). Alcohol and drugs account for about 50% of motor vehicle accidents, accounting for another $54 billion. In addition, welfare expenses to sustain individuals who are either imprisoned or on treatment due to substance abuse is another source of expenditures.

Table 1 is not an exhaustive survey of all the expenditures due to drugs and alcohol, but gives a sense of how this epidemic drains our national financial resources. The funds that would be available from reducing the problem even by half could more than pay off the national debt in a few years.

The Implementation of the Stress-Immunization Program: Maharishi (1986b) has offered to the national governments of the world a three-step plan for reducing stress in world, national and city consciousness in order to create world peace: (1) create a group of 10,000 experts to create coherence for the whole world; (2) create a national coherence creating group; and (3) create coherence for each city. This plan can be adapted to the problem of immunizing the population against drug and alcohol abuse because drugs, alcohol, and international conflicts are different symptoms of the same worldwide stress epidemic. It does not matter for which immediate purpose the program is implemented; it will also take care of all other stress-related problems as a side effect.

Coherence is needed on the world level because the drug-alcohol epidemic is a worldwide problem. A group of 10,000 is needed because that exceeds the square root of one percent of the world population, the number needed to create global coherence. It is logical that a large group to create world coherence be located in the U.S. because of the U.S.'s uniquely powerful position in the post-Soviet era. In addition, a 10,000 group located in the U.S. would also take care of the national level, step 2 of the plan.

What remains is to implement a program for the city level. In late 1992, a group of experts in this technology based in the Netherlands representing business corporations and universities in 32 countries offered a plan to reduce and eliminate crime to the city governments of 60 major American cities. The plan, presented to the public in newspaper ads appearing in the cities, outlined a two to six month trial period of evaluating the effects on reducing crime of groups of approximately 1,000 TM and TM-Sidhi participants per million population. We recommend that 50 such coherence creating groups be established in the major urban areas of the U.S.

Thus the *Stress-Immunization Program* for stress-immunization of the United States consists of one large group of 10,000 experts in the Transcendental Meditation technique and TM-Sidhi program and 50 groups of 1,000 each located in the major urban areas. The financial benefit analysis presented in the next section is a conservative estimate based on the results of previous research of the effects of this Stress-Immunization Program.

Savings from the Stress-Immunization Program: Research on collective consciousness shows that the Stress-Immunization Program would affect virtually all problems of society because they are all symptoms of stress in collective consciousness. The cost-benefit calculated from its effects on the economy, health, defense, crime, and automobile insurance alone is $614 billion a year.

Unemployment: Drug and alcohol abuse increase unemployment and unemployment increases drug and alcohol abuse. Three separate researchers in seven studies have found highly significant effects of TM and TM-Sidhi groups on unemployment. In the most rigorous of these studies, Cavanaugh and King (1988) have shown that the coherence creating group at MIU was responsible for 54% of the total decline in the United States misery index (an aggregate of inflation and unemployment) from its peak in 1980 to the end of the sample period in 1988. (In recent years the participation in the program at MIU has declined. In 1992 it was at the lowest level since 1982, with a daily average of only 1,362 participants, well below the predicted threshold of 1,600 needed for the U.S.). During the period of Cavanaugh's study (1980 to 1988), the misery index dropped a total of 14.1 points. The amount of the change in unemployment that can be attributed to the coherence creating group of 1,600 can be estimated to be 0.384 points. With a group of 10,000, which should have over 6 times the effect, it can conservatively be estimated that unemployment would drop 1% per year until a basic minimum level of about 4.5% unemployment is reached. (This minimum level is estimated by economists to be from 3.5% to 5.5 %, below which it is difficult to go because of people changing jobs, etc.) Given the current unemployment rate of over 7.5%, there is now room for a 3% decrease in unemployment, which would increase the GDP 2.5% each year over four years for an increase of $728.8 billion. Table 2 shows the results of a 1% decrease in unemployment projected for the first year of the Stress-Immunization Program. The GDP would increase $156.4 billion. Based upon federal figures, it is assumed that the financial benefit to the private sector in wages, corporate profits, and other taxable income would account for slightly over $120.4 billion (CBO Report, 1990). This would result in a $51 billion benefit to the Federal government due to increased tax revenues, decreased federal outlays, and decrease in the deficit. Moreover, state governments would benefit by $6.9 billion due to sales and gross receipts, income tax revenues, and decreased outlays for unemployment.

Health: Since 1970, US medical expenditures have grown 11.6% annually, 2.9 percentage points faster than the GNP (Jencks & Schieber, 1991). In the late 1940s medical payments were less than 5% of the GNP. By 1991 these expenses rose to 13.5% of the GNP or $838.5 billion. In 1993 medical costs are likely to exceed $900 billion. Rising medical expenditures impose severe strains on public budgets, business expenses, and individual solvency.

A published study by Orme-Johnson (1987) showed that 2,000 individuals practicing the TM program over a five-year period consistently had less than half the number of doctor visits and hospitalizations than other groups of comparable age, gender, profession, and insurance terms. In addition, the TM practitioners had markedly

TABLE 2. Savings from a 1% Reduction in Unemployment Due to the Stress-Immunization Program.

Source	**1993 ($ Billions)**
Private Sector: 2.5% increase in GDP (U.S. 1993 GDP = $6,255 billion)	$156.4
Private Sector: Increased Wages, Corporate Profits, and other Taxable Income from Increase in GDP	**$120.4**
Federal Government: Increased Tax Revenues[1]	43.0
Federal Government: Decreased Federal Outlays[1]	8.0
Federal Government: Decrease in Deficit[1]	51.0
Federal Government: Total Increase	**$ 51.0**
State Government: Sales and Gross Receipts[2]	3.4
State Government: Income Tax Revenues[2]	3.4
State Government: Decreased Outlays[3] (Unemployment Benefit)	.1
State Government: Total Increase	**$ 6.9**
Total (Private, Federal and State)	**$178.3**

1. Source: The Economic and Budget Outlook: Fiscal Years 1994-1998. Congressional Budget Office Report.
2. Source: U.S. Bureau of the Census, State Government Tax Collections in 1985.
3. Source: U.S. Employment and Training Administration, Unemployment Insurance Statistics and Annual Report of the Secretary of Labor.

fewer incidents of illness in *all* medical treatment categories, including 87% less hospitalization for both heart disease and nervous system disorders, 55% less for cancer, and 73% less for nose, throat, and lung problems.

A number of studies on the Maharishi Effect and quality-of-life indicators have found that the incidence of disease can be decreased simply by increasing coherence in collective consciousness. For example, one result of the three-week coherence creating assembly of over 7,000 participants, which began in December 1983, was a

15% drop in incidence of infectious diseases compared to the three-week periods just before and after the assembly. Moreover, an analysis of the same three-week period for the previous 5 years revealed a 32% drop in the total number of infectious diseases during the assembly compared to the median number of cases for that period in the previous 5 years (Orme-Johnson et al., 1989).

Still other studies on the Maharishi Effect have shown reductions in disease, accident rates, hospital admissions, infant mortality, and so on, with decreases ranging from just under 5% to 11% (reviewed in Orme-Johnson & Dillbeck, in press). Moreover, the long-term effects of having a 10,000 group as well as groups for the major urban areas of the U.S. could be several times greater than indicated by these short-term studies, which used much smaller groups, because sustained larger groups would also have the effect of increasing health promotion/disease prevention awareness and would thereby contribute to the prevention of disease.

Based on all of the foregoing, a projected 33% reduction in disease is chosen as a conservative, realistic estimate of the potential long-range impact of a sustained group of 10,000 and 50 groups of 1,000 people in urban areas collectively practicing the TM and TM-Sidhi program. Based on information from experts at the Congressional Budget Office, a 33% reduction in incidence of disease would translate into a 30% reduction in different areas of health payments. Table 3 summarizes the financial benefit from such a reduction in disease.

Crime: Our penal system is strained both in financial terms and in terms of the human tragedy involved in warehousing hundreds of thousands of potentially productive human beings. Bureau of Justice data reveal that at the end of 1988, more than 3.7 million adults in the United States–2 percent of the adult population–were under the care or custody of probation, parole, jail, or prison authorities (BJS Bulletin, 1989: *Probation and Parole in 1988*). The number of prisoners under the jurisdiction of federal and state correctional authorities at year-end 1989 reached a record 703,687, an increase of 113.4% since 1980. The number of inmates increased at a rate of 12.1% in the first half of 1989, requiring the addition of 1,500 new beds per week nationally (BJS Bulletin, 1989: *Prisoners in 1989*). In addition, as of June 30, 1988, local jails throughout the United

TABLE 3. Savings from a 30% Reduction in Health Care Expenditures per Year Due to the Stress-Immunization Program.

Source of Health Care Expenditures	Expenses ($ Billions)	Expenses with 30% Savings	Savings ($ Billions)
Private Sector Projected Health Care Claims (1993)[1]	$469.7	$328.8	**$140.9**
Federal Government Medicare[2]	$128.8	$90.2	$38.6
Federal Government Health Care Services[2]	$96.9	$67.8	$29.1
Federal Government Total			**$67.7**
State and Local Projected Health Care Costs[3]	$115.2	$80.6	**$34.6**
Total Savings			**$243.2**

1. These figures were calculated using information from the following source: Health Care Financing Administration, Office of the Actuary: Data from the Office of National Cost Estimates. The average increase of 8.5% for past years 1986-1988 was assumed for years after 1988, using the 1988 base amount of $312.4 billion.
2. These figures are from The Budget for Fiscal Year 1993, CBO Report 1992, Table 1-2.
3. These figures were calculated using information from the following source: Health Care Financing Administration, Office of the Actuary: Data from the Office of National Cost Estimates. The average increase of 10.6% for years 1986-1988 was assumed for years after 1988, using the 1988 base amount of $69.6 billion.

States held 343,569 prisoners, 54% more than in 1983 (BJS Bulletin, 1989: *Census of Local Jails*). The total number of American citizens now incarcerated at any one time well exceeds one million.

Occupancy in federal prisons is currently 60% over capacity. Construction is now underway to provide 67,347 more beds in existing prisons or new prisons. In addition, 88,847 more beds are being planned. The national average cost per bed in a new facility is

$53,663; in an existing facility, $24,881 (Corrections Yearbook, 1989).

In 1988, agencies spent more than $20,000 a year per inmate, including legal fees (Corrections Yearbook, 1989). This figure excludes law enforcement costs, court costs, welfare and other social programs for the family of inmates, and costs to victims. Most of the costs of crime are borne at the state and local level. The federal share was between one-eighth and one-ninth of the total $12.6 billion in 1991, and is expected to rise to $14.6 billion in 1995. It costs over $100 billion annually to maintain the U.S. criminal justice system. The impact of violent crime cannot, of course, be measured in monetary loss alone. This tremendous financial burden only represents a fraction of the human expense of criminal activity and does not take into account the intangible costs resulting from loss of life, threat of force, serious personal injury, fear, and psychological trauma.

In 1987, state and federal prisons released 232,871 prisoners (BJS, 1989, *Sourcebook of Criminal Justice Statistics, 1988*). Approximately 30% of those released from prison commit new offenses and are returned to prisons within the first three years of parole. Within the next seven years, an additional 16.25% are predicted to return to prison (BJS Bulletin: *Examining Recidivism*). Once inmates are returned to prison, they will cost taxpayers an annual $16,315 per inmate.

More than 2,000 adult inmates in U.S. correctional institutions and several hundred incarcerated juveniles in eight facilities have learned Maharishi's Transcendental Meditation. The TM program has been found in controlled studies with inmates to reduce anxiety, increase autonomic stability–a physiological indicator of resistance to stress, decrease neuroticism and psychopathology, increase ego development, and reduce recidivism (Alexander, 1982; Bleick & Abrams, 1987; Dillbeck & Abrams, 1987, review).

A recent nationwide application of TM in the prisons of Senegal showed particularly dramatic results. Between 1987 and 1988, 12,000 prisoners in Senegal were instructed in the TM technique. After a general amnesty to relieve prison overcrowding, only 2% recidivated over a six-month period, compared to the usual 90%. The government was able to close three prisons as a result. In addition, the TM program has been cited by the World Health Organization as an effective strategy for treating mental illness and enhancing mental health.

Of greatest relevance are the 17 studies on the Maharishi Effect indicating that crime rate decreases more than 10% when the requisite numbers gather together to practice the TM and TM-Sidhi program. The effect of coherence creating groups on crime is the most documented of the Maharishi Effect findings (reviewed in Orme-Johnson & Dillbeck, in press).

The average crime drop seen in the 17 studies assessing the impact of the Maharishi Effect was 10.5%, in most cases using a group that is just over the square root of one percent of the population. Given that the Stress-Immunization Program calls for a 10,000 group, which is six times larger the square root of one percent of the U.S. population, as well as 50 smaller groups of 1,000, it is conservatively estimated that the effects of the Stress-Immunization Program would be a 50% reduction of crime and eventual elimination of crime in five years.

Assuming the average 50% drop in crime from the Stress-Immunization Program produces an equivalent 50% drop in new incarcerations, then the expected $6 billion in new expenditures would be reduced by $3 billion at the federal and state level. Also, assuming that the average 150,000 new incarcerations per year are reduced by 50% and that the average cost per inmate per year is $20,000, there would be a savings of $1.5 billion dollars at the federal and state level. In addition, private financial losses suffered by crime victims total approximately $15 billion per year. We should see the most immediate impact of a lower crime rate in reducing the private costs of crime. With a 50% decrease in crime, we can estimate that savings in this area would amount to $7.5 billion per year. The total savings from crime reduction from the program would be $12 billion (see Table 4).

Automobile Accidents: The benefits of the Stress-Immunization Program to the United States life, property, and liability insurance industry would be sizable. Such benefits would, sooner or later, be passed on to the public as a whole in the form of decreased premiums.

A number of studies have shown that the Maharishi Effect results

TABLE 4. Savings Due to a 50% Reduction in Crime per Year from the Stress-Immunization Program.

Source	**Projected New Expenses ($ Billions)**	**Savings ($ Billions)**
New Prison Beds	$6.0	$3.0
New Incarcerations	$3.0	$1.5
Private Sector	$15.0	$7.5
Total		**$12.0**

in decreases in traffic accidents, traffic fatality rates, air fatalities, and other fatalities. In the area of automobile insurance alone, nine research studies have shown that when a population has the required number of people in the coherence creating group, the Maharishi Effect produces significant decreases in automobile accidents, including traffic fatalities. This analysis will focus on the projected benefits from decreased automobile accidents because research statistics are available in this area. The Maharishi Effect should, however, account for equal reductions in all other types of accidents as well.

Three studies have found decreases in traffic accidents when the coherence creating group in the area was large enough, for an average decrease of 17.6%. Six other studies have found decreases in traffic fatalities correlated with coherence creating groups. These studies found decreases ranging from 6.5% to 41.6% with the average decrease found being 16.61% (reviewed in Orme-Johnson & Dillbeck, in press).

We can therefore conservatively estimate a decrease of 50% in automobile accidents from a sustained coherence creating group of 10,000. Table 5 shows the premium earned and losses paid by automobile insurers in 1987, and then projected to 1993 at a 10% annual increase. The savings enjoyed by these companies (50% of those losses paid) from the Stress-Immunization Program is then shown.

TABLE 5. Savings from a 50% Reduction in Automobile Accidents Due to the Stress-Immunization Program.

	1993
Premiums earned[1]	136.23
Losses Paid[1]	107.89
Savings	**$53.9**

Source: Extrapolated from 1987 figures in The National Underwriter Co., Cincinnati. Found in *Statistical Abstracts.*

TABLE 6. Summary of Financial Benefit per Year Due to the Stress-Immunization Program

	Private	Federal	State	Total
Economy	$120.4	$51.0	$6.9	**$178.4**
Health	$140.9	$67.7	$34.6	**$243.2**
Crime	$7.5	$.6	$3.9	**$12.0**
Auto Insurance	$53.9	$0.0	$0.0	**$53.9**
Total Savings from a 10,000 Group	**$322.7**	**$119.3**	**$45.4**	**$487.5**

Summary of Financial Benefits from the Stress-Immunization Program: Table 6 summarizes the savings to the private sector, federal government, and state governments from the Stress-Immunization Program. The savings from the program would be $322.7 billion for the private sector, $119.3 billion for the federal government, and $45.4 billion for the state governments, for a total saving of $487.5 billion (see Table 6).[2]

The expense of the Stress-Immunization Program can be derived from the proposal that the group of businessmen and educators based in the Netherlands made in 1992 to reduce crime in American cities. This proposal specified a cost of 10 cents per citizen per day for a group of 1,000 experts in the Transcendental Meditation technique and TM-Sidhi program per one million population. This comes to a total expenditure of $36,000 per expert per year, a modest amount for trained specialists, considering that it would also cover administrative expenses. At this rate, a group of 10,000 would require $.36 billion per year, and the 50 groups of 1,000 would require $1.8 billion, for a total program requirement $2.16 billion. Thus the financial savings from the program, minus the expense of the program, is $485.34 billion.

Level of Public Interest in the Program: A recent national survey by the Bruskin/Goldring Research company indicates that 52% of the population felt that government, insurance agencies and private companies should provide more information on the use of Transcendental Meditation to reduce stress-related problems, such as crime, in the larger population, encourage research on it, and/or encourage greater use of this technique (Bodeker, 1992).

CONCLUSION

Prior to the rise of epidemiology as the basic science of preventive medicine, epidemics of infectious diseases desolated huge populations. Then the causes of these epidemics were identified, new technologies to prevent the problem were discovered, experimental field trials were carried out, and practical public health programs were implemented, saving millions of lives (Friedman, 1985). The present proposal to use the Transcendental Meditation and TM-Sidhi program to control and eventually eliminate the drug and alcohol epidemic has followed this classical pattern.

First, epidemiological analytic research strongly supported the hypothesis that social stress is a causative factor in the drug-alcohol epidemic. A new theory that extended previous concepts of social influence was postulated, holding that stress is transmitted systemically through an underlying field of collective consciousness. It was proposed that Transcendental Meditation is a powerful means of stress reduction, and its ability to reduce stress has been convincingly demonstrated at the behavioral/psychological level (Alexander et al., 1991; Eppley et al., 1989), physiological level (e.g.,

Dillbeck & Orme-Johnson, 1987; Jevning et al., 1992), and molecular level (e.g., Walton & Levitsky, this volume). Retrospective, observational research then found that in urban areas in which 1% of the population practiced Transcendental Meditation, the multiple symptoms of stress in collective consciousness were significantly reduced (e.g., Dillbeck et al., 1981, 1988). Resorting to an even more powerful technology, the TM-Sidhi program, field experiments were then conducted in which coherence creating groups were introduced into populations, and it was found that symptoms of social stress were consequently reduced (e.g., Dillbeck, 1990; Dillbeck et al., 1987, 1988; Orme-Johnson et al., 1988). Now, over 40 studies have demonstrated the effectiveness of this technology to reduce the societal correlates of drug and alcohol abuse such as crime, traffic accidents, and unemployment, and in some studies, to directly reduce alcohol and tobacco use as part of quality of life indices (Orme-Johnson & Dillbeck, in press). The financial analysis indicates an enormous financial savings from implementation of the Stress-Immunization Program.

NOTES

1. The word Veda means knowledge. Vedic means pertaining to knowledge.
2. *Defense:* The studies reviewed in the Research section indicate that decreased stress and rising coherence in world consciousness produced by the Maharishi Effect precipitated the most dramatic political reorientation of the past 50 years. The extensive political changes in Eastern Europe and the Soviet Union have virtually put an end to the Cold War and have great potential for reducing defense expenditures.

Nevertheless, the current crises in the Middle East, the Balkans, and Somalia demonstrate the urgent need for the immediate establishment of a 10,000 group to continue these very positive trends. The Stress-Immunization Program of a permanent group of 10,000 experts and 50 groups of 1,000 in the U.S. would secure world peace and would thus bring significant but at present incalculable benefits to the United States' ability to fulfill the goals of our nation's military at an ever decreasing cost.

REFERENCES

Alexander, C. N. (1982). Ego development, personality, and behavioral change in inmates practicing the Transcendental Meditation technique or participating in other programs: A cross-sectional and longitudinal study (Doctoral dissertation, Harvard University). *Dissertation Abstracts International 43*:539B.

Alexander, C. N., Rainforth, M. V., & Gelderloos, P. (1991). Transcendental Meditation, self-actualization and psychological health: A conceptual overview and statistical meta-analysis. *Journal of Social Behavior and Personality, 6*, 189-247.

Alexander, C. N., Robinson, P., & Rainforth, M. V. (this volume). Treating and preventing alcohol, nicotine, and drug abuse through Transcendental Meditation: A review and statistical meta-analysis. *Alcoholism Treatment Quarterly.*

Assimakis, P. D. (in press). Change in the quality of life in Canada: Intervention studies of the effect of the Transcendental Meditation and TM-Sidhi program. *Psychological Reports.*

Azar, E. E. (1982). *Conflict and peace data bank (COPDAB): A computer-assisted approach to monitoring and analyzing international and domestic events.* College Park, MD: Center for International Development and Conflict Management, University of Maryland.

Bleik, C. R. & Abrams, A. I. (1987). The Transcendental Meditation program and recidivism in California. *Journal of Criminal Justice, 15*, 211-230.

Bodeker, G. (1992). *Alternative treatments: An Omnitel national telephone survey.* North Bethesda, MD: Lancaster Foundation.

Borland, C. & Landrith III, G. S. (1977). Improved quality of life through the Transcendental Meditation program: Decreased crime rate. In D. W. Orme-Johnson & J. T. Farrow (Eds.), *Scientific research on the Transcendental Meditation program: Collected papers, Vol. 1.* Rheinweiler, Germany: Maharishi European Research University Press.

Box, G. E. P. & Jenkins, G. M. (1976). *Time series analysis: Forecasting and control.* San Francisco: Holden-Day.

Bureau of Justice Statistics Bulletin (January 1993). *Drugs, crime and the custice system. National update. Criminal victimization in 1991.*

Bureau of Justice Statistics Bulletin (January 1992). *National update.*

Bureau of Justice Statistics Bulletin (1989). *Probation and parole in 1988.*

Bureau of Justice Statistics Bulletin (1989). *Prisoners in 1989.*

Bureau of Justice Statistics Bulletin (1989). *Census of local jails.*

Bureau of Justice Statistics (1989). *Sourcebook of criminal justice statistics, 1988.*

Bureau of Justice Statistics Bulletin (1989). *Examining recidivism.*

Campbell, J. (1949). *The hero with a thousand faces.* Princeton: Princeton Univ. Press.

Cavanaugh, K. L. (1987). Time series analysis of US and Canadian inflation and unemployment: A test of a field-theoretic hypothesis. Presented at the Annual Meeting of the American Statistical Association, San Francisco, California, August 17-20, 1987, and published in *Proceedings of the American Statistical Association, Business and Economics Statistics Section.* Alexandria, Virginia: American Statistical Association, 799-804.

Cavanaugh, K. L. & King, K. D. (1988). Simultaneous transfer function analysis of Okun's misery index: Improvements in the economic quality of life through Maharishi's Vedic Science and technology of consciousness. Paper presented at the Annual Meeting of the American Statistical Association, New Orleans, Louisiana, August 22-25, 1988. An abridged version of this paper appeared in

Proceedings of the American Statistical Association, Business and Economics Statistics Section: 491-496.

Cavanaugh, K. L., King, K. D., & Ertuna, C. (1989). A multiple-input transfer function model of Okun's misery index: An empirical test of the Maharishi effect. Paper presented at the Annual Meeting of the American Statistical Association, Washington, D. C., August 6-10, 1989. An abridged version of this paper appears in *Proceedings of the American Statistical Association, Business and Economics Statistics Section* (Alexandria, Virginia: American Statistical Association): 565-570.

Children's Defense Fund. (1991). *The state of America's children 1991.* Washington, DC: Children's Defense Fund.

Chrousos, G. P. & Gold, P. W. (1992). The Concepts of stress and stress system disorders: Overview of physical and behavioral homeostasis. *Journal of American Medical Association, 267,* 1244-1252.

Cohen, M. A. (1990). A note on the cost of crime to victims. *Urban Studies,* 27, 139-146.

Congressional Budget Office Report (January 1990). The economic and budget outlook: Fiscal years 1991-1995. A Report to the Senate and House Committees on Budget Part I.

Corrections Yearbook (1989). Criminal Justice Institute.

Davies, J. L. & Alexander, C. N. (1989). Alleviating political violence through enhancing coherence in collective consciousness: Impact assessment analyses of the Lebanon war. Presented at the 85th Annual Meeting of the American Political Science Association. (Refer also to *Dissertation Abstracts International 49*(8): 2381A, 1988.)

D'Espagnat, B. (1979). The quantum theory and reality. *Scientific American, 24,* 158-181.

Dillbeck, M. C. (1990). Test of a field theory of consciousness and social change: Time series analysis of participation in the TM-Sidhi program and reduction of violent death in the US. *Social Indicators Research 22,* 399-418.

Dillbeck, M. C. & Abrams, A. I (1987). The application of the Transcendental Meditation program in corrections. *International Journal of Comparative and Applied Criminal Justice, 11,* 111-132.

Dillbeck, M. C., Banus, C. B., Polanzi, C., & Landrith III, G. S. (1988). Test of a field model of consciousness and social change: The Transcendental Meditation and TM-Sidhi program and decreased urban crime. *The Journal of Mind and Behavior, 9,* 457-486.

Dillbeck, M. C., Cavanaugh, K. L., Glenn, T., Orme-Johnson, D. W., & Mittlefehldt, V. (1987). Consciousness as a field: The Transcendental Meditation and TM-Sidhi program and changes in social indicators. *The Journal of Mind and Behavior, 8,* 67-104.

Dillbeck, M. C., Landrith III, G. S. & Orme-Johnson, D. W. (1981). The Transcendental Meditation program and crime rate change in a sample of forty-eight cities. *Journal of Crime and Justice, 4,* 25-45.

Dillbeck, M. C. & Orme-Johnson, D. W. (1987). Physiological differences between Transcendental Meditation and rest. *American Psychologist, 42,* 879-881.

Dossey, L. (1989). *Recovering the soul.* New York: Bantam Books.

Durkheim, E. (1951). *Suicide: A study in sociology* (John A. Spaulding & George Simpson, Trans.). New York: The Free Press.

Eddington, A. (1984). Defense of mysticism. *In Quantum questions: Mystical writings of the world's great physicists.* Ken Wilbur (Ed.) Boston: New Science Library.

Elliot, G. R. & Eisendorfer, C. (Eds.) (1982). *Stress and human health: Analysis and implications of research.* New York: Springer Publishing Co.

Eppley, K., Abrams, A., & Shear, J. (1989). The differential effects of relaxation techniques on trait anxiety: A meta-analysis. *Journal of Clinical Psychology, 45,* 957-974.

Friedman, G. D. (1985). Epidemiology. In Kuper and Kuper (Eds.). *The Social Science Encyclopedia.* Boston, MA: Routledge and Kegan Paul,.

Garfinkle, S. A., Riley, G. F., & Iannacchione, V. G. (1988). High-expenditure users of medical care. *Health Care Financing Review, 9*(4), 867-870.

Gelderloos, P., Cavanaugh, K. L. & Davies, J. L. (1990). The dynamics of US-Soviet relations, 1979-1986: Effects of reducing social stress through the Transcendental Meditation and TM-Sidhi program. In *Proceedings of the American Statistical Association.* Alexandria. VA: American Statistical Association.

Gelderloos, P., Frid, M. J., & Xue, X. (1989). Improved US-Soviet relations as a function of the number of participants in the collective practice of the TM-Sidhi program. Abstract insert in *Journal of the Iowa Academy of Science, 96,* A33.

Gelderloos, P., Walton, K. G., Orme-Johnson, D. W., & Alexander, C. N. (1991). Effectiveness of the Transcendental Meditation program in preventing and treating substance misuse: A review. *International Journal of Addiction, 26,* 293-325.

Hagelin, J. S. (1987). Is consciousness the unified field? A field theorist's perspective. *Modern Science and Vedic Science, 1,* 29-87.

Hagelin, J. S. (1989). Restructuring physics from its foundation in light of Maharishi's Vedic Science. *Modern Science and Vedic Science, 3,* 3-72.

Harris, W. H. & Levey, J. S. (Eds.). (1975). Sociology. *The New Columbia Encyclopedia.* New York: Columbia Univ. Press.

Harwood et al. (1984). *The economic costs of alcohol and drug abuse and mental illness.* Research Triangle Park, NC: Research Triangle Institute.

Hazelden Foundation. (1991). *Hazelden news and professional update.* Minneapolis: Hazelden Foundation.

Horton, L. (1985). *Adolescent alcohol abuse.* Bloomington, IN: Phi Delta Kappa.

James, W. (1898/1977). *Human immortality: Two supposed objections to the doctrine.* Boston: Houghton Mifflin.

Jeans, J. (1981). *Physics and philosophy.* New York: Dover.

Jencks, S. F. & Schieber, G. J. (1991). Containing U.S. health care costs: What bullet to bite? *Health Care Financing Review.* Annual Supplement: 1-12.

Jevning, R., Wallace, R. K., & Beiderbach, M. (1992) The physiology of meditation: A review. A wakeful hypometabolic integrated response. *Neuroscience and Biobehavioral Reviews, 16*, 15-424.

Johnson, B. D., Goldstein, P. J., Preble, E., Schmeidler, J., Lipton, D., Spunt, B., & Miller, T. (1985). *Taking care of business: The economics of crime by heroin abusers.* Lexington, MA: Lexington Books.

Jöreskog, K. G. & Sörbom, D. (1979). *Advances in factor analysis and structural equation models.* Cambridge, MA: Abt Books.

Jöreskog, K. G., & Sörbom, D. (1986). *LISREL user's guide, version VI.* Mooresville, IN: Scientific Software.

Klein, D. B. (1984). *The concept of consciousness: A survey.* Lincoln, NE: University of Nebraska Press. (Reference cited is facing the book title page.)

Linsky, A. S. & Strains, M. A. (1986). *Social stress in the United States: Links to regional patterns in crime and illness.* Dover, MA: Auburn House Publishing Company,.

Linsky, A. S., Straus, M. A., & Colby, J. P. (1985). Stressful events, stressful conditions, and alcohol problems in the United States: A partial test of the Bale's theory of alcoholism. *Journal of Studies on Alcohol, 46*, 72-80.

Linsky, A. S., Colby, J. P., & Straus, M. A. (1986). *Social stress, smoking behavior and respiratory cancer: A macro-social analysis.* 2nd National Conference on Social Stress Research, Durham, University of New Hampshire.

Long, J. S. (1983). *Covariance structure models.* Beverly Hills, CA: Sage.

Maharishi Mahesh Yogi. (1966). *Science of being and the art of living.* New. York, NY: Signet.

Maharishi Mahesh Yogi. (1977). *Creating an ideal society.* Rheinweiler, Germany: Maharishi European Research University Press.

Maharishi Mahesh Yogi. (1979). *World government news #11.* Rheinweiler, Germany: Maharishi European Research University Press.

Maharishi Mahesh Yogi. (1986a). *Life supported by natural law.* Washington, DC: Age of Enlightenment Press.

Maharishi Mahesh Yogi. (1986b). *Maharishi's program to create world peace: Removing the basis of terrorism and war.* Washington, DC: Age of Enlightenment Press.

McDougall, W. (1920/1973). *The group mind.* New York: Arno Press.

McGinnis, J. M., & Foege, W. H. (1993). Actual causes of death in the United States. *Journal of the American Medical Association, 270*(18), 2207-2212.

Oates, Jr., R. M. (1976). *Celebrating the dawn.* New York: G. P. Putnam's Sons.

Orme-Johnson, D. W. (1987). Medical care utilization and the Transcendental Meditation program. *Psychosomatic Medicine, 49*, 493-507.

Orme-Johnson, D. W., Alexander, C. N., & Davies, J. L. (1990). The effects of the Maharishi Technology of the unified field: Reply to a methodological critique. *Journal of Conflict Resolution, 34*, 756-768.

Orme-Johnson, D. W., Alexander, C. N., Davies, J. L., Chandler, H. M., & Larimore, W. E. (1988). International peace project in the Middle East: The effect of the Maharishi technology of the unified field. *Journal of Conflict Resolution, 32*, 776-812.

Orme-Johnson, D. W., Cavanaugh, K. L., Alexander, C. N., Gelderloos, P., Dillbeck, M. C., Lanford, A. G., & Abou Nader, T. M. (1989). The influence of the Maharishi technology of the unified field on world events and global social indicators: The effects of the Taste of Utopia Assembly. In R. A. Chalmers, G. Clements, H. Schenkluhn, & M. Weinless (Eds.), *Scientific Research on Maharishi's Transcendental Meditation and TM-Sidhi Programme: Collected Papers*, Vol. 4. Vlodrop, Holland: Maharishi Vedic University Press.

Orme-Johnson, D. W., & Chandler, H. M. (1993). Crime rate in Fairfield, Iowa. Research in progress.

Orme-Johnson, D. W. & Dillbeck, M. C. (in press). Higher states of collective consciousness: Theory and research. In J. Gackenbach, C. N. Alexander, & H. T. Hunt (Eds.). *Higher states of consciousness: Theoretical and experimental perspectives*. New York: Plenum Press.

Orme-Johnson, D. W., Dillbeck, M. C., Alexander, C. N., Chandler, H. M., & Cranson, R. W. (1989). Time series impact assessment analysis of reduced international conflict and terrorism: Effects of large assemblies of participants in the Transcendental Meditation and TM-Sidhi program. Presented at the 85th Annual Meeting of the American Political Science Association, Atlanta, Georgia. Also presented at the Annual Conference of the American Psychological Association, Boston, Massachusetts, 1990.

Orme-Johnson, D. W., Dillbeck, M. C., Wallace, R. K., & Landrith III, G. S., (1982). Intersubject EEG coherence: Is consciousness a field? *International Journal of Neuroscience 16*:203-209.

Orme-Johnson, D. W. & Gelderloos P. (1988). Topographic EEG brain mapping during "Yogic Flying." *International Journal of Neuroscience, 38*, 427-434.

Orme-Johnson, D. W., Gelderloos, P., & Dillbeck, M. C. (1988). The long-term effects of the Maharishi technology of the unified field on the quality of life in the United States (1960 to 1984). *Social Science Perspectives Journal, 2*, 127-146.

Peto, R., Lopez, A. D., Boreham, J., Thum, M., & Heath Jr., C. (1992). Mortality from tobacco in developed countries: Indirect estimation from national vital statistics. *The Lancet*, 339, 1268.

Prasada, R. (Trans). (1912/1978). *Yoga sutras* [of Patanjali]. New Delhi: Oriental Books Reprint Corporation.

Pugh, N. D. C., Walton, K. G., & Cavanaugh, K. L. (1988). Can time series analysis of serotonin turnover test the theory that consciousness is a field? Poster presented at the 18th annual meeting of the Society for Neuroscience, Toronto, November 13-18.

Reeks, D. L. (1990). Improved quality of life in Iowa through the Maharishi effect. (Doctoral Dissertation, Maharishi International University).

Rice et al. (1990). *Economic costs to society of alcohol and drug abuse and mental illness: 1980*. San Francisco: Institute for Health and Aging, University of California-San Francisco.

Sapolsky, R. M. (1992). *Stress, the aging brain, and mechanisms of neuron death.* A Bradford Book, The MIT Press, Cambridge, MA.

Scheffler, R. M, & Pringer, L. A. (1980). A review of the economic evidence on prevention. *Medical Care, 18,* 473-484.

Straus, M. A., Linsky, A. S., & Bachman-Prehn, R. (1989). Change in the stressfulness of life in American states and regions from 1976 to 1982. *Social Indicators Research, 21*, 229-257.

Travis, F. T., & Orme-Johnson, D. W. (1989). Field models of consciousness: EEG coherence changes as indicators of field effects. *International Journal of Neuroscience, 49*, 203-211.

Travis, F. T., & Orme-Johnson, D. W. (1990). EEG coherence and power during yogic flying. *International Journal of Neuroscience, 54*, 1-12.

U.S. Department of Health and Human Services (1990a). *Healthy people 2000: National health promotion and disease prevention objectives.* Washington, DC: Government Printing Office.

U.S. Department of Health and Human Services (1990b). *Prevention '89/'90: Federal programs and progress*. Public Health Service. Washington, DC: Government Printing Office.

U.S. Department of Health and Human Services (1991). No. ADM 91-1835. Washington, DC: Government Printing Office.

Walton, K. G. & Levitsky, D. (this volume). Role of Transcendental Meditation in reducing drug abuse and addictions: Neurochemical evidence and a theory. *Alcoholism Treatment Quarterly.*

Walton, K. G., Pugh, N. D. C., Gelderloos, P. & Macrae, P. Mechanisms of prevention through stress reduction: Suggestive results on corticosteriods, salt excretion and negative emotions. *Journal of Hypertension.*

Yoder, B. (1990). *The recovery resource book.* New York: Simon and Schuster.

Zook, C. J. & Moore, F. D. (1980). High-expenditure users of medical care. *The New England Journal of Medicine, 302*(18), 996-1002.

Spirituality, Recovery, and Transcendental Meditation

Father Diarmuid O'Murchu, MSC

In this essay, I would like to consider the relationship between spiritual growth and recovery from addictive behavior, giving special attention to the role that the Transcendental Meditation program (TM) can play in recovery. I would like to make clear that for me, this is a very personal statement. I am writing it purely from my own individual perspective and experience as a priest who has practiced Transcendental Meditation and seen its relevance to the problem of addiction and other problems we face as individuals and as a society. I have drawn on the teachings of Maharishi Mahesh Yogi to explain the mechanics and value of Transcendental Meditation in this context, but the connections I have drawn between TM, spirituality, recovery, and religion reflect my own views on the subject.

SPIRITUALITY AND RELIGION

What precisely do we mean by spirituality? In my view, spirituality is about the human search for meaning and fulfillment in life.

Father Diarmuid O'Murchu is a Catholic priest and member of the Missionaries of the Sacred Heart, counselor and social psychologist working in London, England.

[Haworth co-indexing entry note]: "Spirituality, Recovery, and Transcendental Meditation." O'Murchu, Father Diarmuid. Co-published simultaneously in the *Alcoholism Treatment Quarterly* (The Haworth Press, Inc.) Vol. 11, No. 1/2, 1994, pp. 169-184; and: *Self-Recovery: Treating Addictions Using Transcendental Meditation and Maharishi Ayur-Veda* (ed: David F. O'Connell and Charles N. Alexander) The Haworth Press, Inc., 1994, pp. 169-184. Multiple copies of this article/chapter may be purchased from The Haworth Document Delivery Center [1-800-3-HAWORTH; 9:00 a.m. - 5:00 p.m. (EST)].

Deep within each one of us is an indescribable desire to make sense and meaning out of life, to discover one's ultimate true nature and relationship to the universe. This desire is active in the new-born infant in its various attempts to master the environment; it is active in the young adult through his/her relationships with people and with the world of work and achievement; and, it underpins the elderly person's desire to enjoy his or her later years in love and peace.

A critical problem in today's world is that most of us are not in touch with our inner spirituality, we do not experience a deep inner meaning to life that integrates all our diverse activities and relationships. Instead, life is experienced in a fragmented and unsatisfying way. Lack of inner meaning and subsequent lack of fulfillment often expresses itself in the inordinate pursuit of wealth, power, and pleasure, and can lead to warfare, religious fanaticism, etc. When life becomes fragmented, sickness and suffering result. But true spirituality is about a search for meaning and fulfillment that every human being pursues, although this pursuit may be misguided or poorly informed. The ultimate purpose of this search, I maintain, is always genuine, no matter how misguided the means may be. Unknown to ourselves, sometimes in spite of ourselves, we are always pursuing meaning.

Given this orientation, I feel it is important to differentiate between religion and spirituality. The confusion of these two realities has caused considerable damage to our world and to its peoples. The term "religion" refers to systems of belief and worship that people inherit or adopt, and that they understand to be means leading to ultimate happiness and fulfillment. The purpose of religion is to provide a framework in which we can develop our spiritual awareness, but today, strange as it may sound, religion as it is commonly practiced often becomes an obstacle to the growth and development of genuine spirituality.

There are a number of reasons for this. First, the framework of religion–its formal teaching, laws, forms of worship, etc.–may no longer seem meaningful for many people. Second, it is all too easy to fall into a destructive trend within some streams of Christian teachings (and other traditions as well), namely, "dualisms." In dualistic thinking, we divide everything into pairs of opposites, such as heaven-earth, grace-nature, God-man, good-evil. Dualisms are inventions or constructs of the human mind, and were widely used for much of the Christian era when humans in general tended to think and act out of those simple opposing categories. Some theologians have suggested in the past few decades that dualisms can be highly dangerous. They oversimplify, create false divisions, and fail to recognize the "gray area" in between the opposites, where people live most of their daily lives.

But the biggest problem with dualisms is that they present a false picture of life at every level. Life does not consist of "either/or," but of "both/and." Earth and heaven are not opposites, they are two aspects of the one reality of life. God is not the opposite of man, because God lives primarily in people, not outside of them. This truth gave rise to the great Christian conviction that God (in the person of Jesus) assumed the fullness of our humanity; therefore it follows that, in the oft-quoted words of St. Iraneus (130-200 AD): "The glory of God is a person fully alive." More recently, a similar thought has been expressed by the theologian Gregory Baum: "God is what happens to a person on the way to becoming human."

A great danger for any of us is to internalize one particular narrow understanding or belief about God and cling rigidly to it. This limits our ability to expand our understanding and experience of God. We all grope for a sense of the Divine, and come most close to understanding it as a *life-force* within, rather than some powerful figurehead above or outside us. God is something that is felt in the heart rather than understood in the mind or figured out by the human brain.

In today's world, many people think that to be "spiritual" means to be "religious," but there are millions of very spiritual people who have no link with, nor affiliation to, a formal religion. It is one of the primary functions of religion to awaken, nurture, and sustain this inner spiritual dimension of life, but at the present time, many people feel that religion is failing at this task. Moreover, religion as commonly understood has never been the sole instrument used by people for spiritual nurturance. Many other methods, sometimes referred to as spiritual disciplines, mystical experiences, or saintly practices have always been available.

Religion *can* help to deepen one's spiritual awareness because, as mentioned above, it tries to provide a framework in which we can develop our spiritual consciousness. It is not so much that people have "abandoned religion" or "given up the faith," rather, there seems to be a new period in our evolution as a species in which people are outgrowing the need for religion as typically practiced. In this process we are rediscovering, in a whole new way, what it means to be *spiritual* people (see also Bancroft, 1990; Bockl, 1988; Macy, 1991; Powell, 1987).

MEDITATION AND PRAYER IN CONTEMPORARY SOCIETY

Because contemporary religion is not fulfilling its goal and because the desire for spiritual growth is built into life, since around 1960, our Western world has been fascinated with yoga, peace of mind, meditation, interiority, anything to do with the "inner journey." Thus ancient techniques and practices of the East began to have a powerful impact in the West. They seemed to offer something that was right for the time, and with this movement came a renewed spiritual upsurge. Addressing a conference in 1976, theologian Anthony Padovana said: "Faith is not dying in the West. It is merely moving inside." To that observation, I would like to add: moving to its original center and encountering in a new way the Spirit who dwells within.

Today, the word *meditation* is used in a range of different meanings and thus merits further description. In the West, "prayer" and "meditation" tend to be understood in the more traditional religious sense of word-formulas used to address God (prayer), or silent reflection on scriptural texts (meditation). But the terms carry a potentially deeper significance, namely the cultivation of one's spiritual nature whereby we become more open, receptive, and attuned to the divine power within. In its deeper meaning, *meditation* is about experiencing a deeper *level* of conscious awareness, more open and receptive, and more attuned to the still voice within. This deepening of awareness may take place systematically through methods not typically practiced in the West.

In the West, meditation has been conceived almost exclusively as a *thinking* exercise, with the head playing the major role. Its usefulness has been further jeopardized by conceiving of it as a specialized feature of life in a monastery or convent, involving reflection on Sacred Scripture. Although this approach may be meritorious, it does not fully capture the deeper meaning of meditation, which properly applies to methods which cultivate experience of the pure inner spiritual content of life. Whereas these approaches seem to have been virtually lost in the West, some of them appear to have been continuously maintained in the East, most clearly in the ancient Vedic tradition of India.

People are now beginning to describe meditation as the technology (the "know-how") for a new "age of consciousness." Each scientific breakthrough throughout history has had a corresponding set of technological skills to articulate and apply the new information. For the electronic age, we invented televisions, videos, etc. For the information age we invented computers. For the forthcoming era, we need a new global, supramaterial technology which can fully enliven the pure spiritual content of consciousness within each of us. Such an approach should be capable of taking one's attention to the center of one's being, of facilitating an inward movement of awareness (*interiority* rather than *introspection*) (cf. Starcke, 1974).

Many approaches to meditation exist either in a spiritual or secular context, but these categories tend to become superfluous in the realm of pure spirit. In its deepest sense, the capacity to meditate is first and foremost a *natural birthright*, a potency within every human being. Today many people objectify meditation, seeing it as a highly specialized practice designed for the religiously oriented, or, conversely, as a generic remedy to be purchased or learned from a textbook. We are thus in danger of trivializing this precious innate capacity of the human psyche to experience inner wholeness and peace, which needs tender and careful nurturing by trained instructors of meditation.

THE TRANSCENDENTAL MEDITATION TECHNIQUE AND THE SEARCH FOR GENUINE SPIRITUALITY

The Transcendental Meditation (TM) technique is a simple yet profound mental technique from the ancient Vedic tradition of knowledge brought to light by Maharishi Mahesh Yogi over 30 years ago. TM is now practiced by more than 4 million people worldwide, and is the most thoroughly researched technology for developing consciousness, with over 500 studies documenting its physiological, psychological and sociological effects. This research confirms that it is a distinctively rich resource for cultivating health, longevity, and wisdom in contemporary society (Alexander, Robinson, & Rainforth, this volume; Walton & Levitsky, this volume). Several chapters in this volume also recount subjective experiences in which meditators describe the benefits they have obtained from regular TM practice (Bleick, this volume; Ellis & Corum, this volume).

TM effortlessly promotes the sense of inner harmony and integration that enables people to grow spiritually, thus reclaiming the essential unity and oneness of their selves, and the interconnectedness to the "sacred" at every level of their existence. Unfortunately, there have been certain misunderstandings about the spiritual/religious nature of TM. It needs to be stated quite categorically that TM is NOT a religion in any way, shape, or form. It does not require adoption of any belief or lifestyle. It is a virtually mechanical technique that provides a profound psychophysiological state of restful alertness that prepares one for more successful activity in whatever spheres of life in which one engages. TM is practiced in every culture by members of all religious faiths and their clergy–including priests, ministers, rabbis, and Buddhist monks. Also, many people who do not subscribe to any particular religion, or may be quite skeptical about religion, cherish the technique for its unfoldment of their inner potential.

Although not a system of religion, the TM technique cultivates a sense of inner calm, well-being, harmony, and attunement with life that provides a natural basis for greater appreciation of others and the universe as a whole. What in fact is happening for many TM practitioners is a *rediscovery* of their inner spiritual nature. How? As a technique, TM works in a very effortless and spontaneous way. During Transcendental Meditation, awareness experiences increasingly refined or settled states of the mind until the mind "transcends" (goes beyond) the subtlest state of the thinking process and one experiences a completely silent, unified state–called pure consciousness–in which awareness is fully awake to itself, with no objects of thought or perception (Maharishi, 1969, p. 470). Maharishi (1966) explains that this unified state of wholeness is the universal field of Being, or pure intelligence, underlying all of creation. As the mind settles down to experience this field, the body also experiences deep physiological rest that normalizes deep-rooted stresses that block the natural unfoldment of full human development (Maharishi, 1969).

As a result of this process, with the practice of TM, we find that the spiritual capacity (like the physical, social and mental aspects) begins to flow according to its innate, God-given propensity. We do not become "Godly," or "mystical." We simply become ourselves, and gradually realize that there is, deep within each and all of us, a holy and spiritual dimension that enriches rather than damages our humanity. In his own writings, Maharishi (1966) has emphasized that TM is a simple method to help fulfill the shared aspiration of all religions to develop this innate spiritual capacity. He explains how various religions arose in different historical eras and geographical locations to provide guidance on how to live life in accord with "natural law" (in the language of modern science) or in accord with the "Will of God" (in the language of religion). He emphasizes that TM is not meant to substitute for any religion's practices or precepts but rather to provide a means by which they may be more effortlessly realized (Maharishi, 1991).

I myself learned the TM technique out of intellectual curiosity. Within weeks, I noticed that my digestive problems had abated considerably and that my compulsiveness towards work had waned. But what fascinated me most of all were the spiritual changes. For eight years previously, as a priest I had led a semi-monastic lifestyle of regular prayer, formal meditation (reflection on Sacred Scripture), and frequent spiritual reading. And I was diligent in carrying out these *duties,* but rarely achieved that inner sense of peace and "being at one" that became so apparent when I started TM. The presence of God–in myself and in the world–came alive in a whole new way. By shifting the focus *within,* religious observances *without* became quite secondary. Everything shifted into a new perspective. Rather than effortfully having to follow my religious precepts, I found myself spontaneously behaving on the basis of feeling good deep within.

What I have attempted thus far is a brief outline of what spirituality is about, and what I feel the TM technique has to offer in that context. Of course, people learn the technique for a whole range of reasons, but those who practice TM regularly tend to confirm my personal experience as outlined above–namely, the reawakening of an inner sense of value, worth, purpose, meaning, and closer bonds with nature and/or the universe, and a deepening sense of the sacred (whether or not the name "God" is used in describing it).

RECOVERY AND SPIRITUALITY

Many years ago, the eminent psychiatrist Carl Jung wrote to Bill Wilson, co-founder of Alcoholics Anonymous, saying that he thought alcoholism was a search for spiritual wholeness, a misguided attempt to achieve "union with God." Recovery from addictions or compulsions, as envisaged in the Twelve Steps of Alcoholics Anonymous (AA), demands that we acknowledge our drug "problem," the inability to rectify it on our own, and the consequent need to allow a "higher power" to come to our aid. In my opinion, this orientation toward going beyond individual limitations to draw upon a higher or deeper source of power and wisdom is fundamental to all human growth, not just to recovery. It is captured in the Biblical invitation to "lose (let-go-of) one's life in order to find it" (Mk. 8:35), or to quote the words attributed to Jesus himself, "I lay down my life in order that I may take it up again" (Jn. 10:17).

The eleventh of the Twelve Steps of AA states this perspective as follows:

> We sought through prayer and meditation to improve our conscious contact with God, as we understood Him, praying only for knowledge of His will for us and the power to carry that through.

The reference to God here is immediately followed by the words "as we understood Him." The same qualifying phrase is used in the third step of the AA program which reads: "We made a decision to turn our will and our lives over to God, as we understood Him," suggesting that different people may recognize God or the higher power in their own way.

People with addictive behavior patterns sometimes exhibit compulsive tendencies towards "perfectionism." Everything must be perfect, clearly understood, in its right place. When it comes to God, and matters relating to the "higher power" to which we try to hand over our lives, this perfectionist streak can become quite an obstacle. This can be complicated by the perspective of dualisms that we discussed earlier in which God is viewed as separate from ourselves. In a sense, of course, we cannot "hand over" our life to God because God is within us. It should be understood that "handing over" our life does not mean abandoning our responsibility to use our inherent capabilities in the recovery process (cf. the Parable of the Talents, Matt. 25:124ff).

Rather, the challenge is to cooperate with the divine power within us–our spiritual selves–in a more positive and creative way. Instead of using *ego-power*–trying to dominate and control everything for selfish gain, the type of compulsiveness that drives people to drink, drugs, and other destructive forms of behavior–each of us must come to be aware that we are accountable to an "inner dimension" that continuously invites us to be more loving, caring and responsible. A type of inner freedom–freedom from fear, guilt, and inordinate compulsion–needs to be cultivated to allow us to trust ourselves and also God, without feeling that we must box God into one or another limited category of human understanding.

While encouraging meditation, Twelve Step programs have not made specific recommendations on how to practice it. In the absence of a systematic, effortless meditation technique to direct awareness deep within, many recovering addicts have felt frustrated in their attempts to become attuned to this profound inner dimension of life. I have found in my own personal experience that long-term practice of the TM technique does cultivate that inner "letting go." And with it comes the progressive awakening deep within us that, whoever or whatever God is, we are forever held in the love of what, in the Christian tradition, is referred to as the mysterious embrace. It is a feeling of being loved and accepted unconditionally–and I believe this is the type of God to which alcoholics and others are being encouraged to hand over their lives. And in that handing over, we do not lose ourselves; in fact, we often (re)discover our true selve–perhaps, for the first time. (For a new and more holistic Christian understanding of God, see Shield and Carlson, 1990.)

HEALING ILLNESS FROM WITHIN

Like many programs of recovery, the Twelve Steps encourage us to think of illness as an opportunity for spiritual growth. This idea is not entirely new, but with the increasing popularity of multi-dimensional or holistic approaches to health and well-being, the notion has assumed greater significance (e.g., Siegal, 1990). Some health experts claim that illness is fed by fear, a fear that our deeper needs for love, affirmation, approval, and worth will not be met (e.g., Harrison, 1984). Consequently, some of us become ill to elicit care and attention of significant others. However, if we can find a means to foster inner well-being and increase self-worth, then a natural process of inner healing takes place that can overcome such illness. Indeed, scientific research indicates that TM not only increases well-being and self-esteem but substantially decreases the incidence of serious physical illnesses (Orme-Johnson, 1987).

In the absence of such inner growth, we tend to become shrouded in our problems, struggling to keep afloat, at times oblivious to the needs of others. In contrast, when we grow in inner fulfillment, this inner fullness starts to overflow into the environment, and we become capable of spontaneously caring for others with tenderness and compassion. Thus, the TM technique is a helpful tool to cultivate a more self-sufficient yet compassionate quality of thought, attitude and outlook. As inner well-being grows, we naturally no longer have the compulsive need to seek artificial outer means to induce well-being.

Thus, we can see that while illness can provide an opportunity for growth by signaling that change is needed, it is not the case that continual suffering is required during the recovery process. Although the nervous system must be purified of stress to fully experience inner Being, Maharishi (1966) points out that this does not mean that it is necessary to "glorify" the role of suffering in human development. Indeed, he states that TM heals using the "principle of the second element" during the technique. Rather than confronting our stress, we transcend to experience the everpresent inner light of Being, pure consciousness, which is our own inner nature. Contact with Being is said to be inherently blissful and fulfilling. However, as a spontaneous by-product of experiencing this healing inner silence, impurities are automatically released and the nervous system is "normalized."

Thus, while suffering may be a pervasive characteristic of everyday living, it is not intrinsic to the ultimate nature of life which is characterized by wholeness, peace, and happiness (Maharishi, 1966). Through contact with this inner dimension of life through TM, one begins to experience what the Christian gospels call "the fullness of life." Regaining inner fullness, suffering automatically dissolves and need no longer be avoided (or medicated) through addictive behavior. The value of this inner approach to healing is supported by findings of higher abstinence rates among abusers who learn TM than those who participate in standard drug abuse programs relying on external approaches to behavior change and social support (Alexander, Robinson, & Rainforth, this volume).

ON HEALING THE SYSTEM AS WELL AS THE PERSON

This chapter would be incomplete without some consideration of the social and systemic dimensions of addiction and spirituality.

Many alcoholics today go through the painful experience of having to confront family members and loved ones in recovery centers. This approach is now standard in recovery work, and not without its rewards for the alcoholics themselves. Although the "disease" model still dominates our understanding and treatment of alcoholism, we can no longer exclude the unique and complex interaction between family members that increasingly seems to be a contributory factor to the alcoholic illness in the first place. We have abundant examples of the alcoholic being a scapegoat for much of the unresolved pain and conflict of a dysfunctional family system. Thus, it may be that the system, e.g., the family and community in which the alcoholic functions, also is sick and in need of healing (cf. Small, 1991; Wegscheider-Cruse, 1989).

This means that as a society, we cannot simply blame the individual, rather we must acknowledge the reciprocal relationship that exists between individual and society as a whole. Our Western culture prides itself in being person-centered and strongly augments individual human rights. However, the flip-side of this virtue is the tendency to perceive wrongdoing as the fruit of individual failure and irresponsibility. Consequently, the religious notion of sin tends to be portrayed in terms of the individual; but there is overwhelming evidence to suggest that systemic or social sin occurs in abundance and damages the quality of individual life. Thus, a negative downward spiral occurs, with unhappy, unhealthy individuals contributing to and, in turn, influenced by the larger unhealthy society (e.g., Wilson-Schaef, 1987). To reverse this downward spiral, a totally new approach that simultaneously heals the whole society as well as its individual members needs to be adopted.

How to bring about change in a social or political system is an issue of much debate today. In the 1970s, researchers investigating the sociological effects of TM found that if only 1% of a population practices TM, or the square root of that number practices the advanced TM-Sidhi program, the benefits experienced by individuals practicing these mental techniques will spill over into the whole community. Scientists named this phenomenon the Maharishi Effect after Maharishi who predicted it as early as 1960. The Maharishi Effect has been replicated in over forty studies in many geographical locations. A comprehensive review of this research is presented by Dr. David Orme-Johnson (this volume). This theory proposes that, at the deepest level of our inner Nature–Being or pure consciousness–we are all profoundly interconnected and if even relatively few of us enliven this level through direct experience, we can create a healing influence that spreads throughout the larger community. This approach has been tested in urban settings, and the results were that the overall quality of urban health improved in the sense that violent crime and suicides diminished, and road accidents decreased (e.g., Dillbeck, Banus, Polanzi, & Landrith, 1988). Because the majority of violent crimes and fatal car accidents are committed under the influence of alcohol or drugs, these findings suggest that group practice of these techniques may be lowering substance abuse in society as well.

To date, the scientific community, largely locked into a mechanistic mode of operating, has paid far too little attention to this discovery. But the cumulative sociological evidence–along with the ancient spiritual wisdom of the Vedic tradition which has long acknowledged such possibilities–suggests we can no longer dismiss or ignore this important development.

Thus far we have explored the meaning and interconnectedness of spirituality and recovery at both the individual and societal levels. Spirituality and recovery are intimately related because true recovery–the letting go of life-destructive behaviors and the adoption of more mature and responsible patterns of activity–goes hand in hand with the growth of a more meaningful, spiritually mature life. In my view, TM can enhance both the growth of spirituality and the process of recovery at both the individual and societal level, and therefore naturally accelerates a return to optimal functioning.

THE MOTIVATION TO LEARN TRANSCENDENTAL MEDITATION

Spirituality, recovery and TM may interact in many ways. Motivation to learn TM may come from at least three sources: (1) The recovery process itself, (2) the desire for spiritual growth, or (3) the insight of health care professionals.

First, the impetus toward growth may arise from the recovery process itself. An acceptance of addiction as a spur to recognizing the problem and moving toward positive change is a first step in recovery. The person trying to break an addictive habit, or one who has already taken the first steps, hears about TM, learns the technique, and proceeds to practice it twice daily. TM will certainly enhance the recovery process, improving the health of body, mind, and behavior. With the heightened mental clarity and increased self-worth gained through TM, recovering addicts become disposed to see more clearly and deeply what is happening in the environment, and by the same token, come to realize the inappropriateness of the social/systemic context in which they formerly lived. And, instigated by this new awareness, in time, they may make significant changes at both personal and social levels.

Second, the thirst for spiritual realization may create the original impetus towards growth. Often in the struggle with an addiction, people still may be experiencing a very real sense of the God who loves them despite their many failures. Even before recovery work begins, the addict may be filled with a sincere desire to experience more of God's love and support in daily life. A spiritual orientation can aid the choice to work for recovery, and it can help sustain and enhance that process in significant ways.

Third, the person in the healing profession who works with addicts is challenged to provide a discerning and supportive presence. For the health care professional as well as the person in recovery, TM can be a powerful tool for maximizing spiritual growth. With the experience of TM, the high level of stress and consequent "burn-out" so frequently experienced in the service professions can be profoundly alleviated. Once professionals experience for themselves inner happiness and vitality through this technique, they know its benefits first-hand. Consequently, it is quite natural to recommend to clients that which has helped the helper.

CONCLUSION

So why learn and practice TM? TM will help to deepen spiritual growth, and it will augment the process of integrating the spiritual with the other dimensions of one's life. In the process of spiritual growth, it may also help heal old wounds and alleviate the burden of past guilt. Very likely it will help to broaden the horizon of self-awareness, shifting the focus from just a personal problem to a dis-ease that may need to be understood in a wider social/systemic context. Even more than this, as Maharishi explains, TM can facilitate growth to the highest realms of human evolution, with a profoundly transforming effect not merely on self-awareness but on one's perception of all reality. These higher levels of awareness–known to the enlightened for millennia and described in a wide range of spiritual and religious expressions–are known in the literature on TM as higher states of consciousness; the sequential unfoldment of these higher states results in complete spiritual union with the Divine (Maharishi, 1969; see also Alexander, Robinson, & Rainforth, this volume; O'Connell, this volume).

In religious parlance, we use the term *discernment* to distinguish between true and false spiritualities. A person who talks a lot about God is not necessarily in tune with God. And perception of God as only an external agent of power and influence may also be accompanied by feelings of fear and guilt, rather than by feelings of genuine trust and faith. Perhaps what people in recovery need most of all is the ability to trust their own spiritual intuitions, especially those that arise from within the spiritual awakening that may accompany recovery. This awakening is about life, about the recovery of meaning and fulfillment. Within this awakening is the "God" who waits, who loves, who seeks us out. We do not need rituals, laws, or even religions to encounter this inner presence; what we do need is a listening heart and the humility to accept that, despite everything, we are loved unconditionally.

I believe it is this awakening which is cultivated through TM. It builds on what is already present in a gentle but powerful way. And it augments growth, not in a piecemeal fashion, but in a rounded, holistic way. So if a person in recovery expresses an interest in TM, explore this option with them. And for the person who may be already undergoing a spiritual awakening, TM has much to offer to enhance that development.

It is difficult to appreciate what a technique like TM has to offer in terms of growth and integration without having had the experience for oneself. Having had that experience, I offer it to you–not as a solution from the head, but as a gift from the heart.

REFERENCES

Alexander, C. N., Robinson, P., & Rainforth, M. (this volume). Using Transcendental Meditation to treat alcohol, nicotine, and drug abuse: A review and statistical meta-analysis. *Alcoholism Treatment Quarterly*.

Bancroft, A. (1990). *The spiritual journey*. Element, MA: Element Books.

Bleick, C. R. (this volume). Case histories: Using the Transcendental Meditation program with alcoholics and addicts. *Alcoholism Treatment Quarterly*.

Bockl, G. (1988). *God beyond religion: Personal journeyings from religiosity to spirituality*. Marina del Rey, CA: Devors & Co.

Dillbeck, M. C., Banus, C. B., Polanzi, C., & Landrith III, G. S. (1988). Test of a field model of consciousness and social change: The Transcendental Meditation and TM-Sidhi program and decreased urban crime. *The Journal of Mind and Behavior, 9*, 457-486.

Ellis, G. A., & Corum, P. (this volume). Removing the motivator: A holistic solution to substance abuse. *Alcoholism Treatment Quarterly.*

Harrison, J. (1984). *Love your disease.* London and Melbourne: Angus and Robertson.

Macy, J. (1991). *World as lover: World as self.* Berkley, CA: Parallax Press.

Maharishi Mahesh Yogi (1966). *Science of being and art of living.* New York, NY: Signet.

Maharishi Mahesh Yogi (1969). *On the Bhagavad Gita: A translation and commentary, Chapters 1-6.* Baltimore, MD: Penguin.

Maharishi Mahesh Yogi (1991). Maharishi's plan to create heaven on earth. Vlodrop, Holland: Maharishi Vedic University Press.

O'Connell, D. F. (this volume). Possessing the self. *Alcoholism Treatment Quarterly.*

Orme-Johnson, D. W. (1987). Medical care utilization and the Transcendental Meditation program. *Psychosomatic Medicine, 49*, 493-507.

Orme-Johnson, D. W. (this volume). Transcendental Meditation as an epidemiological approach to drug and alcohol abuse: Theory, research and financial impact evaluation. *Alcoholism Treatment Quarterly.*

Powell, J. (1987). *Through seasons of the heart.* London: Faber & Faber.

Sheldrake, R. (1988). *The presence of the past.* London: Collins.

Shield, B. and Carlson, R. (1990). *For the love of God.* Fallbrook, CA: New World Library.

Siegal, B. (1990). *Peace, love and healing.* London and Sydney: Rider/Century Hutchinson, Ltd.

Small, J. (1991). *Awakening in time: The journey from co-dependence to co-creation.* New York: Bantam Books.

Starcke, W. (1974). *The gospel of relativity.* Boerne, TX: Guadalupe Press.

Walton, K. G., & Levitsky, D. (this volume). Role of Transcendental Meditation in reducing drug use and addictions: Neurochemical evidence and a theory. *Alcoholism Treatment Quarterly.*

Wegscheider-Cruse, S. (1989). *Another chance: Hope and health for the alcoholic family.* Palo Alto, CA: Science and Behaviour Books.

Wilson-Schaef, A. (1987). *When society becomes an addict.* New York: Harper and Row.

SECTION II: ORIGINAL RESEARCH ON TRANSCENDENTAL MEDITATION AND ADDICTIONS TREATMENT

Effectiveness of Broad Spectrum Approaches to Relapse Prevention in Severe Alcoholism: A Long-Term, Randomized, Controlled Trial of Transcendental Meditation, EMG Biofeedback and Electronic Neurotherapy

Edward Taub, PhD
Solomon S. Steiner, PhD
Eric Weingarten, PhD
Kenneth G. Walton, PhD

Edward Taub (to whom correspondence should be addressed) is affiliated with the Department of Psychology, 201 Campbell Hall, University of Alabama at Birmingham, Birmingham, AL 35294. Solomon S. Steiner is affiliated with the Pharmaceutical Discovery Corp., Elmsford, NY. Eric Weingarten is at Trumansburg, New York. Kenneth G. Walton is in the Departments of Chemistry and Physiology, Maharishi International University, Fairfield, IA. The authors wish to acknowledge Ray B. Smith, PhD, for his involvement in this research project.

This work was supported in part by Public Health Service Grant AA 01279. The authors would like to thank Drs. Linda and Mark Sobell for consultation on important aspects of the experimental procedures, particularly on techniques for maintaining frequent follow-up contact with the subjects.

[Haworth co-indexing entry note]: "Effectiveness of Broad Spectrum Approaches to Relapse Prevention in Severe Alcoholism: A Long-Term, Randomized, Controlled Trial of Transcendental Meditation, EMG Biofeedback and Electronic Neurotherapy." Taub, Edward, Solomon S. Steiner, Eric Weingarten, and Kenneth G. Walton. Co-published simultaneously in the *Alcoholism Treatment Quarterly* (The Haworth Press, Inc.) Vol. 11, No. 1/2, 1994, pp. 187-220; and: *Self-Recovery: Treating Addictions Using Transcendental Meditation and Maharishi Ayur-Veda* (ed: David F. O'Connell and Charles N. Alexander) The Haworth Press, Inc., 1993, pp. 187-220. Multiple copies of this article/chapter may be purchased from The Haworth Document Delivery Center [1-800-3-HAWORTH; 9:00 a.m. - 5:00 p.m. (EST)].

INTRODUCTION

Alcohol and drug related problems place a large burden on American society. The yearly cost due to alcohol abuse alone, including increases in health care, accidents and crime, and reductions in productivity, is projected to be $150 billion by 1995 (U.S. Department of Health and Human Services, 1986). The toll in pain and suffering cannot be rendered in dollar amounts, but is also very large (Marlatt & Gordon, 1985; Yoder, 1990). While approaches to treatment of alcoholism abound, their effectiveness is far from the level that would be desirable, with the result that relapse to alcoholism is recognized as one of the most intractable problems in the alcoholism field (Hunt, Barnett & Branch, 1971; Marlatt & Gordon, 1985). To address this problem, more research, and in particular more long-term follow-up research, is needed to facilitate identification of the most useful rehabilitation therapies.

In general, the causes of relapse to alcoholism appear similar to those of initial addiction. Thus, the wide range of treatment strategies in use today stem from the variety of concepts of the causes of alcohol addiction as well as from the multidimensional nature of the condition. Despite the existence of many treatment approaches, little research is available on the relative efficacy of individual therapies (Greenstreet, 1988). Furthermore, the number of studies employing long-term (one year or longer) follow-up is even smaller.

Among the concepts of the cause of alcoholism (see Miller & Hester, 1989), long-standing models such as the "temperance" model (abuse due to the pernicious nature of alcohol itself), the "disease" model (alcoholism as a unique and progressive condition), the "educational" model (abuse arising from a knowledge deficit), "characterological" models (rooted in abnormalities of the personality) and the "biological" model (emphasizing genetic and physiological processes), appear to be giving way to more integrative models such as the "public health" and "biopsychosocial" models. The public health formulation (see Miller & Hester, 1989) is a type of disease model which holds that study of three classes of causal factors can give a relatively complete understanding of alcoholism: (1) the *agent* (usually a microorganism, but in this case, ethyl alcohol), (2) *host* factors (individual differences influencing susceptibility and potential for recovery), and (3) *environment* (in this case, mainly social context). Similar factors are assembled under the biopsychosocial model, which holds that a dynamic interaction of biological, psychological and social processes underlies alcoholism (see Donovan, 1988). One key point brought out by proponents of the biopsychosocial model is that all addictions, including eating disorders, drinking, drug use, gambling and smoking, appear to share the same spectrum of behaviors and characteristics (Donovan, 1988). This may imply that any treatment addressing the common features of addiction will be useful regardless of the specific addiction to which it is applied.

Whatever conceptual view is adopted concerning the cause of alcohol addiction and relapse, the practical application of techniques for relapse prevention and rehabilitation must address a multitude of interdependent symptoms and conditions. After the acute withdrawal stage, most addicts are left with memory problems, inability to think clearly, emotional numbness (or its opposite, emotional overreactivity), sleep disturbance, poor physical coordination and increased sensitivity to stress (Gorski & Miller, 1986; Stockwell & Town, 1989). Also important are lingering dysfunctional behaviors and a high frequency of depression and antisocial, anxiety and personality disorders–which may or may not have predated the addiction (Spotts & Shontz, 1991). Most treatment modalities are not suited to simultaneously affecting the full range of these problems. However, broad spectrum approaches, including techniques for reducing stress and improving self-efficacy, appear to be the most useful (Greenstreet, 1988), perhaps because their effects cover the widest range of factors contributing to addiction and relapse (Alexander, Robinson & Rainforth, this volume; Staggers, Alexander & Walton, this volume).

Studies on factors contributing to relapse have often focused on measures of problem severity and social stability (for reviews see Marlatt & Gordon, 1985; Miller & Hester, 1986a). For example, patients who lack a stable home or job, and have a severe drinking problem, tend to fare especially poorly in outpatient treatment programs (Miller & Hester, 1986a). Another major factor contributing to relapse and addiction is that alcohol appears to give the individual an alternate form of coping with problems and perceived control over life (Donovan, 1988). In a review of the reasons for alcohol use given by adolescents and young adults, Segal (1983) said:

> it was found that a major motive for such use was to relieve sadness, loneliness, anger, and pressure, as well as to help deal with problems. Alcohol is also used to feel better, to forget problems, to overcome feelings of low self-esteem, and to deal with frustration . . . . Another set of reasons related to alcohol use is that drinking is associated with relaxation, with relief of fatigue, with hot weather, and with overcoming boredom.

According to these studies, "drinking as a social function" is soon joined or replaced by "drinking as a means of coping with needs and problems."

Gorski and Miller (1986) noted similar associations in the recovering adult alcoholic. Stress is a particularly important issue because it appears to worsen other symptoms experienced during the months or years following acute withdrawal. Furthermore, recovering addicts often fail to distinguish between low-stress situations and high-stress situations, and may exhibit excessive reactions to events that would be of small consequence to most people (Gorski & Miller, 1986). Thus, a major need in relapse prevention is to improve a person's coping ability and to find some healthier way to relieve stressful emotions than relapse to alcohol consumption (Segal, 1983; Stockwell & Town, 1989). Along the same lines, Greaves (1980) pointed out that we ask the addict to give up something that seems to relieve stress or give pleasure without offering an immediate replacement for these functions.

Recognizing these problems, many researchers have begun to explore ways to fill the legitimate needs of the recovering addict. Segal (1983), Greaves (1980) and others (e.g., Clarke & Saunders, 1988; Marlatt & George, 1984) have recommended either meditation or relaxation, usually in combination with other active regimens that promote "self-regulation" or "self-control," such as expressive art therapy or physical exercise. Other researchers, inspired primarily by the "tension-reduction" hypothesis of the cause of alcohol abuse (Conger, 1956), have focused on muscle-relaxation techniques (Parker, Gilbert & Thoreson, 1978; Rohsenow, Smith & Johnson, 1985; Strickler, Tomaszewski, Maxwell & Suib, 1979). Meditation and relaxation are of particular interest since they may be candidates for effective broad spectrum approaches to treatment.

The purpose of this experiment was to evaluate the relapse prevention efficacies of one meditation and two relaxation techniques when these are added to the routine treatment program of a municipal alcoholism treatment center (primarily counseling and Alcoholics Anonymous (AA) programs). The four conditions assessed were routine treatment alone (AA and counseling) and routine treatment coupled with either Transcendental Meditation (TM), electromyographic (EMG) biofeedback, or electronic neurotherapy. AA and counseling by alcoholism professionals are widely used treatments, but their success rates tend to be low, especially among severe alcoholics (Miller & Hester, 1986b).

Relaxation and meditation programs have not often been objectively compared with each other in the same experiment. However, recent randomized, longitudinal studies (Alexander, Langer, Newman, Chandler & Davies, 1989; Schneider, Alexander & Wallace, 1992) and meta-analyses (Alexander, Rainforth & Gelderloos, 1991; Alexander, Robinson, & Rainforth, this volume; Dillbeck & Orme-Johnson, 1987; Eppley, Abrams & Shear, 1989) appear to indicate major differences in the physiological and psychological effects of different types of meditation and relaxation.

Transcendental Meditation, a type of meditation originating in the ancient Vedic tradition of India, is taught in a uniform manner through personal instruction by trained teachers (Maharishi Mahesh Yogi, 1963). This form of meditation elicits a state of restful alertness distinctly different from simple eyes-closed rest, as indicated by higher basal skin resistance, lower respiratory rate, lower plasma lactate and differences in an assortment of hormones (reviewed in Dillbeck & Orme-Johnson, 1987; Jevning, Wallace & Beidebach, 1992). Practice of this technique appears to have been helpful in reducing alcohol and drug use in each of 24 studies (reviewed by Alexander et al., this volume; Gelderloos, Walton, Orme-Johnson & Alexander, 1991). These studies varied widely in methodological rigor, but a quantitative meta-analysis adjusting for these and other variables suggests the effectiveness of this technique compared to a number of other treatments (Alexander et al., this volume). There are also over 500 studies which indicate TM has beneficial effects at the physiological, psychological and social/environmental levels–each of the areas identified as important to relapse prevention and recovery from addictions. Such effects have been found to occur across the full range of age, gender, race, severity of drug involvement, and personality variables. [For summaries, see Gelderloos et al. (1991), Alexander et al. (this volume), Walton & Levitsky (this volume).]

Since alcohol is often perceived as "relieving pressure" and producing "relaxation" (Segal, 1983; Stockwell & Town, 1989), there is also a rationale for using muscle relaxation techniques as a component of relapse prevention and alcoholism treatment. Evidence supports EMG biofeedback as a means of reducing tension and anxiety (Budzynski, Stoyva & Adler, 1970; Budzynski, Stoyva, Adler & Mullaney, 1973; Hurley & Meminger, 1992) and apparently alcohol consumption (Denney, Baugh & Hardt, 1991). In the above-mentioned quantitative meta-analysis (Alexander et al., this volume), biofeedback had a larger effect on alcohol abuse than other relaxation techniques studied. Thus, it also was considered to be a reasonable candidate therapy for reducing alcohol abuse.

A third type of technique employed in this experiment was electronic neurotherapy (NT), also known as electrosleep and cerebral electrotherapy (Clemente, 1970; Rosenthal, 1973; Wageneder & St. Schuy, 1966; Wageneder & St. Schuy, 1970). The mechanism of this therapy is not well known, but the procedure has come into use primarily because of considerable enthusiasm in the former USSR, starting in the latter half of the 1940's, over its clinical effects in promoting sleep and relaxation. A preliminary report suggested that the technique had promise in alcoholism treatment (Smith & O'Neil, 1975), but this has not been confirmed.

In this controlled trial of relapse prevention efficacy, severe, chronic, highly transient alcoholics at a residential facility were randomly assigned, following detoxification, to groups who were to receive either TM, EMG biofeedback or electronic neurotherapy along with the routine AA and counseling services of the rehabilitation center. The results from these groups were compared with those of patients who had volunteered for one of the therapies but were subsequently randomly assigned to a "general comparison" group receiving AA and counseling alone. Severe, transient alcoholics of the type studied are known to be among the most prone to relapse as well as the most difficult to follow after release from an institution (Miller & Hester, 1986a). Using intensive follow-up procedures, information was collected on amount of alcohol consumption and a variety of other parameters from over 90% of the subject sample, both at the time of admission and over an 18-month period of follow-up after departure from the institution. (This article is based on a comprehensive progress report to the Institute of Alcohol Abuse and Alcoholism written 10 months before the last subjects taken into the project had completed the study.)

METHODS

Research Site and Subjects

The experiment was conducted on the premises of the Rehabilitation Center for Alcoholics and District of Columbia Veterans Home, Occoquan, Virginia (recently relocated to the D.C. General Hospital), a large facility which draws its patients from the District of Columbia. The subjects were male, inner-city, highly transient, "skid-row"-type alcoholics with long histories of alcohol abuse. (Only males were studied because they represented over 95% of the Center's patient population.) Eighty percent were African Americans. Approximately one-third of the volunteers who were tested and interviewed were excluded from eligibility on the basis of severe brain damage, serious medical problems, IQ's below 80 (Beta Intelligence Test), a diagnosis of psychosis, or previous exposure to one of the special therapies.

Subject selection (Figure 1) was accomplished approximately one week following detoxification. Eligible patients were assigned randomly to hear one of three lectures, each describing a different special therapy and the follow-up procedures of the project. Patients had the option of accepting or rejecting the described therapy; if they rejected the therapy, they were excluded from the study. Two-thirds of those who accepted were given the therapy, while one-

FIGURE 1. Experimental design. As subjects presented for the study they were randomly offered the chance to accept one of the three special treatments. One-third of those who accepted each treatment were then randomly assigned to a control group receiving only routine therapy. Approximately half of each group accepting a special treatment were repeated admissions.

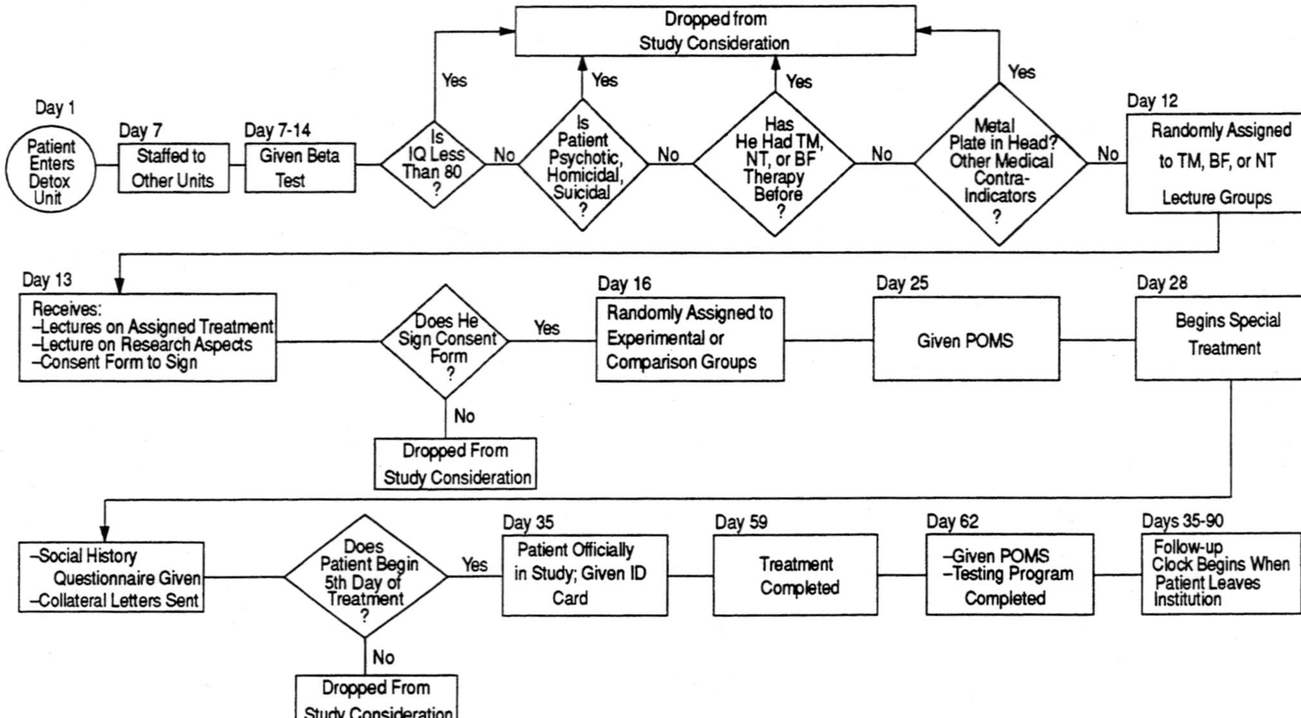

third who accepted were assigned to a control group which received only the routine therapeutic services of the Center. This procedure controlled for the self-selection factor in patient distribution by randomly assigning subjects to all experimental conditions and the routine therapy group.

The patient flow and timeline chart is shown in Figure 2. By the end of the subject intake period (19 months), 913 of the patients who had volunteered for the study had been offered one of the three special therapies; 457 had agreed to participate; and 250 had become subjects in the study by completing the first week of therapy, approximately 10 days after agreeing to participate. The principal reason for the high pre-therapy attrition rate is the short period that most patients usually elected to stay at the institution. Since therapy did not begin until two weeks after moving from the detoxification unit to one of the recovery units, many of the patients (presumably those less committed to recovery) had "eloped" (i.e., prematurely left the Center) prior to initiation of the study treatments. Of the 250 who became subjects, half were randomly assigned to a once-per-month follow-up assessment protocol and the other half to a once-per-six-month protocol; only the data from the former will be discussed here. Although all patients were asked to remain in the institution for the full 90 days, some study participants eloped over the period between 35 and 90 days after admission. The follow-up clock began on the day patients left the institution.

Subject characteristics for each group are summarized in Tables 1-4. For all subjects, average age and years of education were 44.3 and 10.7, respectively. Average IQ was 97.5. The starting number of subjects in each group differed somewhat due to the inability to process more than 6-10 subjects per month in the biofeedback group, while the other groups were not limited in this fashion. Volunteers were allowed to hear the lectures for the other two special therapies at a rate approximately equivalent to that for biofeedback, but some differences in subject intake rate across treatment groups were unavoidable.

Therapeutic Procedures

Each of the special treatments was administered by personnel who enthusiastically believed in its efficacy. In addition, the sched-

FIGURE 2. Patient flow-chart and time line for the experiment, from day one to start of follow-up.

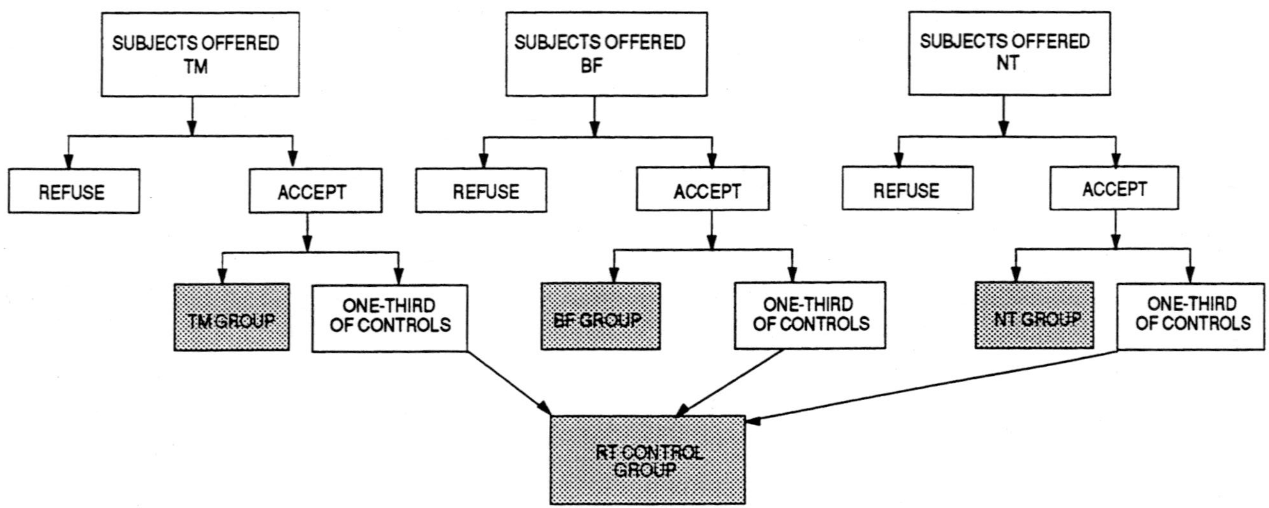

uling and procedures of the three techniques were kept as similar as possible, consonant with valid administration of the treatment. Thus, the three involved similar amounts of training time and a similar amount of personal contact between client and therapist while the subjects were in the institution. Patients in the three special therapy groups received all the routine therapeutic services of the Center (primarily AA and alcoholism counseling) in addition to their special regimen. The routine therapy comparison group received only the routine therapy.

An after-care program was made available to all patients in the three special therapy groups; after leaving the Center, they could receive one "booster" session of their therapy each week, if they wished to. None of the subjects in any of the groups chose to do this. Electronic neurotherapy cannot be practiced independently, and since none of the subjects in this group chose to return for "booster" treatment, this treatment was procedurally the same as the routine treatment comparison group after the patients left the institution. The extent to which subjects continued to participate in AA after leaving the institution was not determined, but Center staff members did not perceive it as high for this population.

Transcendental Meditation. Instruction in the TM technique was provided by certified teachers of TM in the same, uniform manner in which it is taught elsewhere (Roth, 1987). There are seven steps, beginning with the introductory lecture, which briefly discusses the nature of the practice and the benefits that have been observed. Step 2 is a preparatory lecture, giving a person information necessary to prepare for personal instruction. Steps 1 and 2 are conducted on a group basis. Step 3, which usually occurs at the end of the preparatory lecture, is a personal interview by the teacher to ascertain details important for instruction. At this time the pupil can ask any questions which he might have felt uncomfortable asking in the group. Step 4 is the individual instruction in the technique of TM. At the end of a traditional ceremony performed by the teacher, a special sound, or "mantra," is imparted to the pupil, along with the correct procedure for using it. Correct practice does not involve concentration or contemplation. It is a simple technique that emphasizes lack of effort, and can be practiced effectively by persons with less than average intelligence. After instruction, three more steps, consisting of nightly meetings for group practice and feedback from the teacher concerning the specific experiences of each pupil, are carried out. Each meeting requires about one and one-half hours. The total time spent with the teacher during these seven steps is nine to ten hours. Thereafter, Transcendental Meditation is practiced for 15 to 20 minutes twice a day.

In this study, while the patients were in the institution, meditations took place in group sessions at scheduled times, once before breakfast and once before dinner. This procedure began after personal instruction and continued for 20 consecutive weekdays under the supervision of a TM instructor. On the intervening weekends there were also group meditations, but these were unmonitored and were outside the Center's official program. Group meditation (which is available in local TM centers for persons who have time to attend) was viewed as having several advantages, namely: (1) promoting regularity in participation, (2) enabling quantification of frequency of practice, and (3) providing social facilitation for the practice of meditation. In addition to conducting the group meditations twice a day, the TM teachers were available for "checking" the technique of the individual patients. Frequent use of this service was encouraged to insure that each patient's practice remained correct.

EMG Biofeedback (BF). Electromyographic biofeedback was used in training subjects to relax muscular tension. It provides clear information (feedback) on the tension level in special muscle groups as an aid in teaching individuals to relax those muscles. The goal was then to generalize that muscle control: first from the training site to other muscles, and then from the training session to everyday situations in the patient's life.

In each feedback session, the patient was seated in a comfortable chair with bioelectrically sensitive electrodes affixed to the forehead by means of a headband. Signals from these sensors were fed into the biofeedback apparatus and were converted into a series of clicking sounds which the patient heard via a pair of earphones. Click rate was directly related to the amount of tension in the frontal area. The patient's task was to sit back and relax, and by relaxing to reduce the frequency of clicking sounds. When he had become proficient at this, his attention was focused on the various proprioceptive and interoceptive sensations that accompanied the decrease in feedback clicks.

BF was given to individual subjects in 20 daily, one-hour sessions, with the time of day depending on where a person fell in the sequence of subjects treated in a day by the therapist (E.W.). The patients were instructed to practice what they had learned for one additional 20-minute period before dinner on training days and for one 20-minute period in the morning and one in the evening on weekends and after the conclusion of training. Thus, the instructed frequency and duration of BF was the same as for TM. In training session numbers 5, 10, 15 and 20, patients listened to tapes containing suggestions promoting the relaxation of individual muscle groups. They were not given feedback at these times, but were connected to the recording portion of the apparatus so that the biofeedback therapist could determine muscle tension levels. The patients learned the suggestions so that they could be self-administered during relaxation periods outside of the training environment. Group practice of BF was not part of the protocol.

Neurotherapy (NT). Electronic neurotherapy consists of the application of low-intensity pulses of interrupted direct current, usually at a frequency of 100/sec, with a pulse duration of one msec through electrodes carried on a headband. The cathodes are placed over the orbits, and the anodes over the mastoid processes. NT was administered using the Neurotone 101 (Neuro Systems, Inc., Garland, Texas). Before beginning the session, the current is adjusted to the point where a person just begins to feel a tingle, and is then decreased to just below the awareness threshold. A dial and lights continue to register the passage of current. Patients were treated in daily sessions five days a week for three weeks. Sessions were 30 minutes in length. Since the technique requires the use of laboratory equipment, it cannot be self-administered. As in the case of TM and BF, this therapy was administered by therapists enthusiastic about its effects. An aftercare program for booster treatments was offered, but no subject took advantage of it after leaving the Center. This means that any benefits derived would have to come from the 15 treatments given at the beginning of the study. Thus, in effect, this group may have been more of a placebo control than a special treatment group. It is not possible to say what the outcome might have been had these subjects continued with a treatment frequency similar to the frequency of the independent practice of TM and BF.

Routine Therapy (RT). The routine therapy in the Center included counseling by professionals experienced in alcoholism treatment (who were available in the institution every weekday), attendance at frequent meetings of Alcoholics Anonymous, and optional instruction in occupational therapy in shop facilities, which few patients took advantage of. Physical exercise was encouraged in those whose physical condition permitted it. Subjects in the RT group received only routine therapy.

Data Gathering Instruments

Data gathering instruments were as follows: (1) the Social History Questionnaire or intake interview, (2) a Follow-Up (abbreviated) Version of the Social History Questionnaire, which was filled out by the interviewer at each of the planned monthly interviews, (3) the Beta Intelligence Test, and (4) the Profile of Mood States.

The Social History Questionnaire (SHQ) and its Follow-Up Version. These were revised from an instrument developed for the Bureau of Alcoholism of the Department of Mental Health of the City of New York by one of us (S.S.S.). The Pretreatment SHQ was administered before each patient began therapy. It collected data on a variety of objective measures for assessing patient history, with emphasis on the past year and on present status. The areas of interest were amount and pattern of drinking (e.g., days not drinking, days having 1-2 drinks, days having 3-6 drinks, days having 6+ drinks), employment record, income level, previous hospitalizations and incarcerations, residential stability, and family status. The forms were precoded and could be machine scored. A shortened version of the Pretreatment SHQ, which could be filled out by an interviewer in 10 minutes, was employed in the monthly follow-up sessions. This form was appropriate for either telephone interviews (the large majority) or interviews in person (only when a patient could not be located by phone). It covered the same categories as the Pretreatment SHQ, but was shorter because it involved only the previous month.

Beta Intelligence Test. This easily administered, culture-fair, intelligence test was employed as a basis for excluding some individuals from the study (scores below 80). It was anticipated that persons with scores below 80 might be incapable of practicing the special techniques.

Profile of Mood States (POMS). The Profile of Mood States is a factor-analytically derived adjective checklist designed to collect information on mood or emotional state. It is scored for six different dimensions: tension-anxiety, depression-dejection, anger-hostility, vigor-activity, fatigue-inertia, and confusion-bewilderment. The test was developed in the 1960's (McNair, Lorr & Droppleman, 1971) and has been used for assessing mood change in alcoholics and marijuana users (Mirin, Shapiro, Meyer, Pillard & Fisher, 1971; Nathan, Titler, Lowenstein, Solomon & Rossi, 1970; Nathan, Zare, Ferneau & Lowenstein, 1970).

Follow-Up Procedures

The most important aspect of the project's data collection was the intensive follow-up program. The follow-up techniques were based on procedures devised by Sobell and Sobell (1973; 1976) that enabled them to maintain contact with 69 out of 70 subjects over a 2-year period. The most helpful practice for maintaining frequent contact was that of obtaining information during the pretreatment interview about who the patients were in contact with, where they tended to stay during different parts of the year, and the phone numbers and addresses of as many significant people in their lives as possible. Patients were questioned to determine daily drinking disposition and, where applicable, frequency of practice of their special therapy, as well as the major dimensions tapped by the Pretreatment SHQ. All follow-up interviews were recorded, with prior permission of the subjects, and were randomly spot-checked by one of us (E.T.) for interrogative neutrality by the interviewer and for the accuracy with which information on the follow-up form matched that in the spoken record. Friends and relatives whose names were provided by the patients were contacted at semiannual intervals as one means of verifying the subjects' reports. These collateral sources were asked questions similar to those on the Follow-Up SHQ administered to the subjects, and were also asked to give their opinion of the patients' status.

Project patients were not interviewed by phone when it was apparent that they had been drinking. The veracity of the self-reports was checked in the following three ways. (1) When interviews were conducted in person (i.e., when the patient could not be reached by phone), in-field breath tests (Sober Meter 5M6, Luckey Laboratories) were administered at the end of the interview to determine blood alcohol concentration, as long as this procedure did not compromise the subject (e.g., job situation). (2) The dates of all reported incarcerations and hospitalizations were verified with the institutions in question. (3) When information supplied by a collateral was markedly different from that supplied by a subject, further contacts were made with one or both of the individuals to resolve the disparity. Disagreement between the patients' self-report concerning alcohol consumption and alcohol-related events (e.g., incarcerations, hospitalizations) was less than 5% for each of the three methods employed for verification. It is worth noting that the amount of disagreement between self-reports and sources of verification dropped markedly during the first several interviews. It seems clear that in some cases the subjects' observation of the verification process in operation served to increase the accuracy of self-reports.

Once subjects had officially entered the study, the overall loss rate (i.e., subjects not contacted within six months of their last scheduled interview) was only 5%. Contact with patients within one month of the time they were scheduled for an interview was 81%. Although Tables 1-4 indicate that there was a decreasing number of subjects for whom data were available at successive follow-up points, this was *not* due to increased drop-out rate or progressive loss of contact with subjects over time. The reason for the decreasing numbers of subjects at 12 and 18 months was that the follow-up was not yet complete when the progress report providing the data for this paper was written. There is no apparent selection bias which might have produced a difference in subjects at the beginning of project intake (for whom follow-up data were complete) compared to subjects taken into the study at a later time (for whom follow-up data were incomplete). The missing data were approximately evenly distributed across groups.

TABLE 1. Effects of Transcendental Meditation on Alcohol Consumption at Pretreatment and at 1-6, 7-12, and 13-18 Months of Follow-Up

	Pretreatment	1-6 Mo. Post		7-2 Mo. Post		13-18 Mo. Post	
	% Days	% Days (or opp.[c])	Pre-Post Difference	% Days (or opp.[c])	Pre-Post Difference	% Days (or opp.[c])	Pre-Post Difference
Alcohol Consumption							
Days Not Drinking[a,b]	26.2	71.7[d]	+45.5	64.6[d]	+38.4	76.3[e]	+50.1
Days Having 1-2 Drinks	6.7	0.4	– 6.3	0.8	– 5.9	0.5	– 6.2
Days Having 3-6 Drinks	11.3	3.3	– 8.0	5.0	– 6.3	3.4	– 7.9
Days Having 6+ Drinks	55.8	24.6	–31.2	29.6	–26.2	19.8	–36.0
Practice of TM[c]	N/A	(41.0)	N/A	(33.0)	N/A	(26.0)	N/A
Sample Characteristics							
Sample Size	35	35		32		18	
Mean Beta (I.Q.)	96.4						
Mean Age	44.3						
Mean Years of Education	10.7						

[a]Drinks defined as 1 oz. of 86-proof beverage or equivalent in other beverages. [b]Data are percentage of "drinking opportunity days" (i.e., days when subject was not in an institution). [c]Percentage of total opportunities (two per day) that subjects actually practiced the therapy. [d]Significantly ($p < .05$) different from RT group. [e]Significantly different from both the RT and the NT groups.

TABLE 2. Effects of EMG Biofeedback on Alcohol Consumption at Pretreatment and at 1-6, 7-12. and 13-18 Months of Follow-Up

	Pretreatment	1-6 Mo. Post		7-12 Mo. Post		13-18 Mo. Post	
	% Days	% Days (or opp.[c])	Pre-Post Difference	% Days (or opp.[c])	Pre-Post Difference	% Days (or opp.[c])	Pre-Post Difference
Alcohol Consumption							
Days Not Drinking[a,b]	21.3	68.0[d]	+46.7	66.8[d]	+45.5	79.2[e]	+57.9
Days Having 1-2 Drinks	7.2	0.5	– 6.7	0.7	– 6.5	0.5	– 6.7
Days Having 3-6 Drinks	12.1	3.7	– 8.4	4.7	– 7.4	2.9	– 9.2
Days Having 6+ Drinks	59.4	27.8	–31.6	27.8	–31.6	17.4	–42.0
Practice of BF[c]	N/A	(29.0)	N/A	(32.0)	N/A	(20.0)	N/A
Sample Characteristics							
Sample Size	24	24		22		13	
Mean Beta (I.Q.)	98.4						
Mean Age	44.3						
Mean Years of Education	10.7						

[a]Drinks defined as 1 oz. of 86-proof beverage or equivalent in other beverages. [b]Data are percentage of "drinking opportunity days" (i.e., days when subject was not in an institution). [c]Percentage of total opportunities (two per day) that subjects actually practiced the therapy. [d]Significantly ($p < .05$) different from RT group. [e]Significantly different from both the RT and the NT groups.

TABLE 3. Effects of Neurotherapy on Alcohol Consumption at Pretreatment and at 1-6, 7-12. and 13-18 Months of Follow-Up

	Pretreatment	1-6 Mo. Post		7-12 Mo. Post		13-18 Mo. Post	
	% Days	% Days	Pre-Post Difference	% Days	Pre-Post Difference	% Days	Pre-Post Difference
Alcohol Consumption							
Days Not Drinking[a,b]	28.1	59.8	+31.7	55.3	+27.2	60.5	+32.4
Days Having 1-2 Drinks	3.6	9.3	+ 5.7	3.6	0	3.3	– 0.3
Days Having 3-6 Drinks	8.0	9.8	+ 1.8	13.2	+ 5.2	11.8	+ 3.8
Days Having 6+ Drinks	60.3	21.1	–39.2	27.9	–32.4	24.4	–35.9
Sample Characteristics							
Sample Size	28	28		26		18	
Mean Beta (I.Q.)	97.5						
Mean Age	44.4						
Mean Years of Education	10.8						

[a]Drinks defined as 1 oz. of 86-proof beverage or equivalent in other beverages. [b]Data are percentage of "drinking opportunity days" (i.e., days when subject was not in an institution).

TABLE 4. Effects of Routine Therapy on Alcohol Consumption at Pretreatment and at 1-6, 7-12, and 13-18 Months of Follow-Up

	Pretreatment	1-6 Mo. Post		7-12 Mo. Post		13-18 Mo. Post	
	% Days	% Days	Pre-Post Difference	% Days	Pre-Post Difference	% Days	Pre-Post Difference
Alcohol Consumption							
Days Not Drinking[a,b]	31.8	50.5	+18.7	52.9	+21.1	45.7	+13.9
Days Having 1-2 Drinks	3.4	11.3	+ 7.9	3.8	+ 0.4	4.4	+ 1.0
Days Having 3-6 Drinks	7.5	11.9	+ 4.4	13.9	+ 6.4	16.1	+ 8.6
Days Having 6+ Drinks	57.3	26.3	–31.0	29.4	–27.9	33.8	–23.5
Sample Characteristics							
Sample Size	31	31		25		18	
Mean Beta (I.Q.)	97.5						
Mean Age	44.4						
Mean Years of Education	10.8						

[a]Drinks defined as 1 oz. of 86-proof beverage or equivalent in other beverages. [b]Data are percentage of "drinking opportunity days" (i.e., days when subject was not in an institution).

RESULTS

Validation of Self-Report Drinking Data with an Objective Measure

Validity of self-report data concerning the drinking behavior of alcoholics is often a problem, especially in a severely alcoholic population such as the present one (e.g., Maisto, McKay & Connors, 1990). One might anticipate greater self-report accuracy from individuals maintaining sobriety than from those who are currently drinking. Consequently, an effort was made to determine the agreement between the self-report data collected and an objective index of drinking (in-field breath test). Portable in-field breath tests were administered to determine blood alcohol level at the end of 52 consecutive in-field interviews (i.e., those subjects who could not be reached by phone). While giving their self-report data, the subjects were unaware that they were going to receive a breath test. Of the 52 subjects administered the breath test, it was found that 24 had ingested alcohol on that day, and 28 had not. There was close agreement between self-report data and blood-alcohol level in 83% of the cases. Of the nine cases not showing close agreement, seven were within the accepted measurement error of the breath test. Only two cases (4%) involved a major disagreement. Both these instances occurred when the subjects had been drinking on the day of the interview. In the other 22 cases where there had been drinking on the day of the interview, there was no serious disagreement between the self-report and objective measures of alcohol consumption. Furthermore, any selection factor that might have resulted from using, for in-field breath tests, only those subjects most difficult to track might be expected to mitigate against the veracity of the reports obtained. As mentioned above, there was also less than 5% disagreement between subject self-reports, collateral reports and institutional records of incarcerations and hospitalizations.

These data suggest that, with this subject population, with the monthly interview technique employed, and with the rapport established by the interviewers during the frequent contacts, these self-report data on alcohol consumption are sufficiently reliable to support the accuracy of the outcomes reported below.

Increase in Percent Days Not Drinking

The main findings from the drinking parameters studied–percent nondrinking days and percent of the subjects completely abstinent–are presented here. Percent Days Not Drinking was arrived at by dividing drinking opportunity days (number of days not in a treatment facility, hospital or jail) into the number of days in the preceding six months on which no alcohol was ingested. All groups, control as well as experimental, showed a large reduction in drinking after leaving the Center, compared with their reported level prior to entry (Tables 1-4).

The data shown in Tables 1-4 indicate that 6, 12 and 18 months after leaving the Center the TM and BF groups had considerably more non-drinking days than the RT and NT groups, both in absolute terms and in terms of mean individual pre-post-treatment differences. With individual pre-post-treatment differences as the measure, the TM and BF groups showed from 24 to 39 percent fewer drinking days than the NT and RT groups. Separate analyses of variance were performed on the groups at each follow-up point. (Because data compilation was not complete for all subjects at the 12-and 18-month follow-up points at the time of data analysis, it was not feasible to perform a single trend analysis of variance on all of the data.) The analyses of variance showed a significant difference in treatment effect between the four groups at each follow-up point (at 6 mo., $p < .01$; at 12 mo., $p < .05$; at 18 mo., $p < .01$). *Posthoc* comparisons (Duncan's Multiple Range Test) were performed for the analyses at each follow-up point. At 6 and 12 months, the TM and BF groups were both drinking significantly less than the RT control group. The NT group fell in between the RT group and the TM and BF groups, and it was not significantly different from any of these groups. At 18 months, the TM and BF groups were drinking significantly less than not only the RT group but also the NT group. Neither the NT and RT groups nor the TM and BF groups were significantly different from each other.

Increase in Percentage of Subjects Completely Abstinent

Figure 3 compares for each group the number and percentage of subjects who were completely abstinent and had opportunities to

FIGURE 3. Average percentage of subjects given routine therapy (RT) alone or along with one of three special treatments, Transcendental Meditation (TM), EMG biofeedback (BF), or neurotherapy (NT), who were completely abstinent from 1-6, 7-12, and 13-18 months.

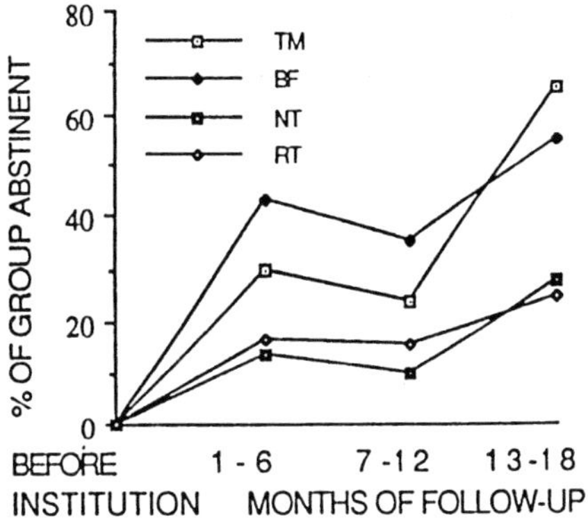

drink (i.e., were hospitalized or incarcerated on less than half of follow-up days). The percentage of subjects completely abstinent in the TM and BF groups was from 1.5 to 2.5 times as great as in the NT and RT comparison groups at each follow-up interval. The largest improvement was seen at 18 months for both the TM group and the BF group, presumably a reflection of cumulative benefit from continued practice of the techniques in the life situation. At each follow-up point, a chi-square test for proportions was performed, with the Pearson correction for continuity. These initial omnibus tests, simultaneously comparing all four groups, fell short of significance: *p*'s = 0.08, 0.22, 0.07. However, given the similarity of results on the percent non-drinking days measure for the two active treatment groups (TM and BF) and in order to increase the power of the tests, the results for these two groups were combined; similarly the results for the control group (RT) were combined with those for the NT group (which was essentially a placebo control–see Discussion). The combined TM and BF groups had more subjects who had been completely abstinent since leaving the treatment center than the combined RT and NT groups; for 6, 12 and 18 months, *p*'s = 0.02, 0.057, and 0.009, respectively, using the Z test for difference between two proportions (one-tailed). Using this test, the proportions abstinent in the TM and BF groups were not significantly different from each other at any follow-up point, nor were those for the RT and NT groups different from each other.

Psychological Change

Responses on the Profile of Mood States given before the special techniques (institutional day 25) and after completion of the institutional phase of instruction and practice of these techniques (institutional day 62) indicated a different degree of elevation of mood and decrease in negative affect with the different treatments. This pre-post-treatment change reached significance ($p < .05$) on five of six scales for the TM group and two of six scales for the BF group. None of the changes was significant for the NT and RT groups.

Adherence with TM and BF Practices

In the institutional phase of the study, the twice-daily group meditation sessions were therapist-monitored on weekdays. For the unmonitored weekend sessions, subjects were admitted to the meditation room by an alcoholism counselor. Attendance was recorded unobtrusively for both types of sessions. Attendance at the monitored group sessions was 90.2%, and was equally high (89.6%) for the unmonitored sessions. Attendance at BF and NT therapy sessions was similarly high (88.6% and 94.8%, respectively). Adherence to the special practices after leaving the institution is given in Tables 1-4. The TM subjects reported adherence with opportunities to practice their technique after leaving the treatment center (Table 1) that compares favorably with that observed for the general population (e.g., Delmonte, 1980; Williams, Francis & Durham, 1976). At six months, for example, the TM group reported practicing the technique 41% of the total opportunities (twice per day). The breakdown, in terms of regularity of individuals, was that 27% practiced TM more than 75% of the opportunities, 27% practiced an average of half the opportunities, and 45% practiced irregularly or not at all. BF subjects reported similar rates (Table 2), suggesting that adherence with the regimen is not an impediment to the use of these techniques with this severely impaired patient population. Moreover, adherence rates for the two groups appear sufficiently close to warrant direct comparison of the groups throughout the study, and they are high enough to permit evaluation of the long-term effect of practice of these two procedures on drinking behavior.

DISCUSSION

In the present study, the TM and BF (active treatment) groups exhibited significant increases in percent non-drinking days that were considerably larger than those recorded for the two control groups (RT and NT). The NT group did not differ from the RT group at any of the follow-up points on this measure, and similarly, there were no differences between the TM and BF groups.

Many in alcohol relapse prevention consider the number of subjects completely abstinent to be the most important indicator of therapeutic success (see for example Gorski & Miller, 1986). Sixty-five percent of the Transcendental Meditation group and 55% of the EMG biofeedback group reported complete abstinence 18 months after leaving the treatment center, compared to 25% for the routine therapy and 28% for the neurotherapy comparison groups. The rates for the routine therapy and neurotherapy groups are comparable to those reported for all adults completing treatment for alcohol and drug dependence, i.e., about one-third remain abstinent after the first 90 days of follow-up (Hunt et al., 1971; Surgeon General, 1988). Thus, the complete abstinence rates for the TM and BF groups represent large improvements (1.5 to 2.5 fold) over those in this study who received counseling and AA therapy alone as well as those in the general population who complete similar routine treatment.

Both TM and BF were associated with improvements on subscales of the Profile of Mood States during the institutional phase of these treatments. The TM group showed significant improvement on five of the six subscales, while the BF group improved significantly on two. These changes are consistent with the treatment outcome data in follow-up.

These results appear to support the usefulness of Transcendental Meditation and EMG biofeedback in alcohol relapse prevention. They suggest that even seriously deteriorated alcoholics with little social or financial support are capable of deriving benefit from these continuing, primarily self-administered, programs. However, a number of methodological questions deserve special consideration.

The validity of self-report in the area of substance abuse is known to vary widely. This is due mainly to differences in both methodological and contextual variables (Maisto et al., 1990). However, some researchers have found that the self-reports of alcoholic persons can be accurate, especially when they are corroborated by other sources (Sobell & Sobell, 1973; Sobell & Sobell, 1976). The present study used methods previously found by the Sobells [one of whom (L.S.) consulted on this aspect of the project] to be most helpful in verifying and increasing the accuracy of self-reports in alcoholism studies. Three types of checks were employed: (1) in-field breath tests, (2) verification of the dates of all reported incarcerations and hospitalizations with the institutions in question, (3) the reports of significant others, including further contacts with both collaterals and subjects when there was apparent disagreement. Disagreement between the patients' self-report concerning alcohol consumption and alcohol-related events was less than 5% for each of the three methods of verification. Moreover, the amount of disagreement between self-reports and sources of verification dropped markedly during the first several interviews (probably, as noted, as a result of the subjects' observation of the verification process in operation). The loss rate (i.e., subjects not contacted within six months of their last scheduled interview) was approximately 5%. Contact with patients within one month of the time they were scheduled for an interview was 81%. This success rate in making scheduled monthly contacts reduces the possibility that a selective trait bias associated with patient unreliability in maintaining contact may have significantly influenced the outcome.

The similarity of results for the routine therapy and neurotherapy groups is another factor supporting the conclusion of therapeutic efficacy for the TM and BF procedures. Electronic neurotherapy involves the use of an impressive-appearing piece of apparatus. Electrodes are fitted onto a patient's head. A dial and lights register the passage of current. Subjects were told that the device promotes relaxation and sleep, and indeed most of them were observed to sleep or drowse through most of the sessions. Thus, for this event, NT constituted a useful attention-placebo control for TM and BF, at least during the period immediately following departure from the institution. Inspection of the data indicates that NT subjects did not drink appreciably less than the RT comparison subjects for any time period, including the first month after leaving the institution (not shown in graphs above). This may strengthen confidence that the therapeutic effect observed for TM and BF was not due to attentional or expectancy differences, especially for the first follow-up period.

To prevent self-selection bias, subjects were assigned by a random process to the subject pool for one of the three special therapies. In addition, the routine therapy group was formed by a second process of random assignment so that it consisted of equal numbers of subjects who had agreed to participate in the special therapies but instead were placed in the control group.

Three precautions were taken to guard against experimenter/subject expectancy bias. First, an explicit effort was made to present the experiment to the subjects as a study of the effects of the therapy which they received (including the routine-therapy comparison group). Second, in the institutional phase, each of the therapies was administered by individuals who were enthusiastic about their technique. BF and NT were administered at the Center well before the project began, and they were provided by persons who strongly believed in their respective effectiveness (e.g., for NT see Smith & O'Neil, 1975). Third, once the subjects left the institution, the only relationship they had with the study was with follow-up interviewers. Although not blind to the general hypotheses of the study, these interviewers were mainly students specializing in alcoholism studies in the mental health program of a local community college who had little interest in the special therapies as such. Their objective was to develop skill in interacting and maintaining contact with the project's population of highly transient, severe alcoholics. Thus, the accuracy of the data-gathering procedures, the low loss and high contact rates, the agreement in results between the routine therapy and neurotherapy groups, and the precautions taken to avoid subject self-selection, unequal expectations and experimenter bias, all reduce the likelihood that observed abstinence differences between groups were due to artifacts introduced by the experimental methodology.

It should be noted that, following departure from the institution, a relatively large reduction in drinking days was found even in the RT and NT groups. This effect was not as prominent for the complete abstinence measure. This result probably reflects a selection factor which resulted from accepting for the study only those subjects who remained in the institution for three or more weeks past release from the detoxification unit and successfully completed the first week of special treatment. Presumably, only the subjects most committed to overcoming their drinking problem made the extra effort to stay for this period of time.

Treatment adherence for the two techniques was similar both within and outside the institution. Adherence while outside the institution was lower than when inside, probably due to the absence of organized group support for the specific therapies once patients were released. If such support could be provided, the therapeutic result might be even larger than that observed here.

The factors promoting relapse are thought to be largely the same as those underlying the original addictive behaviors. Paramount are the reinforcing properties of the addictive experience, the perceived control it provides the individual, and its function as an alternate form of coping (Donovan, 1988). Other, related factors known to predict addiction and relapse include negative emotional states, interpersonal conflicts, social pressure and difficulty dealing with stress, or, more broadly, poor self-efficacy (Cummings, Gordon & Marlatt, 1980; Gorski & Miller, 1986; Marlatt, 1985; Marlatt & George, 1984). Thus, the major goal in relapse prevention is to provide a positive way to relieve stress and negative affect while also improving a person's self-esteem and ability to deal effectively with a changing environment, including his or her ability to act from a more established internal locus of control (Greenstreet, 1988; Klajner, Hartman & Sobell, 1984; Marlatt, 1985; Segal, 1983).

Evidence exists for the ability of either EMG biofeedback, other relaxation techniques or electronic neurotherapy to relieve anxiety (e.g. Budzynski et al., 1970; Budzynski et al., 1973; Cole, Pomerleau & Harris, 1992; Denney et al., 1991; Ford, Stroebel, Strong & Szarek, 1983; Hurley, 1980; Hurley & Meminger, 1992; Smith &

O'Neil, 1975). A review of earlier research concluded that the effects of these types of relaxation on alcoholism were difficult to interpret due to a variety of methodological problems (Klajner et al., 1984). However, results of a more recent statistical meta-analysis (Alexander et al., this volume) which controlled for methodological differences clearly suggests that some of these procedures are effective in reducing addictions and relapse.

A body of research on the effects of the Transcendental Meditation technique on a number of factors relevant to the hypothesized causes of addiction and relapse exists. [For recent results and reviews see Alexander et al. (1991), Alexander et al. (this volume), Dillbeck & Orme-Johnson (1987), Eppley et al. (1989), Gelderloos et al. (1991), Jevning et al. (1992), Walton & Levitsky (this volume).] These studies indicate that TM has a beneficial effect on these variables.

The present study indicates the acceptability of the types of treatments tested here for severe, skid-row-type alcoholics. Each of the three special treatments was embraced by the groups assigned them. The majority of patients and staff were unfamiliar with TM at the outset of the project, unlike BF and NT, which were already practiced at the Center. However, by the end of the project, TM was widely accepted and received a large number of staff referrals of subjects who did not meet the project's inclusion criteria.

Based on considerations of cost and effectiveness, Greenstreet (1988) has argued for the superiority of broad spectrum approaches in alcoholism treatment. While he focused most attention on the community-reinforcement approach, an outpatient treatment based on behavior modification (Azrin, Sisson, Meyers, & Godley, 1982; Hunt & Azrin, 1973), the present study suggests that the Transcendental Meditation technique or EMG biofeedback might also become the basis of cost-effective, outpatient approaches. Alternatively, either of these procedures could be incorporated easily into other successful programs, with a reasonable likelihood of improving the outcome. Certainly, further testing of Transcendental Meditation and EMG biofeedback in prevention of relapse to alcoholism is justified.

Summary and Conclusions

Percent nondrinking days and abstinence rates, determined by monthly interviews and a "convergent validity" approach involving in-field breath tests and reports of collaterals and institutions with whom the patients had contact, were compared in 118 low-resource, transient, severe, chronic alcoholics at 6, 12 and 18 months after they left a treatment facility. Two to three weeks after completion of detoxification, randomly assigned patients received routine treatment alone or along with one of three special treatments: Transcendental Meditation, EMG biofeedback, or electronic neurotherapy. The main outcome was that addition of Transcendental Meditation or biofeedback to the routine AA and counseling treatment produced large improvements in relapse prevention beyond AA and counseling alone or AA and counseling plus neurotherapy. The effectiveness of Transcendental Meditation and biofeedback was roughly equal, but neurotherapy had no significant effect on relapse at any time point. These results indicate that Transcendental Meditation and EMG biofeedback are capable of increasing the effectiveness of routine therapies such as AA and counseling at preventing relapse to alcoholism.

REFERENCES

Alexander, C. N., Langer, E. J., Newman, R. I., Chandler, H. M., & Davies, J. L. (1989). Transcendental Meditation, mindfulness, and longevity: An experimental study with the elderly. *Journal of Personality and Social Psychology, 57*, 950-964.

Alexander, C. N., Rainforth, M.V., & Gelderloos, P. (1991). Transcendental Meditation, self actualization and psychological health: A conceptual overview and statistical meta-analysis. *Journal of Social Behavior and Personality, 6*, 189-247.

Alexander, C. N., Robinson, P., & Rainforth, M. (this volume). Transcendental Meditation: A comprehensive approach for the treatment and prevention of substance dependence. *Alcoholism Treatment Quarterly.*

Aron, A., & Aron, E. N. (1980). The Transcendental Meditation program's effect on addictive behavior. *Addictive Behaviors, 5*, 3-12.

Azrin, N. H., Sisson, R.W., Meyers, R., & Godley, M. (1982). Alcoholism treatment by disulfiram and community-reinforcement therapy. *Journal of Behavior Therapy and Experimental Psychiatry, 13*, 105-112.

Budzynski, T., Stoyva, J., & Adler, C. (1970). Feedback-induced relaxation: Application to tension headache. *Journal of Behavior Therapy and Psychiatry, 1*, 205-211.

Budzynski, T. H, Stoyva, J. M., Adler, C. S., & Mullaney, M. A. (1973). EMG biofeedback and tension headache: A controlled outcome study. *Psychosomatic Medicine, 35*, 484-496.

Clarke, J. C., & Saunders, J. B. (1988). *Alcoholism and Problem drinking: Theories and treatment.* New York: Pergamon Press.

Clemente, C. D. (1970). Basal forebrain structures and the electrical induction of sleep. In N. L. Wulfsohn, & A. Sances (Eds.), *The nervous system and electric currents: Proceeding of the Annual National Conference of the Neuroelectric Society, 1*, 135-136.

Cole, P. A., Pomerleau, C. S., & Harris, J. K. (1992). The effects of nonconcurrent and concurrent relaxation training on cardiovascular reactivity to a psychological stressor. *Journal of Behavioral Medicine, 15*, 407-414.

Conger, J. J. (1956). Reinforcement theory and the dynamics of alcoholism. *Quarterly Journal of Studies of Alcohol, 17*, 296-305.

Cummings, C., Gordon. J., & Marlatt, G. (1980). Relapse: Strategies of prevention and prediction. In W. Miller, (Ed.), *The addictive behaviors.* Oxford: Pergamon Press.

Delmonte, M. M. (1980). Personality characteristics and regularity of meditation. *Psychological Reports, 46*, 703-712.

Denney, M.R., Baugh, J. L., & Hardt, H. D. (1991). Sobriety outcome after alcoholism treatment with biofeedback participation: A pilot inpatient study. *The International Journal of the Addictions, 26 , 335-341.*

Dillbeck, M. C., & Orme-Johnson, D.W. (1987). Physiological differences between Transcendental Meditation and rest. *American Psychologist, 42*, 879-881.

Donovan, D. M. (1988). Assessment of addictive behaviors: Implications of an emerging biopsychosocial model. In D.M. Donovan, & G.A. Marlatt, (Eds.), *Assessment of addictive behaviors* (pp. 3-47). New York: The Guilford Press.

Eppley, K., Abrams, A., & Shear, J. (1989). The differential effects of relaxation techniques on trait anxiety: A meta-analysis. *Journal of Clinical Psychology, 45*, 957-974.

Ford, M. R., Stroebel, C. F., Strong, P., & Szarek, B. L. (1983). Quieting response training: Long-term evaluation of a clinical biofeedback practice. *Biofeedback and Self-Regulation, 8*, 265-278.

Gelderloos P., Walton, K. G., Orme-Johnson, D.W., & Alexander, C. N. (1991). Effectiveness of the Transcendental Meditation program in preventing and treating substance misuse: A review. *International Journal of the Addictions, 26*, 293-325.

Gorski, T. T., & Miller, M. (1986). *Staying sober.* Independence, Missouri: Independence Press.

Greaves, G. B. (1980). An existential theory of drug dependence. In D. Lettieri, M. Sayers, & H. Pearson (Eds.), *Theories of drug abuse.* Washington, DC: National Institute on Drug Abuse.

Greenstreet, R. L. (1988). *Cost-effective alternatives in alcoholism treatment.* Springfield, Illinois: Charles C Thomas.

Hunt, G. M., & Azrin, N. H. (1973). A community-reinforcement approach to alcoholism. *Behavior Research and Therapy, 11*, 91-104.

Hunt, W. A., Barnett, L. W., & Branch, L. G. (1971). Relapse rates in addiction programs. *Journal Clinical Psychology, 27*, 455-466.

Hurley, J. D. (1980). Differential effects of hypnosis, biofeedback training, and trophotropic responses on anxiety, ego strength, and locus of control. *Journal of Clinical Psychology, 36*, 503-507.

Hurley, J. D., & Meminger, S. R. (1992). A relapse-prevention program: Effects of electromyographic training on high and low levels of state and trait anxiety. *Perceptual and Motor Skills, 74*, 699-705.

Jevning, R., Wallace, R. K., & Beidebach, M. (1992). The physiology of meditation: A review. A wakeful hypometabolic integrated response. *Neuroscience and Biobehavioral Reviews, 16*, 415-424.

Klajner, F., Hartman, L. M., & Sobell, M. B. (1984). Treatment of substance abuse by relaxation training: A review of its rationale, efficacy and mechanisms. *Addictive Behaviors, 9*, 41-55.

McNair, D. M., Lorr, M., & Droppleman, L. F. (1971). *Profile of mood states.* San Diego, CA: EdITS/Educational and Industrial Testing Service, Inc.

Maharishi Mahesh Yogi (1963). *Science of being and art of living: Transcendental Meditation.* New York: Signet.

Maisto, S. A., McKay, J. R., & Connors, G. J. (1990). Self-report issues in substance abuse: State of the art and future directions. *Behavioral Assessment, 12*, 117-134.

Marlatt, G. A. (1985). Cognitive factors in the relapse process. In G. A. Marlatt, & J. R. Gordon (Eds.), *Relapse prevention: Maintenance strategies in the treatment of addictive behaviors.* New York: The Guilford Press.

Marlatt, G. A., & George, W. H. (1984). Relapse prevention: Introduction and overview of the model. *British Journal of the Addictions, 79*, 261-272.

Marlatt, G. A. & Gordon, J. R. (Eds.). (1985). *Relapse prevention: Maintenance strategies in the treatment of addictive behaviors.* New York: The Guilford Press.

Miller, W. R., & Hester, R. K. (1986a). Inpatient alcoholism treatment: Who benefits? *American Psychologist, 41*, 794-805.

Miller, W. R., & Hester, R. K. (1986b). The effectiveness of alcoholism treatment: What research reveals. In W. R. Miller, & N. Heather (Eds.), *Treating addictive behaviors.* New York: Plenum.

Miller, W. R., & Hester, R. K. (1989). Treating alcohol problems: Toward an informed eclecticism. In R. K. Hester, & W. R. Miller (Eds.), *Handbook of alcoholism treatment approaches: Effective alternatives* (pp. 3-13). New York: Pergamon.

Mirin, S. M., Shapiro, L. M., Meyer, R. E., Pillard, R. C., & Fisher, S. (1971). Casual versus heavy use of marijuana: A redefinition of the marijuana problem *American Journal of Psychiatry, 127*, 1134-1140.

Nathan, P. E., Titler, N. A., Lowenstein, L. M., Solomon, P., & Rossi, A. M. (1970). Behavioral analysis of chronic alcoholism: Interaction of alcohol and human contact. *Archives of General Psychiatry, 22*, 419-430.

Nathan, P. E., Zare, N. C., Ferneau, E. W., & Lowenstein, L. M. (1970). Effects of content differences in alcoholic beverages on the behavior of alcoholics. *Quarterly Journal of Studies on Alcoholism, Suppl. No. 5*, 87-100.

Parker, J. C., Gilbert, G. S., & Thoreson, R. W. (1978). Anxiety management in alcoholics: A study of generalized effects of relaxation techniques. *Addictive Behaviors, 3*, 123-127.

Rohsenow, D. J., Smith, R. E., & Johnson, S. (1985). Stress management training as a prevention program for heavy social drinkers: Cognitions, affect, drinking and individual differences. *Addictive Behaviors, 10*, 45-54.

Rosenthal, S. H. (1973). Alterations in serum thyroxine with cerebral electrotherapy (electrosleep). *Archives of General Psychiatry, 28*, 28-29.

Roth, R. (1987). *Transcendental Meditation*. New York: Donald I. Fine Inc.

Royer, A. (this volume). An evaluation of the Transcendental Meditation technique's role in promoting smoking cessation. *Alcoholism Treatment Quarterly*.

Schneider, R. H., Alexander, C. N., & Wallace, R. K. (1992). In search of an optimal behavioral treatment for hypertension: A review and focus on Transcendental Meditation. In E. H. Johnson, W. D. Gentry, & S. Julius (Eds.), *Personality, elevated blood pressure, and essential hypertension*. Washington, DC: Hemisphere Publishing Corporation.

Segal, B. (1983). Drugs and youth: A review of the problem. *The International Journal of the Addictions, 18*, 420-433.

Smith, R. B., & O'Neil, L. (1975). Electrosleep in the management of alcoholism. *Biological Psychiatry, 10*, 675-680.

Sobell, M., & Sobell, L. (1973). Alcoholics treated by individualized behavior therapy: One-year treatment outcome. *Behavioral Research and Therapy, 11*, 599-618.

Sobell, M., & Sobell, L. (1976). Second year treatment outcome of alcoholics treated by individualized behavior therapy: Results. *Behavior Research and Therapy, 14*, 195-215.

Spotts, J. V., & Shontz, F. C. (1991). Drug misuse and psychopathology: A meta-analysis of 16PF research. *The International Journal of the Addictions, 26*, 923-944.

Staggers, Jr., F., Alexander, C. N., & Walton, K. G. (this volume). Importance of reducing stress and strengthening the host in drug detoxification: The potential offered by Transcendental Meditation. *Alcoholism Treatment Quarterly*.

Stockwell, T., & Town, C. (1989). Anxiety and stress management. In R. K. Hester, & W. R. Miller (Eds.), *Handbook of alcoholism treatment approaches: Effective alternatives*, (pp. 222-230). New York: Pergamon Press.

Strickler, D. P., Tomaszewski, R., Maxwell, W. A., & Suib, M. R. (1979). The effects of relaxation instructions on drinking behavior in the presence of stress. *Behavior Research and Therapies, 17*, 45-51.

Surgeon General. (1988). *The health consequences of smoking & nicotine addic-*

tion: A report of the Surgeon General. U.S. Department of Health and Human Services.

United States Department of Health and Human Services. (1986). *Toward a national plan to combat alcohol abuse and alcoholism: A report to the US Congress by the Secretary of Health and Human Services.* Rockville, MD: Author.

Wageneder, F. M., & St. Schuy, G. (Eds.). (1966). *First International Symposium on Electrotherapeutic Sleep and Electroanesthesia.* Graz, Austria: Excerpta Medica.

Wageneder, F. M., & St. Schuy, G. (Eds.). (1970). *Second International Symposium on Electrotherapeutic Sleep and Electroanesthesia.* Graz, Austria: Excerpta Media.

Walton, K. G., & Levitsky, D. (this volume). A neuroendocrine mechanism for the reduction of drug use and addictions by Transcendental Meditation. *Alcoholism Treatment Quarterly.*

Williams, P., Francis, A., & Durham, R. (1976). Personality and meditation. *Perceptual and Motor Skills, 43*, 787-792.

Yoder, B. (1990). *The recovery resource book.* New York: Simon & Schuster.

The Role of the Transcendental Meditation Technique in Promoting Smoking Cessation: A Longitudinal Study

Ann Royer, PhD

INTRODUCTION

There is strong and growing evidence of the health risks and high costs of smoking, yet more than 51 million Americans are regular cigarette smokers (US Health and Human Services, 1988). Although approximately 90% of smokers desire to quit (Orleans, 1985), 80% of those who attempt to quit, fail on their first effort (US Health and Human Services, 1984). One reason for failure seems to be that quitting smoking causes physiological and psychological distress. Another reason some smokers may not quit is because they believe smoking helps them to think better, to feel better (less tense or anxious), to cope with stress, and to keep their weight under control (Health and Human Services, 1988; Charlton, 1984; Klesges & Klesges, 1988).

In order to adequately address the many factors associated with smoking behavior, multicomponent programs have been developed

Ann Royer is an independent researcher in the field of smoking cessation programs, Lac Beauport, Quebec, Canada.

[Haworth co-indexing entry note]: "The Role of the Transcendental Meditation Technique in Promoting Smoking Cessation: A Longitudinal Study." Royer, Ann. Co-published simultaneously in the *Alcoholism Treatment Quarterly* (The Haworth Press, Inc.) Vol. 11, No. 1/2, 1994, pp. 221-239; and: *Self-Recovery: Treating Addictions Using Transcendental Meditation and Maharishi Ayur-Veda* (ed: David F. O'Connell and Charles N. Alexander) The Haworth Press, Inc., 1994, pp. 221-239. Multiple copies of this article/chapter may be purchased from The Haworth Document Delivery Center [1-800-3-HAWORTH; 9:00 a.m. - 5:00 p.m. (EST)].

that incorporate behavior modification, self-control techniques and social support. In some cases, these appear to produce encouraging outcomes (Health and Human Services, 1988); however, since relatively few smokers (around 5%) will participate in formal cessation clinics (Health and Human Services, 1988), it is important to look for alternate treatment approaches.

There is a large body of evidence documenting that the Transcendental Meditation (TM) technique has a wide range of effects that contribute to the psychological and physiological well-being of the individual. Research conducted on the TM program has shown its value in reducing stress and anxiety (Eppley, Abrams, & Shear, 1989), decreasing illness rates (Orme-Johnson, 1987), enhancing psychological well-being (Alexander, Rainforth, & Gelderloos, 1991), increasing creativity (Travis, 1979) and normalizing hypertension (Schneider, Alexander, & Wallace, 1992).

Several studies (e.g., Benson & Wallace, 1972; Monahan, 1977; Lazar, Farwell, & Farrow, 1977) have also investigated the effects of the TM technique on smoking behavior. These studies suggest that the TM technique may be effective in increasing smoking quit rates. However, since these studies were retrospective in nature and/or without control groups they were unable to fully test this hypothesis.

A most remarkable feature of these studies, however, is the unique time-course of smoking cessation following adoption of the TM technique. In conventional smoking cessation programs, virtually all participants quickly stop smoking during the early phase of the program, but 75% to 80% return to smoking within a few months (Hunt & Matarazzo, 1973; Schwartz, 1987). In contrast, the studies on the TM technique and smoking consistently suggest that smoking tends to gradually decrease and then cease within a few months to one to two years after beginning to practice the TM technique. As the TM technique is a program of self-development and not presented as a smoking cessation intervention, at no point are subjects asked to stop smoking. Instead, smoking cessation appears to occur spontaneously without experience of withdrawal symptoms. Also, it appears that once smoking activity is stopped, little recidivism occurs (cf. Alexander, Robinson, & Rainforth, this volume).

If the above observations regarding TM and smoking quit rates are true, they establish a promising relationship between quitting smoking and a specific procedure that is available to any smoker. The current study was designed to assess prospectively the influence of the TM technique on smoking behavior relative to an untreated control group. It aimed at observing the smoking behavior of a sample of smokers over a period of nearly two years. Since previous studies reported gradual decrease as well as eventual smoking cessation in TM practitioners, the data were analyzed in terms of both decreased smoking and cessation. A decrease or increase was defined as a change of at least 5 cigarettes per day, which accounted for an average of 25% of the cigarettes smoked daily in this sample.

The proposed research program was designed to answer two fundamental questions: First, does the practice of the TM technique promote smoking cessation? Second, is regular participation in the TM program a predictor of smoking cessation? In the case of other substance dependencies (such as opiate dependence) it has been found that length of time practicing a treatment and completion of treatment as prescribed are positively correlated with successful outcomes (McLellan et al., 1983; De Leon, Wexler, & Jainchill, 1982). Similar positive correlations between regularity of practice and positive results were reported in prior TM studies on smoking cessation (cf. Alexander et al., this volume). This study is parallel in design and methodology to prospective studies on risk factors as predictors of incidence of diseases such as cancer and coronary heart disease (e.g., Schlesselman, 1984). In these studies, the progress of already established groups is followed and measured over time. Similarly, this study can be viewed as a test of whether the practice of TM is a positive predictor of smoking cessation.

METHODS

The subjects for this study were made available through cooperation with the organization teaching the TM program (WPEC-US). This organization has conducted public awareness campaigns in major population centers throughout the US in order to inform individuals about the TM technique and to give them the opportunity to learn it.

All subjects attended free introductory lectures on the TM technique following a local TV program or a newspaper ad. Their current smoking status, smoking history, demographic and socioeconomic status as well as their interest in the TM technique was determined through a questionnaire designed by the investigator, which each individual completed, before entering the lecture hall. This questionnaire was administered by the representatives of the TM organization conducting the lecture. The design of the questionnaire was based on questionnaires developed for more traditional smoking interventions and from consultation with an expert in this field (Lando, 1988, personal communication).

The initial questionnaires were screened to obtain the names of those who were currently smoking. This process yielded 226 smokers who subsequently learned the TM technique (Group A) and 850 smokers who attended the lecture but chose not to participate in the TM program at this point (Group B). The latter became the control group.

Standard TM instruction occurred over a 4-day period and involved 7 steps lasting approximately 1 1/2 hours each. No change in life-style or beliefs is required to begin this program. The subjects in the TM group were requested to practice the technique for twenty minutes twice daily. The TM organization provides a follow-up support program for those interested, although participation is not mandatory. Follow-up includes advanced lectures on relevant topics and individual check-ups to see that the program is practiced effortlessly.

A second, follow-up questionnaire (see Appendix A) was mailed to all participants from 20 to 24 months (average 22 months) after the date of the introductory lecture. This questionnaire was accompanied by a self-addressed envelope and a cover letter describing the experiment, requesting the subject's participation, and providing instructions. The follow-up questionnaires used for the TM and the non-TM groups were identical except that Group A also answered questions regarding the regularity of their practice of the TM technique, while Group B answered comparable questions regarding their possible participation in other personal development programs. Three to five weeks later, subjects that did not respond to the follow-up questionnaire were contacted by telephone.

One hundred and ten of the 226 smokers who attended the introductory lecture and subsequently learned TM completed the follow-up questionnaire and agreed to participate. They comprise the TM group (Group A). Of the 850 smokers who attended TM introductory lectures without beginning the practice, 214 completed the questionnaires and agreed to participate in the study. They comprise the control group (Group B). The higher recontact rate for the TM group may have been due in part to the fact that the TM organization was available to help relocate some subjects. The return rate for the control group is more typical for follow-up mail surveys.

Data Analysis

Chi-square analysis was used to assess potential initial differences on demographic and socioeconomic variables between the TM and non-TM groups; smoking activity was also compared via chi square analysis both initially and at the end of the study to assess decrease in smoking and cessation rates. Also, data were analyzed to determine the influence of adherence to the TM program on smoking cessation. Full adherence to TM was defined as the daily practice of the TM technique for the entire length of the study, whereas partial adherence to TM was defined as practicing TM less than daily by the end of the two-year period.

RESULTS

One hundred and ten smokers completed the follow-up questionnaires in the TM group (Group A) while 214 smokers did so in the non-TM control group (Group B). Thirty-three percent of the TM subjects reported that they were fully adherent; 67% reported that they were partially adherent by the end of the study period. To assure that the subjects who responded to the follow-up questionnaire were representative of the larger groups from which they were sampled, demographic information obtained from the initial questionnaire on the 110 smokers was compared to that of the 116 smokers who subsequently learned TM but did not participate in this study. Also, the 214 smokers who comprised the non-TM control group were compared with the other 636 smokers who attended an introductory lecture (and completed the initial questionnaire) but did not begin TM.

There were no significant differences found on any demographic variables between the subgroups who responded to the follow-up questionnaire (and agreed to participate) and the larger groups from which they were sampled. Also no significant differences were found at pretest between Group A and Group B on demographic variables or smoking habits. Table 1 presents the initial profiles of the smokers in both groups. Both groups were composed of approximately half men and half women in their mid-to-late thirties, with slightly over half of each group married (unmarried status was defined as single, divorced/separated, or widowed). About 70% of both Group A and Group B had attended some college or graduated from college. Although differences at pretest in smoking behavior did not reach significance, prior to learning TM, Group A smoked slightly more cigarettes per day (24 vs. 21) and had been smoking for a longer period of time (20 vs. 18 years) than the smokers in Group B.

Although similar in their pretest smoking behaviors (with 100% smoking in both groups), the TM group (Group A) showed a significantly higher smoking cessation rate at the two-year posttest than the controls (Group B): 31% quit in the TM group vs. 21% in the controls (df = 1, $\chi^2 = 3.85$, $p < .05$). Among those that quit, on the average, meditators produced a 12-month continuous abstinence from smoking period (SD = 7.57) compared to a 10-month continuous abstinence period (SD = 8.54) for the non-meditators; however, the differences between the groups did not reach significance ($t = .609$; $p = .54$).

Changes in the smoking behavior of Group A were then further examined to determine the influence of adherence to the TM technique on cessation rate throughout the two-year period. The time course was determined from the subjects' response to the question "When did you quit smoking?" asked in the follow-up questionnaire. As Figure 1 shows, there is a strong relationship between full

TABLE 1. Initial Profile of Smokers in the Transcendental Meditation (TM) and Non-TM Groups.

	TM Group				Non-TM Group			
		N = 110	%	% Responding		N = 214	%	% Responding
Gender	Male	57	52	100	Male	100	47	100
	Female	53	48		Female	114	53	
Marital Status	Single	38	34	100	Single	49	23	100
	Married	57	52		Married	117	54	
	Div/Sep	12	11		Div/Sep	44	21	
	Widowed	3	3		Widowed	4	2	
Education Level	No HS Deg	4	4	100	No HS Deg	13	6	100
	HSD Deg	22	20		HSD Deg	51	24	
	Some College	39	35		Some College	88	41	
	College	33	30		College	43	20	
	Postgrad	12	11		Postgrad	18	8	
Average Age		39		100		37		100
# Cig/Day		24		90		21		97
# Yrs Smoking		20		92		18		100

FIGURE 1. Time-course for quitting smoking for TM subjects fully adhering to the program, for the partially adhering TM subjects, and for non-TM controls over a two-year period.

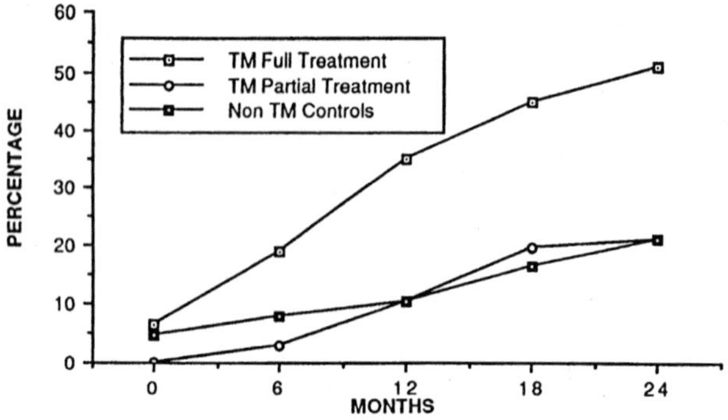

adherence to the TM practice and abstinence levels throughout the two-year follow-up period. Fifty-one percent of those who were fully adherent to TM had quit smoking by two years as compared to a 21% cessation rate for both the partially adherent and the controls (df = 2, $\chi^2 = 16.5$, p = .0003).

Table 2 presents the data illustrated in Figure 1 for the time-course of smoking cessation for the subjects who quit smoking in the full adherence TM group, the partial adherence TM group, and the non-TM control group at 6-month intervals from 0-24 months. While the percentage who successfully quit smoking increased steadily over time in all three groups, the largest rate of increase occurred in the full adherence TM group whose cumulative quit rate was almost 2 1/2 times that of the partial TM adherers and the non-TM control group after the two-year period.

Figure 2 summarizes the results at two years, not only for quit rates but also for decreased smoking levels. Eighty-one percent of those who fully adhered to the TM intervention had quit or decreased smoking after an average of 22 months. Those who partially adhered had a quit/decrease rate of 55% while the controls showed a 33% quit/decrease rate (df = 2, $\chi^2 = 34.30$, p = .0001). Although those who adhered partially to the TM intervention had the same quit rate as the non-TM group, they had a significantly

TABLE 2. Time-course for quitting smoking for TM subjects fully adhering to the program, for partially adhering TM subjects, and for non-TM controls.

Months	TM Full Adherers % Quit	TM Partial Adherers % Quit	Non-TM Controls % Quit
0	6.4%	0%	4.6%
6	19%	3%	7.7%
12	35%	10.5%	10.2%
18	45%	19.5%	16.3%
24	51%	21%	21%

FIGURE 2. Quit and decreased smoking rates for the TM subjects fully adhering to the program, for the partially adhering TM subjects, and for non-TM controls after a two-year follow-up.

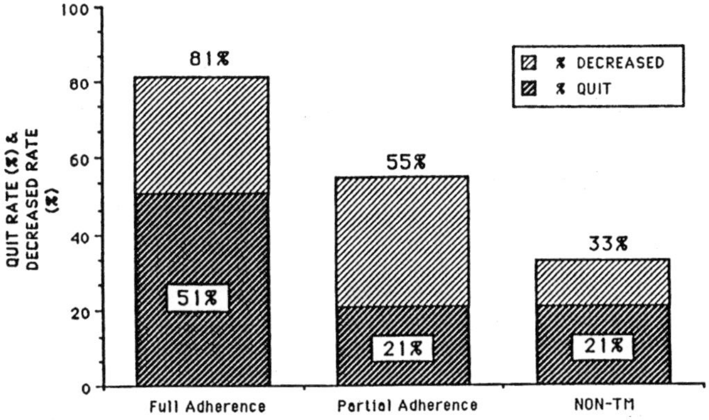

higher proportion decrease in the number of cigarettes smoked daily compared to the non-TM controls: 34% vs. 12% (df = 1, χ^2 = 18.19, p = .0001).

In addition, the TM group as a whole (including partial adherers) showed a significant decrease in the number of cigarettes smoked per day from the beginning to the end of the study (mean reduction = 6.03 cigarettes) (paired t = 5.68; p < .0001). In contrast, the non-TM group showed a slight but nonsignificant increase in the number of cigarettes smoked daily (mean increase = .35 cigarettes) (paired $t = -.63$; $p < .53$).

Table 3 summarizes the frequency of use of different methods of quitting smoking among those who quit for both Groups A and B. No significant differences were found between the groups. A large majority of both the TM and non-TM groups (78.1% and 79.5%, respectively) attempted quitting smoking on their own, while approximately 20% in each group tried professional methods such as smoking cessation programs, doctor recommendations, hypnosis, or other procedures.

The follow-up questionnaire also assessed the smokers' motivation to quit in both the TM and non-TM groups. Table 4 summarizes these results. No significant differences were found between the groups in terms of the following: (1) level of motivation to quit smoking ($df = 2$, $\chi^2 = .217$, $p = .897$); (2) number of quit attempts in the past year ($df = 4$, $\chi^2 = 3.463$, $p = .483$); and (3) number of quit attempts made during their life ($df = 4$, $\chi^2 = 3.462$, $p = .483$). Interestingly, only about 50% of both the TM and non-TM groups expressed a strong interest in quitting smoking.

Another issue of concern is smokers' compliance: smokers tend to be less likely to stay with any self-improvement programs that they begin, including smoking cessation programs (Health and Human Services, 1988). To evaluate possible differences in compliance rate for the practice of TM, compliance levels of meditation practice for the 110 TM smokers were compared to the levels of 288 non-smoking TM practitioners. These non-smokers attended the

TABLE 3. Quitting methods for TM and Non-TM groups.

	TM		Non-TM	
	N = 32		N = 44	
On their own	25	78.1%	35	79.5%
Cessation programs	2	6.2%	0	0.0%
Doctor's advice	2	6.2%	4	9.1%
Hypnosis	1	3.1%	1	2.3%
Other	2	6.2%	4	9.1%

TABLE 4. Recontacted smokers: Motivation to quit and number of quit attempts for the TM and non-TM groups.

How much do you want to quit?

	TM		NON-TM	
Not at all	4	6.3%	13	8.1%
Somewhat	26	41.3%	67	41.6%
Very much	33	52.4%	81	50.3%

Number of quit attempts in past year?

	TM		NON-TM	
None	25	39.7%	63	39.6%
Once	21	33.3%	54	34.0%
Twice	8	12.7%	24	15.1%
Three times	6	9.5%	6	3.8%
More than three	3	4.8%	12	7.5%

Number of quit attempts in your life?

	TM		NON-TM	
0-5	44	78.6%	117	80.7%
5-10	7	12.5%	22	15.2%
10-15	2	3.6%	2	1.4%
15-20	1	1.8%	3	2.1%
More than 20	2	3.6%	1	1.0%

TM introductory lecture and agreed to further cooperate with this study by completing the follow-up questionnaire. No differences were found in terms of compliance between these two groups.

DISCUSSION

This is the first long-term longitudinal study with a control group to assess the role of the TM technique in promoting smoking cessation. It evaluates the effects of the practice of the TM technique on smoking for a period of approximately 2 years. Initially there were no differences in demographic variables or smoking patterns between the TM and non-TM groups. Since the higher rates of abstinence (31% vs. 21%) among the TM practitioners could not be attributed to differences on other smoking variables such as motivation to quit, attempts to quit, or methods of quitting, this suggests the difference was due to practice of the TM technique. Furthermore, there was a consistent relationship between extent of adherence to the TM technique and successful quit rates; 51% of those who were fully adherent to TM had quit vs. 21% for those who partially adhered. When quit and decreased rates were combined the results were even more impressive: 81% of those who were fully adherent to TM had quit or decreased smoking after 24 months. While the quit rate of those who adhered partially to the TM intervention was the same as the non-TM group, they had a significantly higher proportion decrease in the number of cigarettes smoked daily compared to the non-TM controls: 34% vs. 12%. Thus, even partial adherence to the TM practice was sufficient to decrease the level of smoking.

The follow-up questionnaire data on when they quit smoking, as well as anecdotal reports, support previous findings on the time-course of smoking cessation following adoption of the TM technique. Results suggest that effects of TM are cumulative, with smoking continuing to decline or cease up to 24 months after beginning the practice. Moreover, once smoking activity stopped, little recidivism appeared to occur. The quit rates found in the present study (31% total TM group and 51% for full TM adherers) were in the same range as the average cessation rate of 41% found across 8 TM studies on smoking behavior included in a recent meta-analysis (Alexander, Robinson, & Rainforth, this volume). Just as the present study found that quit rates for TM rise linearly over time, the meta-analysis found that effects for TM on quitting or decreasing smoking accumulate over time in a roughly linear pattern. On the other hand, standard smoking cessation programs have been shown via meta-analysis to be smaller in the magnitude of their effects and not sustained over the long term. Average quit rates across 108 interventions in 39 controlled trials (Kottke, Battista,

DeFriese, & Brekke, 1988; Kottke, personal communication, 1993) fell from 30% at 3 months for experimental groups to 18% at 12 months for all types of smoking cessation modalities examined (e.g., nicotine replacement therapy, counseling). Thus the TM quit rate at two years (31%) was 1.7 times higher than for standard programs at one year (18%), and presumably the quit rates for standard programs would have continued to gradually decline over the second year. When treatment outcomes for this study are expressed as effect sizes (a standardized indicator of magnitude of treatment effect measured in standard deviation units), the effect for the TM group (.48) was 2.4 times larger than for Kottke's standard treatments (.20) (Alexander, Robinson, & Rainforth, this volume). Kottke et al. found that for standard programs, quit rates were strongly correlated with duration and frequency of contact with the program. This was similar to the finding in the current study of much higher cessation rates among TM adherers. This "dose-response" relationship is consistent with the conclusion that extent of TM practice is responsible for the observed effects.

Some potential alternative explanations for these promising findings will now be considered, including: initial differences in motivation and expectations, and differential attention from trainers. It is unlikely that these positive results can be accounted for by initial differences on such variables in the TM and non-TM groups because they were highly similar in motivation to quit smoking, number of quit attempts, use of different quit methods, and on smoking-related demographic characteristics. Also, the controls showed sufficiently high motivation or interest in self-development to choose on their own to attend an introductory lecture on the TM program. Expectation of positive smoking results is also unlikely to account for the effect because TM is not presented as a smoking cessation program, and at no time are meditators admonished to quit smoking. Further, attention from trainers is unlikely to account for the effect because the contact hours with the TM teachers are modest, and almost exclusively during the first week of instruction, whereas the most impressive cessation rates were evident after two years. This positive, long-lasting effect is opposite to placebo effects which tend to be short lived. In contrast, conventional smoking cessation programs (Kottke et al., 1988) gave clients explicit expectations and instructions on quitting, as well as attention from trainers specifically directed towards supporting smoking cessation. Also, clients in these conventional programs were highly motivated because they sought outside help to solve their smoking problem (whereas only 50% of the TM smokers indicated some motivation to quit), yet the cessation rates were clearly higher for TM than those reported for standard programs.

The only sampling difference between the TM and non-TM group was the higher response rate to the survey at posttest for the TM group (49% versus 25% for the smoking control group). However, this actually should have worked against the TM group because the lower response rate (which is typical for mailed questionnaires) for the non-TM control group suggests that these selected controls were particularly motivated to respond (without any incentive).

Another possible confound in this study is the use of self-reports whose validity has been previously questioned in the smoking literature (Grabowski & Bell, 1983). Although some studies have reported discrepancies between biochemical indicators and self-reported smoking status (Glasgow, Schafer, & O'Neill, 1981; Kozlowski, 1986; Ohlin, Ludhn, & Westling 1976), other studies have indicated that self-reported smoking status may actually be the more accurate measure, particularly in assessing the number of cigarettes smoked (Bliss & O'Connell, 1984; Pierce, Dwyer et al., 1987; Colletti, Supnick, & Abueg, 1982; Petitti, Friedman, & Kahn, 1981). Moreover, it has been suggested that inaccurate self-reports on smoking are more likely in studies in which the subjects are placed under explicit pressure to quit smoking. Since this was not the case in the present study, it is unlikely that false reporting strongly influenced the data.

Also the external validity or generalizability of the above findings should be considered. This study is composed primarily of individuals who are white, middle class men and women, aged 30-40 years, primarily interested in the TM program for its value in stress reduction and improving psychological well-being. This demographic profile differs somewhat from that of the average American smoker who tends to be lower in socioeconomic status. However, it clearly reflects the white middle class samples used in the vast majority of smoking cessation studies (Health and Human Services, 1988). Although the middle-class population to which this group belongs tends to be better than average at quitting smoking, a substantial percentage of this population still smokes (27% to 29%), and thus could benefit from a program that assists in smoking cessation.

Moreover, there are several reasons why these positive results are likely to generalize to other subpopulations. First, experience of stress has been shown to be a primary factor negatively influencing smoking behavior regardless of socioeconomic status; therefore the smoking cessation shown via this stress-reduction technique should apply to smokers among other socioeconomic subpopulations as well. Second, a large body of research indicates that the TM technique is associated with both immediate physiological changes and long-term psychophysiological effects which contribute to changes observed in the psychological areas of life as well (Eppley, Abrams, & Shear, 1989; Dillbeck & Orme-Johnson, 1987; Schneider, Alexander, & Wallace, 1992; Walton & Levitsky, this volume). It is therefore reasonable to expect that the influence of the TM technique upon smoking behavior is mediated in part by physiological changes that should be similar among all smokers, regardless of socioeconomic status.

Third, although the majority of the more than one million people learning TM in the US has been middle class, other segments of the population such as maximum security prisoners, juvenile delinquents, drug abusers, and chronic alcoholics have experienced substantive benefits from using this technique (e.g., Alexander, 1982; Dillbeck & Abrams, 1987; Taub et al., this volume), suggesting that TM could be an effective smoking cessation method for diverse subpopulations.

Thus, these potential threats to internal and external validity are unlikely to account for TM's effect (or decrease its generalizability). Nevertheless, such potential confounds can only be fully eliminated through the random assignment of a representative sample of smoking subjects to experimental and control conditions. Although such a controlled trial would be ideal, random assignment is oftentimes not a realistic option for clinical and psychosocial research due to logistical and ethical constraints. According to

Schlesselman (1984), cohort studies, similar to that used in the present study, are the typical solution chosen by clinical researchers. The design of this research did have the advantage of making maximal use of resources by interfacing with an ongoing program of the TM organization, and thus it was possible to obtain knowledge that would not have been available otherwise.

Smoking remains the leading cause of avoidable death in the US. In light of the striking difference in smoking cessation between full TM adherers and the non-TM group, large-scale clinical application of this highly cost-effective, nonpharmacological approach to smoking cessation would certainly have important implications for healthcare policy. In this context, further randomized controlled trials comparing TM to other promising treatments would clearly be in the interest of our nation's health and well-being.

REFERENCES

Alexander, C. N. (1982). Ego development, personality, and behavioral changes in inmates practicing the Transcendental Meditation technique or participating in other programs: A cross-sectional and longitudinal study. *Dissertations Abstract International, 43*(2), 539B.

Alexander, C. N., Rainforth, M.V., & Gelderloos, P. (1991). Transcendental Meditation, self-actualization, and psychological health: A conceptual overview and statistical meta-analysis. *Journal of Social Behavior and Personality, 6*, (5) 189-247.

Alexander, C. N., Robinson, P., & Rainforth, M. (this volume). Treating and preventing alcohol, nicotine, and drug abuse through Transcendental Meditation: A review and statistical meta-analysis. *Alcoholism Treatment Quarterly.*

Benson, H., & Wallace, R. K. (1972). Decreased drug abuse with Transcendental Meditation: A study of 1,862 subjects. In C. Zarafonetis (Ed.): *Drug Abuse, Proceedings of the International Conference*. Philadelphia: Lea and Febiger.

Bliss, R. E., & O'Connell, K. A. (1984). Problems with thiocyanate as an index of smoking status: A critical review with suggestions for improving the usefulness of biochemical measures in smoking cessation research. *Health Psychology, 3*, 563-581.

Charlton, A. (1984). Smoking and weight control in teenagers. *Public Health (London), 98*, 277-281.

Colletti, G., Supnick, J. A., & Abueg, F. R. (1982). Association of the relationship between self-reported smoking rate and ecolyser measurement. *Addictive Behaviors, 97*, 183-188.

De Leon, G., Wexler, H. K., & Jainchill, N. (1982). The therapeutic community: Success and improvement rates 5 years after treatment. *International Journal of the Addictions, 17*(4), 703-747.

Dillbeck, M. C., & Abrams, A. I. (1987). The application of the Transcendental Meditation program to correction. *International Journal of Comparative and Applied Criminal Justice, 11*(1), 111-132.

Dillbeck, M. C., & Orme-Johnson, D. W. (1987). Physiological differences between Transcendental Meditation and rest. *American Psychologist, 42*, 879-881.

Eppley, K., Abrams, A., & Shear, J. (1989). The differential effects of relaxation techniques on trait anxiety: A meta-analysis. *Journal of Clinical Psychology, 45*, 957-974.

Glasgow, R. E., Schafer, L., & O'Neill, H. K. (1981). Self-help books and amount of therapist contact in smoking cessation programs. *Journal of Consulting and Clinical Psychology, 49*, 659-667.

Grabowski, J., & Bell, C. S. (Eds). (1983). *Measurement in the analysis and treatment of smoking behavior.* National Institutes on Drug Abuse Monograph #48. Washington DC: Government Printing Office.

Hunt, W. A., & Matarazzo, J. D. (1973). Three years later: Recent developments in the experimental modification of smoking behavior. *Journal of Abnormal Psychology, 81*, 107-114.

Klesges, R. C., & Klesges, L. M. (1988). Cigarette smoking as a dieting strategy in a university population. *International Journal of Eating Disorders, 7*, 413-419.

Kottke, T. T., Battista, R. N., Defriese, G. H. & Brekke, M. L. (1988). Attributes of successful smoking cessation interventions in medical practice: A meta-analysis of 39 controlled trials. *Journal of the American Medical Association, 259*, 2883-2889.

Kozlowski, L.T. (1986). Pack size, self-reported smoking rates and public health. *American Journal of Public Health, 76*(11), 1337-1338.

Lazar, A., Farwell, L., & Farrow, J.T. (1977). The effects of the Transcendental Meditation program on anxiety, drug abuse, cigarette smoking, and alcohol consumption. In D.W. Orme-Johnson & J.T. Farrow (Eds.): *Scientific Research on the Transcendental Meditation Program: Collected Papers Vol. 1.* West Germany: MERU Press.

McLellan, A. T., Luborsky, L., Woody, G. E., O'Brien, C. P., & Druley, K. A. (1983). Predicting response to alcohol and drug abuse treatments: Role of psychiatric severity. *Archives of General Psychiatry 40*, 620-625.

Monahan, R. J. (1977). Secondary prevention of drug dependency through the Transcendental Meditation program in metropolitan Philadelphia. *International Journal of Addictions, 12*(6), 729-54.

Ohlin, P., Ludhn, B., & Westling, H. (1976). Carbon monoxide blood levels and reported cessation of smoking. *Psychopharmacology, 49*, 263-265.

Orleans, C.T. (1985). Understanding and promoting smoking cessation: Overview and guidelines for physician intervention. *Annual Review of Medicine: Selected Topics in the Clinical Sciences, 36*, 51-61.

Orme-Johnson, D.W. (1987). Medical care utilization and the Transcendental Meditation program. *Psychosomatic Medicine, 49*, 493-507.

Petitti, D. B., Friedman, G. D., & Kahn, W. (1981). Accuracy of information on smoking habits provided on self-administered questionnaires. *American Journal of Public Health, 71*, 308-311.

Pierce, J. P., Dwyer, T. et al. (1987). Cotinine validation of self-reported smoking in commercially run community surveys. *Journal of Chronic Diseases, 40*(7), 689-695.

Schlesselman, J. J. (1984). *Case-control studies: Design, conduct analysis*. New York: Oxford University Press.

Schneider, R. H., Alexander, C. N., & Wallace, R. K. (1992). In search of an optimal behavioral treatment for hypertension: A review and focus on Transcendental Meditation. In E. H. Johnson, W. D. Gentry, & S. Julius (Eds.) *Personality, elevated blood pressure, and essential hypertension*. Washington DC: Hemisphere.

Schwartz, J. L. (1987). *Review and evaluation of smoking cessation methods: United States and Canada, 1978-1985*. U.S. Department of Health and Human Services, Public Health Service, National Institutes of Health, NIH publication No.87-2940.

Taub, E., Solomon, S. S., Smith, R. B., Weingarten, E., Alexander, C. N., & Walton, K. G. (this volume). Effectiveness of broad spectrum approaches to relapse prevention: A long-term, randomized controlled trial comparing Transcendental Meditation, muscle relaxation and electronic neurotherapy in severe alcoholism. *Alcoholism Treatment Quarterly*.

Travis, F. (1979). The Transcendental Meditation technique and creativity: A longitudinal study of Cornell University undergraduates. *Journal of Creative Behaviors, 13*(3), 169-180.

United States Department of Health and Human Services. (1988). *The Health Consequences of Smoking: Nicotine Addiction. A report of the Surgeon General*. U. S. Department of Health and Human Services. Public Health Services, Office on Smoking and Health. DHHS publication no. (CDC) 88-8406.

United States Public Health Service. (1984). *The Health Consequences of Smoking: Chronic Obstructive Lung Disease. A report of the Surgeon General*. U. S. Department of Health and Human Services. Public Health Services, Office on Smoking and Health. DHHS publication no. (PHS) 84-50205.

Walton, K. G., & Levitsky, D. (this volume). A neuroendocrine mechanism for the reduction of drug use and addictions by Transcendental Meditation. *Alcoholism Treatment Quarterly*.

APPENDIX A. FOLLOW-UP SMOKING QUESTIONNAIRE

Q-1 Do you smoke? (Circle number of your answer)
1 HAVE NEVER (SKIP TO QUESTION 4)
2 HAVE QUIT (SKIP TO QUESTION 2)
3 STILL SMOKE (SKIP TO QUESTION 3)

(Answer questions Q-2a through Q2-d only if you have quit smoking)

Q-2a How did you quit?

1 ON MY OWN
2 COUNSELING
3 HYPNOSIS
4 DOCTOR'S ADVICE
5 CLINIC
6 OTHER _________

Q-2b How long ago did you quit?

_____ WEEKS _____ MONTHS _____ YEARS

Q-2c How many years did you smoke before you quit?

_____ YEARS

Q-2d How many cigarettes per day did you smoke before you quit?

_____ CIGARETTES

(Answer question Q3-a through Q3-g only is you are currently smoking)

Q3-a For how many years have you been smoking?

_____ YEARS

Q3-b What type of cigarettes do you usually smoke? (Circle one or several numbers)

1 FILTER
2 REGULAR
3 MENTHOL
4 KING

Q3-c How many of the following do you smoke per day?

NOW	ONE YEAR AGO
_____ CIGARETTES	_____ CIGARETTES
_____ CIGARS	_____ CIGARS
_____ PIPE	_____ PIPE

Q-3d If your smoking has changed significantly in the last year, when did that occur?

_____ MONTHS AGO

Q-3e How much do you want to quit smoking?
1 NOT AT ALL
2 SOMEWHAT
3 VERY MUCH

Q-3f How many times have you made a serious attempt to quit smoking during the past year? (Circle number)

1 NEVER
2 ONCE
3 TWICE
4 THREE TIMES
5 MORE THAN THREE TIMES

Q-3g How many times have you made a serious attempt to quit smoking in your life?

_____ TIMES

GENERAL INFORMATION

Q-4 Your present age _____ YEARS

Q-5 Your sex (Circle number)

1 MALE
2 FEMALE

Q-6 Your present marital status

1 NEVER MARRIED
2 MARRIED
3 DIVORCED/SEPARATED
4 WIDOWED

Q-7 What is the highest level of education that you have completed (circle number)

1 DID NOT COMPLETE HIGH SCHOOL
2 COMPLETED HIGH SCHOOL
3 SOME COLLEGE (OR IN COLLEGE)
4 COMPLETED COLLEGE
5 GRADUATE SCHOOL

SELF-DEVELOPMENT

Q-8 When did you learn TM? __/__/__
Mo. day year

Q-9 How often do you practice TM?

1 TWICE A DAY
2 ONCE A DAY
3 OCCASIONALLY
4 NEVER

SECTION III: CASE STUDIES AND CLINICAL APPLICATIONS

Case Histories: Using the Transcendental Meditation Program with Alcoholics and Addicts

Catherine R. Bleick, PhD

INTRODUCTION

A Transcendental Meditation (TM) program for alcoholics and addicts has been operating since autumn of 1986 on the Los Angeles Westside, using the facilities of the CLARE (Community Living for Alcoholics by Rehabilitation and Education) Foundation, an alcohol recovery agency headquartered in Santa Monica. Our inaugural introductory lecture was organized by a CLARE volunteer (see "Steve" below) for a CLARE staff meeting. Thereafter introductory lectures were publicized through posters at CLARE facilities and by word of mouth of meditators at their Alcoholics Anonymous (AA) (see Alcoholics Anonymous World Services, Inc., 1976) or other Twelve Step program meetings, including Narcotics Anonymous (NA) and Cocaine Anonymous (CA). Monthly

---

Catherine R. Bleick is affiliated with the Institute for Social Rehabilitation, P.O. Box 5397 181, Carmel, CA 93921.

The author wishes to express her appreciation to Art Aron, Allan Abrams, and Catherine Davidovich for criticizing the manuscript; to David O'Connell and Charles Alexander for generous editorial suggestions; and to her clients whose kind cooperation with the interviews made these case histories possible.

[Haworth co-indexing entry note]: "Case Histories: Using the Transcendental Meditation Program with Alcoholics and Addicts." Bleick, Catherine R. Co-published simultaneously in the *Alcoholism Treatment Quarterly* (The Haworth Press, Inc.) Vol. 11, No. 3/4, 1994, pp. 243-269; and: *Self-Recovery: Treating Addictions Using Transcendental Meditation and Maharishi Ayur-Veda* (ed: David F. O'Connell and Charles N. Alexander) The Haworth Press, Inc., 1994, pp. 243-269. Multiple copies of this article/chapter may be purchased from The Haworth Document Delivery Center [1-800-3-HAWORTH; 9:00 a.m. - 5:00 p.m. (EST)].

advanced TM meetings consisting of a group meditation, a taped lecture by Maharishi Mahesh Yogi, and discussion, as well as semiannual special events with a guest speaker or videotapes were held for our students between 1986 and early 1991. Regular checking of meditation, a brief procedure designed to insure ease and correctness of TM practice, was provided for students who were willing to participate. By winter of 1992 over 250 alcoholics and addicts had been instructed.

TM is well suited to Twelve Step program adherents, because it helps to fulfill Step Eleven, "Sought through prayer and meditation to improve our conscious contact with God, *as we understood Him*, praying only for knowledge of His will for us and the power to carry that out" (Alcoholics Anonymous World Services, Inc., 1981). Although the founders of AA died before TM reached the U.S., they did not clearly define any specific form of meditation, and TM is thus acceptable in principle.

Since donations cover the TM course fee for alcoholics and addicts at CLARE in case of need, a substantial minority of our clients have learned for free, and nobody has ever been turned away for lack of funds. Also, the TM teachers utilize virtually free facilities and offer their own time as unpaid volunteers. These factors have also assisted us in reducing the course fee.

A review by Alexander, Robinson, and Rainforth (this volume) summarizes previous literature, including both surveys showing a decline in substance abuse by TM meditators and experiments on TM as an adjunct to the treatment of substance abuse. Taub, Solomon, Smith, Weingarten, Alexander, and Walton (this volume) provide the most comprehensive experimental data yet published. Shafii, Lavely, and Jaffe (1975) and Monahan (1977) published important survey data on TM and reduced alcohol and drug use. Bloomfield, Cain, Jaffe, and Kory (1975) and Bloomfield and Kory (1976) published psychiatric case histories, including cases involving chemical dependency and a discussion of TM in spiritual crises; Childs (1977) offered a few case histories of juvenile drug abusers introduced to TM; and O'Connell (1991) provided a detailed case history of a meditating Twelve Step program participant. However, the present paper is the first to give multiple, detailed case histories on adult Twelve Step adherents with long-term histories of substance abuse, and to emphasize their self-reported spiritual growth through TM.

Case histories complement experimental data by adding important information on the natural history and course of recovery from alcoholism when TM is added to traditional recovery programs. They give us insight into the inner psychological workings and specific behavior of meditating alcoholics, indicating exactly how TM may be working to facilitate recovery. They also provide concrete self-report data on how the meditators themselves find TM helpful in recovery. Thus they contribute to our theoretical understanding about how TM works in the treatment of alcoholism and addiction.

The following ten case histories are intended to inform not only clinicians but also alcoholics themselves and any individuals who might like to implement a TM program for substance abusers. Included below are two cases of participants in our program who had learned TM years before the commencement of our program, thus providing an additional long-term perspective. The names used are fictitious.

CASE HISTORIES

Success Stories

The four case histories that follow illustrate how individuals who have practiced TM very regularly have found great benefits.

Tom. Tom is a Caucasian man who learned TM upon the prescription of a physician in September of 1981, at age 27, after about a year of sobriety. Tom became drug free and sober without help, on the strength of his own personal decision. Although he had attended AA meetings since his teens (while using drugs), and continued to attend occasionally, he did not become seriously active in AA until 5 years after his sobriety. He presently attends an average of 2 AA or NA meetings per week. He actively recruited for our TM program for alcoholics for several years, and also helped with introductory lectures.

Tom first got drunk at age 13, and always drank to intoxication to gain relief from mental pain. He was prescribed tranquilizers in his early teens and loved them, and used marijuana daily in high school. He studied classics at his state university, and did part-time cleaning jobs, but frequently missed classes due to drinking and hangovers.

His early post-college years were his worst period. During that time, he abused over 20 prescribed and nonprescribed drugs, either by manipulating doctors to prescribe them or by buying illegally or stealing them. During this period he also drank alcohol, in a binge pattern, with binges lasting a few days to several weeks or months. He tried at times to stop using drugs and alcohol, but his longest period of abstinence was about 1 month. He experienced shakes, blackouts, seizures, and amnesia while sober. He was also hospitalized numerous times for schizophrenia or manic depression rather than for alcoholism or addictions, although his symptoms were likely from the latter cause. He attended a nursing school during this period while on numerous drugs and receiving SSI (Supplemental Security Income, a Social Security benefit available to certain disabled persons). He did a little nurse's aid work, but did not graduate.

After his sobriety, he took a depression control class, assertion training with therapy, and self hypnosis/relaxation. He graduated from a clerical/office technology school while drug free but still on SSI, and he also did intermittent house cleaning during this period.

Before Tom subsequently began TM, he was physically sick, shaky, and exhausted from insomnia, all secondary to detoxification, stress, and a profound inability to relax. TM gave him immediate relief from insomnia, and he still uses it to rid himself of the urge to drink or take a pill. He states, "*Nothing,* including prayer, Twelve Step meetings, talking to other alcoholics, or exercise is so effective as TM in controlling my chemical abuse problem and associated feeling of 'insanity.' I believe all my drug and alcohol abuse can be attributed to a desperate search for inner peace, which I find in TM. TM helps me control anger, bitterness, vindictiveness, and other negative emotions; and helps me deal with family and other social problems with strength, courage, compassion, and energy. It has helped to free me of fear of changing myself, and helps me to make amends" (Step Nine: "Made direct amends to [persons we had harmed] wherever possible, except when to do so would injure them or others" (Alcoholics Anonymous World Services, Inc., 1981)). TM also decreases his arthritis pain.

Tom's earning power increased radically after he learned TM and took up medical transcription. He presently also practices the TM-Sidhi program (advanced TM) twice daily.

Sam. Sam is an African American man who learned TM in our first class, in August of 1986, at age 52, after 4 months of sobriety. His sobriety began when he entered a hospital for mental treatment but was referred to the chemical dependency ward and attended AA meetings there. Since suffering what he describes as a nervous breakdown associated with domestic violence in 1968 he had been depressed and very frequently in and out of mental hospitals, but was never previously diagnosed as alcoholic and actually recalls ordering wine with hospital meals. He began volunteering at CLARE shortly after his sobriety, attends three or four AA or CA meetings weekly, and chairs or assists with AA panels in hospitals, jails, and prisons twice or more monthly.

Sam's education stopped after 11th grade. He learned construction skills from his father, became a partner in a very successful janitorial service, and later a chef. During these days, he had arrests for bad checks, battery in domestic disputes, and DUI ("driving under the influence"), and was incarcerated for some months. Sam asserts that there was no time since 1966 when he could not put his hands on $1/4 million in drugs. However, he was a drug dealer for years before using drugs himself. He also believes he was a social drinker until his mid-thirties.

After the chef job he worked only briefly. He was first on SSI for depression, and then, until several years after learning TM, received disability payments due to back injuries incurred in auto accidents. He was hospitalized on and off for 2-1/2 years starting in 1972 for the back problems, and was prescribed major pain killers. Sam began drinking alcoholically due to depression and domestic problems, which the prescribed medicines did not alleviate. He was a round-the-clock drinker. He was never sober for the 16 years prior to his official sobriety, and could not eat until he had a drink. He started using cocaine, heroin, and other drugs after his alcoholism was firmly established. Prior to his sobriety, he suffered from blackouts, and was suffering increasingly from hot and cold sweats.

Because Sam had practiced a Rosecrucian form of concentration in his youth, which he enjoyed but found difficult, he questioned the ease of TM at his first TM lecture. He did find TM much easier, and has meditated extremely regularly and reported very pleasant experiences from the start. He now attends TM center functions occasionally, and regularly helps with coordinating the instruction of new meditators in our program. He says TM has enabled him to find himself and God, inner peace, and joy. He reports that TM helped him with his divorce, which was finalized recently, and he is now on friendly terms with his former wife. People say he looks younger. CLARE put him on their part-time payroll as a janitor after he learned TM. He also began doing some construction work at that time, and soon began taking classes in such areas as masonry, electrical, plumbing, roofing, etc. He found his back pain bothered him less. After about three years of TM, he became a supervisor for a small construction firm, and he went completely off his disability payments a couple of years before this publication. He is now self-employed doing construction repairs.

In Sam's own words, "I have a lot less anger and a much clearer mind. This has enabled me to make the right decisions, whether it be on the spur of the moment or whether it requires long-term planning. I believe that TM has been a major factor in my being sober today. I cannot express in words the rewards that I receive daily through meditating."

Fred. Fred is a half Native American man who learned TM in January of 1990 at age 40, after 4 months of sobriety and about 1 year drug free. He first got drug free and sober in a 21-day VA treatment program, after being expelled from a VA vocational rehabilitation program due to cocaine use that kept him in bed for a week. He tried beer a half year later, but when he could not stop at a couple of beers, he decided he was alcoholic and remained sober thereafter. He presently attends about two AA and one NA meetings per week.

Fred quit high school in the 12th grade, and received a GED in the Army. During and after high school, Fred worked at a gas station, then in a steel factory, as a file clerk, and as a printer before joining the Army. After the Army, he did printing work, and worked in factories.

Fred first got drunk at age 15. He drank mainly at parties, usually once a week, and always to intoxication. However, drugs were a more serious problem. He used marijuana occasionally in high school, then daily while in the Army in Vietnam. Several years after leaving the Army, he was addicted to cocaine for 2 years. He stopped using cocaine after a suicide attempt which his roommate attributed to the drug. However he started using cocaine again thereafter. He also did drug deliveries at $10 each during this period.

Fred's drug abuse problems were seriously compounded by his schizo-affective disorder, originally diagnosed as paranoid schizophrenia, which dated from use of marijuana apparently spiked with some more dangerous unidentified substance which he took while in Vietnam. He was treated with various anti-schizophrenic medicines, as well as electroconvulsive therapy (ECT), but nonetheless had repeated psychotic breaks. He received VA disability payments, and later SSI. Immediately before learning TM, a Veterans Center counselor suggested he take lithium and Navane, on which he is now stable.

Fred initially learned TM because he hoped it would help with his Third Step of AA ("Made a decision to turn our will and our lives over to the care of God *as we understood Him*" (Alcoholics Anonymous World Services, Inc., 1981)). He has practiced TM very regularly since his instruction date, generally twice daily followed by lying down to rest. He attributes to TM a gradual relief from paranoid thoughts which he associates with a history of being abused by his foster parents in early childhood.

After less than a year of TM, Fred enrolled in a California State vocational rehabilitation program, through which he attended school full-time to study computer-aided drafting. He was the teacher's assistant, and his teacher said he was the best student she has ever had; she planned to use his homework studies format as a model after he finished the program. He attributes his success in school to TM. He feels stronger now, and believes he will not have another psychotic break. He also finds TM excellent for his Eleventh Step.

Although Fred did not find a drafting job, he recently went to work as an apprentice plumber. He reports that he remembers avoiding work in the old days in order to drink, whereas now he enjoys his work, and feels guilty even if he has to stay home briefly with a legitimate cold or flu.

Pedro. Pedro is a Hispanic man who learned TM in April of 1990 at age 35, after 10 months of sobriety. He became drug free and sober at a 90-day residential VA program after being fired from a postal worker job for the second time, a job which had been his link with the world outside of drugs. He was living at the CLARE Adult Recovery Home when he learned TM. He presently attends NA meetings almost every day, occasionally AA meetings, and also has 6 hours weekly answering the NA phone. He is a meeting secretary, and does some AA or NA panels.

Pedro did not graduate from high school, but got a GED after serving in the Army in his late teens, and completed a couple of years of college classes before his sobriety.

Pedro first got drunk at 13 and drank alcoholically from the start, although at first he had to force himself to drink, because it made him sick. He drank because it was "the thing to do" after school, and sometimes used marijuana, uppers, downers, and LSD at school. He was arrested as a juvenile for offenses such as underage purchasing of alcohol. Pedro started using heroin and cocaine right after the Army. He attended an outpatient detoxification and at least 12 short inpatient programs between the Army and his ultimate sobriety. He was fined $300 for his first DUI soon after the Army; and was required to attend DUI school and AA meetings (which did not interest him) after another DUI arrest a few years later. However, he did temporarily stop using drugs, and mostly stopped drinking for 9 months, after incurring injuries in a motorcycle accident.

For the last 5 years before sobriety, he was on methadone dispensed through the VA, but used heroin, other drugs, and alcohol at the same time. His chemical abuse interfered with keeping jobs for any length of time. However, he was able to do routine work for the Post Office for the 6 years preceding sobriety, being fired and rehired once. In the meanwhile, he had been arrested twice for being "under the influence," which led to an unsuccessful VA hospital program. He was able to resign from the Post Office and fulfill the court requirement of the second arrest by entering the 90-day VA program where he attained sobriety. This was immediately preceded by a 6-day methadone detoxification, but he used heroin before entering the subsequent 90-day VA program. At that time he wanted to stop using methadone and get his Post Office job back, but had no plans for staying drug free in the long run. However, he did listen to the counselors.

Pedro came to our TM lecture after seeing one of our posters. He had always been interested in meditation, peace of mind, and finding God; but, except for doing some yoga breathing, had previously turned to hallucinogens instead of meditation, because he "didn't want to work for it." He also learned TM for the sake of his Eleventh Step. He has meditated regularly, since his instruction. He reports having more self-esteem and more energy, and that he exercises, and has a better diet. After a year or more of TM he began living alone instead of, as before, always living with a drinking partner or "moving back to Mom." He had a steady girlfriend, and feels this was the first such relationship in which he has "been there" emotionally, rather than being primarily involved with his drugs. After doing odd jobs, he was rehired by the Post Office a year after learning TM, and has never missed work without prior approval. He says that old postal associates ask him, "What did you do? Did you get younger?" He is attending college classes, which he finds easier, and aims at an M.A. and possibly Ph.D. in psychology in order to counsel recovering addicts. He notes that the progress of friends with whom he got sober appears to have been slower than his. He centers his life around the Eleventh Step, and always puts TM first. He feels that without TM, he would have used drugs by now. He recalls one day when he thought of using drugs, then thought, "If I use, I can't meditate." He feels TM has helped him "just about every way," saying, "TM is one of the most valuable tools in my recovery. At first I meditated in order to stay off drugs, but now I stay off drugs in order to meditate. It keeps me centered–sometimes I feel a blissful state–and allows me to focus on the day, one day at a time."

Comments. Not only did these four individuals indicate to me that TM helped immensely with their sobriety, but also all four experienced great improvements in their quality of life; e.g., success in school, being able to keep a job, and improved interpersonal relationships. Since Tom, Sam, and Fred had all been repeatedly hospitalized for mental disorders prior to learning TM, their greatly improved mental health is particularly noteworthy. Fred in particular noticed relief from psychotic symptoms that had distressed him for over 20 years, despite ECT, hospitalizations, and medications. He did start new medications at the same time he started TM, but he himself attributes his gradually improved state of mind to TM. That such cases responded so well to TM also shows that a very poor past history can be consistent with a very favorable response to TM.

Successes with Irregular Meditation

The standard prescription for regular meditation is 15-20 minutes twice daily. However, not all meditators follow this prescription. This may be particularly true for substance abusers. The three case histories that follow illustrate substantial success even with irregular meditation.

Frank. Frank is a Hispanic man who learned TM in January of 1989 at age 39, after about 1-1/2 months of sobriety. With the aid of AA, NA, and CA meetings, he became sober after a big fight with and separation from his second wife, which were occasioned by his alcohol use. He had been attending twice weekly AA meetings for several years as part of two sequential court-required diversion programs following DUI arrests. He was sober for 11 months of this period, then drank again and stopped attending AA meetings. He had also been drug free and sober for 11 months while in residence at Synanon 20 years ago, but drank immediately upon leaving. Two earlier 21-day detoxification programs in New York had left him drug free and sober only a couple of weeks each time. Thus Frank was definitely relapse-prone before learning TM. He presently attends between three and five AA meetings weekly.

Frank first drank at age 16, and always to intoxication. Although before drinking he was a good student, he repeated 11th grade 3 times, then quit school before completing 12th grade. He married at age 17, and his separation from this first wife about 5 years later was also related to his substance abuse. He used marijuana and heroin mainly in his late teens and early twenties, and used cocaine in his mid-thirties. He was abusive toward his second wife, and she also abused him. He lied to his plumbing customers to explain his failures to meet commitments.

Frank's AA sponsor requested that he learn TM, and Frank complied, despite misconceptions he harbored regarding TM, because he felt desperate. Initially he practiced TM twice daily. At the time he was depressed over the separation from his wife, and was experiencing suicidal thoughts. At first he found in TM a kind of relaxation such as he had sought in drugs. He also mentioned soon after instruction that he was beginning to feel enjoyment and pride in his plumbing work. Presently he meditates only once per day, but does so with great appreciation. He sometimes meditates on a break at work if things are not going well. He says that if he cannot make it to an AA meeting, he can at least meditate. If he does not meditate, he says life does not go so smoothly. He considers that TM is something good to help him stay drug free and sober along with AA. He is not sure whether he is making more money; however, with paying child support for his 5-year-old son, he definitely has more bills, and they are getting paid. After a couple of years of TM he was completely over his depression, has become remarried to a fellow sober alcoholic, and is very happy.

Frank says, "I had some rather hard, difficult times during my first year of sobriety. Facing reality sober is not an easy task. However, through practicing this very natural and easy method of relaxing, the business of living has been easier to handle."

Al. Al is an African American man who learned TM in May of 1990 at age 28, after 14 months of sobriety. He became drug free and sober at a 28-day hospital treatment program after waking up in the hospital intensive care unit due to a heart attack caused by a combination of cocaine, marijuana, beer, amyl nitrate, and whisky–not an unusual combination for him. He attended his first AA meeting there, decided he was an alcoholic after 1 month of sobriety, and currently attends at least one AA meeting daily, plus one AA panel monthly; he sponsors one individual.

He first got drunk at age 6, but drank socially until about age 18. He began drinking daily at age 22. Al graduated from college with a B.A. in art. Until his mid-twenties he lived rent-free with his sister. Then he worked in a warehouse, where he became manager. He abstained from drugs for about 1-1/2 years at about age 23 because he thought he had a problem; then he changed his mind and went back to them. He began drinking heavily at age 24. He drank mainly in the evenings and on weekends, and did not lose his warehouse job due to drinking, although he was sometimes late or failed to show up for work. He also used cocaine, LSD, "speed," and hashish. He sometimes experienced shakes and blackouts. He began his present job, managing a comic book store, in the first year after his sobriety.

Since learning TM, Al has always continued to do TM during the 5-minute meditation at the local 6:45 a.m. AA meditation meeting. However, he has stopped and started his twice daily regular meditations a few times. When he misses the regular meditations, he reports having anxiety attacks, obsessive thinking, and inability to approach problems calmly–just the way he felt before he learned TM. When interviewed, he was meditating regularly, usually on the bus to and from work. He says with TM he is more pleasant to be around, and tackles problems more objectively, one at a time as they arise. He does not take other people's bad humor personally, or try to run other people's lives. With respect to his Eleventh Step, Al finds that with TM his fears about the word "God" are gone. He doesn't have to pray as hard, or struggle to say the right thing in his prayers. He says, "I am more relaxed and feel more open to 'my inside source.' For me, when practiced regularly and diligently, TM is the Serenity Prayer in action. It allows acceptance and access to a power to change."

Jill. Jill is a Caucasian woman who learned TM in July of 1988 at age 37 after 28 months of sobriety. She had previously had 4 years of sobriety from 29 to 33 years of age. Her present sobriety began with a 3-day inpatient detoxification program with 1-month outpatient follow-up. This successful program, when she found she had nothing left, was preceded by 7 previous treatment programs that failed. She had also been in and out of AA, but since her present sobriety is a staunch AA member, not only attending weekly meetings, but also chairing and participating on several AA hospital and institutional panels.

Jill is a high school graduate. She had her first drink at age 14 and started drinking seriously and alcoholically at age 18. She used marijuana and uppers during her teens, and also used amphetamines to alleviate boredom during both long periods of drinking. She was married in her mid-twenties and again, in her early thirties, to another man whom she considers alcoholic and with whom she started drinking again. The second husband threw her out because of drinking. She has worked 20 years for the same attorney, being away from the job only about 6 months prior to each period of sobriety. She had to drink hourly to avoid having shakes in her latter period of inebriety, kept a drink next to her bed, and was blacked out during the last 9 months, but worked part of that time. She had 1 DUI arrest shortly before her present sobriety, resulting in jail, DUI school, and a fine. She also wrecked her car while drunk soon after the DUI school session.

Jill was introduced to TM by a meditating boyfriend who was a sober, recovering alcoholic, and whose stability she admired. She felt that she, although sober, was an "emotional basket case." She now always meditates in the evening, but often misses her meditation in the morning due to being too busy. She views TM as being "the most important thing," next to sobriety, in her life. She says it plays the spiritual role that her Catholicism played during her first sobriety, which slipped away when she began dating drinking men. She feels she is "80% less emotional," rarely cries now, and is able to remain detached from people she helps at AA panels. She reports that she is more harmonious at work, and concentrates better, which helped her to learn to use a computer. Her sleep is often interrupted by AA calls for help, but she feels fresh with less sleep. She says that until learning TM, she did not know how to do the meditation part of the Eleventh Step. Now TM stops her mind from racing and gives her inner quiet. She states that without a spiritual program that includes TM to "go within," she would not have a basis for continuing sobriety.

Jill says, "I truly believe that my last boyfriend was put in my life to lead me to TM, because he and I had virtually nothing in common. However, once I started TM, we had a bond that went beyond our relationship and allowed us to go our separate ways without the usual attendant hysterics and accusations. We basically let go. I had never done that in my life before. I must say that at times I feel so unlike my old self that it scares me. Occasionally my destructive old self comes up and tries to inject negative feelings, but I am curiously detached. I am completely open to strangers and have conversations everywhere I go. I love people of all ages and feel a complete oneness. Clients call me after hours to just talk. I have discovered a part of me that was dormant for 20 years while I was drinking. But I do not believe I could have become this open with just AA and not meditation. I am eternally grateful that I was ready for TM."

Comments. Upon interviewing these individuals, I recommended strongly to them that they meditate regularly. If irregular TM has been so helpful to them, what could more regular practice do?! Al's case shows specifically how TM can help with psychological problems, since he notices that his anxiety, obsessive thinking, etc., all go away when he is meditating regularly, but return when he stops. Jill's story, even though she does not meditate twice daily, is a good example of how the benefits of TM build cumulatively in the direction of not only effectiveness in life but also the state of enlightenment, in which full human potential is said to be utilized (see Discussion, below). Her feelings of detachment from old negative thought patterns, as well as love for her fellow human beings, are characteristic signs of the growth toward this higher state.

A Case with Severe Difficulties but Eventual Progress

Doubtless due to individual variations, response to TM is not uniform. In order to provide a global overview of experiences with TM, one representative case is included of an alcoholic who continued to experience severe problems along with continued but irregular TM practice. This subject's lengthy difficulty with recovery ended only after he found a strong source of external support for sobriety (AA) along with TM.

Steve. Steve is a Caucasian man who learned TM in January of 1968 at age 23 when he believed he was dying from habitual use of 20-30 joints of marijuana per day added to injecting morphine and amphetamines. He was unemployable, had weight loss, poor memory, little sleep, and dreams of death. He had thrown away his syringe many times, but could not stop using drugs. His girlfriend, a TM meditator, threatened to leave unless he learned TM. From the first meditation, he was immediately (although temporarily) relieved of compulsive drug use, and his physical craving was (temporarily) lifted. He tried "speed" 3 weeks later, but had a bad experience, and remained free of drugs with regular TM practice for over 2 years. During this time he married his girlfriend, became a checker of TM, and succeeded extremely well in business, becoming among other things a partner in ownership of shopping centers and a part-time manager in an investment firm.

However, Steve did not take warning from his past history. Steve began drinking alcoholically at 13, stealing his parents' alcohol and drinking on a job with an alcoholic boss. He was subsequently arrested several times for drug-related offenses, and was expelled from college for dealing in drugs. Thus when after 2-3 years of drug free, sober, and successful life with regular TM he began drinking wine with dinner, he quickly slipped into heavy drinking, then drug use and trafficking, and within 6 months had lost his wife and was bankrupt.

For more than 10 years he continued to drink and use drugs periodically, initially being drug free and sober for as much as 3-6 months out of the year while practicing TM regularly to regain his health, but meditating irregularly during periods of drinking and using drugs. Once he overdosed on cocaine, but meditated and survived. He worked at various jobs, but by the end of the 10 years he was virtually never sober and meditated only occasionally. He experienced shakes, DT's, and blackouts. He had arrests for DUI, public drunkenness, driving a stolen car, and credit card forgery, but escaped all convictions except for a probation sentence.

In October 1984, after writing a letter to God during a blackout asking for help, Steve entered a 28-day VA hospital residential drug and alcohol abuse program. Hearing an AA panel his first night there gave him hope. He began meditating regularly again about 4 days into his VA program, and after release began doing both AA service and TM volunteer checking. He worked at restaurant and sales jobs. He started our TM program for alcoholics by setting up the inaugural introductory TM lecture for CLARE staff and by helping give introductory lectures for the next couple of years, before moving away.

Since his lasting sobriety and about 8 years of fairly regular TM, Steve has been twice remarried and divorced, and now has half custody of his infant son. During the last marriage he had four severe attacks of pericarditis (a heart ailment), and lost the house he had been buying while working as a chef. During all of these difficulties, Steve has remained drug free and sober. He attends 5-6 AA meetings weekly, and sponsors about twelve newer AA members. He continues to practice TM, although less regularly since the birth of his son, due to the demands of childcare. He also spent 3-4 years in weekly psychotherapy. Recently, he joined a Christian church. He feels he needed AA and psychotherapy as well as TM to remain sober. But he feels he would not have made it without TM, which he believes helps his spiritual and emotional life, and physical and mental health. He feels TM helped him come through his severe pericarditis with no signs of scar tissue. He feels that TM also helps him to be a good father. He quotes a fellow meditating AA member, who calls TM "the crest jewel in the crown of the Twelve Steps," and he continues to refer AA friends to learn TM.

Comments. This difficult case illustrates that the benefits of TM, while cumulative, may take some time to manifest themselves clearly in some cases where problems are particularly deep and chronic. As indicated by the previous success stories, deeply troubled individuals may well experience rather rapid and lasting relief from many problems through TM. However, for individuals like Steve, although improvements certainly are to be expected, considerable and long-term persistence with TM may be necessary to attain really lasting sobriety and effectiveness in life. In this case, AA was quite complementary to TM, in providing Steve with a supportive environment and education against return to the use of any alcohol whatsoever. Steve lacked these factors until his VA treatment program in 1984. It should be noted that Steve has now been sober for over 8 years.

How TM Helped Individuals Whose Sobriety Was Well-Established

Although our program emphasized improved chances of continued sobriety as a major reason for learning TM, some individuals came to us specifically to improve their Eleventh Step (see Introduction), while feeling well-established in sobriety. The last two cases are representative examples.

Aileen. Aileen is a Caucasian woman who learned TM in November of 1989 at age 41, after 9 months of sobriety. She was sober for 2 days after starting an alcohol-free weight loss diet when she attended a seminar for "women questioning their use of alcohol." She asserts that she would not have attended had the seminar been directed at "alcoholics," but it persuaded her to remain sober. She attended her first AA meeting after 5 days of sobriety, and has remained sober ever since. AA helped her to understand and endure detoxification symptoms such as shakes, sugar cravings, insomnia, and 4 months of amenorrhea. She currently attends three AA meetings weekly, and sponsors three other individuals.

Aileen attended 3 years of college, has been married twice to her present husband, and has two children who were in their teens at the time she became sober. Aileen was a "functioning" alcoholic. She had her first drink at age 12, first became drunk at age 16, and loved alcohol from the beginning. She feels she was initially a social drinker. However, from the time her children entered school until her sobriety, she drank virtually every night until she passed out or blacked out. Her children challenged her to stay sober for three days, but she was never able to do so until after the seminar. She generally consumed 7 or 8 bottles of wine in an evening. (She tried cocaine and marijuana a couple of times, but because they were illegal, she did not continue out of concern for her family.) During at least 12 years of daily drinking she worked part-time at home or at part-time jobs with flexible hours, starting late in the morning. The children got their own breakfast, but she was functional for about 6 hours a day, and always did the household chores and had dinner on the table. However, she was beginning to experience mild jaundice and bladder problems attributable to alcohol before she finally got sober.

Aileen presently practices TM twice daily, sometimes taking a nap after the afternoon session. She feels she was securely sober by the time she learned TM, but needed a stronger spiritual program. Her AA sponsor recommended TM. After 9 months of discovering how to be sober, she found in TM a way to "be still, and experience a loving, positive God." Although she spent the early days of her sobriety simply recovering and later taking care of sick relatives, she has held for a couple of years a full-time job as an administrative assistant for a printer, and also takes care of her parents.

Sue. Sue is a Caucasian woman who learned TM in August of 1989 at age 44, after over 9 years of sobriety. She completed a 3-month residential alcoholism treatment program in early 1980 after what she termed a nervous breakdown that led her to spend time in a psychiatric ward. She entered the treatment program shortly after discharge from the mental hospital because she was afraid she would commit suicide or homicide. She became an AA member, presently attends one or more AA meetings per week and one AA panel per month, and sponsors four or five people.

Sue was abused as a child, and was hospitalized at age 17 for an emotional disorder. She first drank at age 8, drinking leftover drinks after her parents' social parties. She first got drunk at age 11 or 12 and drank alcoholically from that time. She could drink a case of beer alone at night, and had DT's and blackouts in her late teens. She completed 2 years of college, and in her early twenties she drank still more heavily.

She moved to California over 20 years ago, and her daily alcohol consumption decreased at that time by about 50%, but she began abusing prescription drugs, such as diet pills, tranquilizers, and sleeping pills. She also used "speed" and cocaine. Her drug abuse caused weight loss and a hospitalization to drain fluid from her lungs. In her late twenties she worked as a successful manager for a loan company, a bank, and a major credit card company. While working, she drank at lunch. At 31 she was becoming dysfunctional, and was fired. She lived on investments and worked a little, mainly as a hat check girl, continuing to drink and abuse drugs, but trying to stop. She took fewer sleeping pills after a blackout led to driving the wrong way in traffic. Two years before her sobriety she stopped all drugs but Dalmane and marijuana, and cut her alcohol use by 75% and became a periodic drinker because drinking a lot began to make her sick and led to seizures, and interfered with a new, part-time job as a business consultant to her roommate. She had been sober but still used marijuana and sleeping pills for the 4 months before entering the treatment program in 1980.

After her official sobriety, Sue took Elavil (an anti-depressant) by prescription for 6 months, but no drugs thereafter. To her disappointment, however, she continued to function poorly. She did temporary office work on and off for 7 years, then a little business consulting, and was setting up her own travel agency when she learned TM.

Sue initially meditated 15 minutes twice a day, because longer meditations caused her a rush of thoughts accompanied by feelings of panic, or edginess. After a couple of years, she found that if she continued in meditation despite such an experience, it would wane and be replaced by deeper, quiet meditation before the end of the 20 minutes. Presently, she meditates the usually-prescribed 20 minutes twice daily, sometimes lying down to rest afterwards. She says earlier she found solace in therapy, and tried other approaches to meditation during her first 9 years of AA. However she could not do any form of meditation satisfactorily previous to TM. In particular, she found it impossible to control her thoughts, and experienced great relief in finding no control to be necessary in TM.

In Sue's case, after feeling herself a tortured person most of her life, she now feels an overall sense of well-being, inner strength, and harmony. Before TM she could not concentrate, even to read for a couple of minutes. (She asserts that difficulty with concentration is typical of individuals who have suffered child abuse, and TM has helped tremendously with that process of recovery also.) Now her concentration is fine, her travel agency has succeeded as she wished–as a profitable, part-time business that has left her time to fulfill her dream, writing books. She feels TM unblocked her creativity, enabling her to complete the writing of two books. Her formerly negative, obsessive thinking (termed by some AA members "my committee" or "the ghetto between my ears") has improved dramatically. She reports that she is much less judgmental, more accepting, and less upset in reaction to what other people say or do. She says, "My esteem is better; I think of myself as a spiritual being more than I ever have–a part of the universe, and a part of a God consciousness. I have never been able to live in the now as I do today, without terror of the future or self-pity over the past. I am more able to be of service, because I am much more loving, patient, accepting, grateful, peaceful, and creative than I have ever been. I feel now I will be able to fulfill my spiritual life, living my full potential."

Sue believes that TM can be extremely helpful to alcoholics who have been sober for years, but may feel hopeless because they do not feel they are progressing as they should, or even find themselves dysfunctional in practical life after working the Twelve Steps for years. She feels this difficulty can lead to slipping back into active alcoholism.

Comments. Sue's remarks on her ability to do TM after failing with other forms of meditation harken back to Sam's delight with the ease of TM, and Jill's appreciation of how TM enabled her to "go within" and thus fulfilled her need for a spiritual program to sustain her sobriety. Certainly, the ease of TM, and the straightforward instructions for its successful practice provided a welcome relief to many of our Twelve Step clients who were searching for a practical way to spirituality. Aileen, who had not tried any other form of meditation, also welcomed the effectiveness of TM in her Eleventh Step. She seemed to take it for granted that when she became inwardly still with TM, a sense of nearness to God was the natural result.

Since Sue was abused as a child and, like Tom, Sam, and Fred, had been hospitalized for psychiatric treatment, her satisfaction with TM again underscores the holistic relief TM can bring to individuals suffering from multiple problems. Her comments on the failure of long-term sobriety to bring her the relief she expected from deep-seated problems are very telling. It required TM to transform her from being a "tortured" person into a harmonious and creative one. The normalization of stress (see Discussion) she experienced through TM effectively alleviated obsessive thoughts in the same way it alleviated Fred's paranoia. Beyond that, the deep spirituality she now experiences, including her sense of being "part of a God consciousness," living "in the now," and being of "service," "loving," etc., are signs of the growth of enlightenment, as reported by Jill above. Although living "one day at a time" is a tenet of the AA approach to sobriety, surely only a few recovering alcoholics find their desired ability to live in the present extending much beyond abstaining from drinking each day. To the contrary, sorrow over the bygone past and either fear of or yearning about what the future may bring are typical of the lives of almost every unenlightened human being (see Maharishi Mahesh Yogi, 1967).

DISCUSSION

Our program consisted almost entirely of Twelve Step adherents. As indicated by the case histories above, those who continued with TM found it invaluable both as part of their Eleventh Step and also in fulfilling their broader spiritual goals. AA as an organization will not endorse TM or any other outside program; but some AA sponsors sent several sponsees to us for TM instruction, while many AA members sent their friends.

Our nonresidential program did not permit as intensive a follow-up as would have been ideal. Nevertheless, a nonrigorous appraisal of our information on actual TM practice by our meditators indicates that of 225 who had learned TM before I left Los Angeles in early 1991, at the time of last contact (mostly late 1990, or a few months to 4 years after TM instruction), the meditating status of about 20% was unknown, while 46% of the remainder were still meditating. These results may be compared to those of Taub et al. (this volume), who found about 55% of skid row alcoholics who learned TM during a treatment program were still practicing at the time of a 6-month follow-up. Shafii et al. (1975) were able to contact 36% of a sample of 525 individuals who had learned TM at a TM center, and found 70% of those contacted were meditating. Bleick and Abrams (1987) found in a survey of 229 California prison inmates who had learned TM from a few months to 7 years previously that while 32% did not respond to the survey, 87% of the respondents were still meditating. Alexander (1982) found that 64% of Massachusetts prison meditators to be still practicing TM after 1 to 3 years of practice. Alexander, Langer, Newman, Chandler, and Davies (1989) and Schneider, Alexander, and Wallace (1992) found 80%-90% of nursing home meditators and elderly African Americans in a blood pressure study, respectively, to be continuing TM practice after 3 months. These last two studies suggest that a more structured follow-up may assist in maintaining the regularity of TM practice.

Although our program was very successful for alcoholics who are living in the community, it seems likely that the rate of continued TM practice, and therefore the percentage of students who gained long-term benefits from TM, could be greatly increased by teaching TM in the context of a residential alcohol and drug treatment program, preferably lasting 3 months or more. If TM instruction took place as soon as possible after detoxification, and group meditations with checking occurred twice daily for the remainder of the residential period, the habit of regular TM practice would likely be much more firmly established. Also, doubts about experiences could be resolved, and mistakes corrected, before the students had the chance to fall away from TM. A residential program would also provide the necessary structure for the use and testing of Maharishi Ayur-Veda as an auxiliary treatment. Maharishi Ayur-Veda is a revival of the traditional Vedic system of herbal and mineral treatments and the like to balance body and mind. These treatments might be expected to augment TM benefits and help meditators to maintain lasting sobriety. Yoga asanas prescribed by the TM program could also be incorporated in a residential situation. The success of such an intensive, residential program has been illustrated by the teaching of TM to virtually the entire prison population (many of whom were substance abusers) in Senegal, Africa in 1987-1989 (Anklesaria, 1988), which resulted in a dramatic drop in recidivism nationwide.

As a caution to those who may establish such programs, it may be noted from the case histories (see Fred and Sue, above), that some alcoholics cannot meditate comfortably for 20 minutes twice daily, at least initially. This may be due to intensity of what Maharishi calls "normalization of stress." Normalization of stress occurs as a natural by-product of TM practice, typically with no discomfort to the practitioner (see Bloomfield et al., 1975). However, for some individuals who have abused chemicals, or whose psychophysiological imbalances led them to abuse chemicals in the first place, this natural detoxification process may be more intensive at times. This temporary situation can be ameliorated by following the meditation period with lying down rest and by consulting a TM teacher for other special instructions.

The case histories here certainly reveal that, while learning TM may lead to immediate relief from serious chemical dependency and related problems, in most cases the process is a gradual and cumulative one. Thus the AA principle that alcoholics cannot expect a quick cure and a return to social drinking seems likely to hold also when TM is used in treatment. The example of Steve is particularly telling. (However, see the discussion of Maharishi's Vedic

Psychology below.) This gradual and cumulative quality of the decline in substance abuse measured in surveys and experimental studies is mentioned in the major review papers on the subject (Aron & Aron, 1980; Gelderloos, Walton, Orme-Johnson, & Alexander, 1991; Alexander et al., this volume). Considering the magnitude of the alcoholism and drug abuse problem in the U.S. today, it is not surprising if a solution takes time. On the other hand, Frank, Al, and Jill found TM greatly helpful in maintaining sobriety even when practiced irregularly.

Benefits attributed to TM as mentioned by the subjects in their case histories include the following categories:

1. Reduced craving for drugs and alcohol, or otherwise helped with sobriety (Tom, Sam, Pedro, Frank, Jill, Steve).
2. Helped with Eleventh Step, experience of God, or other spiritual sense (Sam, Fred, Pedro, Al, Jill, Steve, Aileen, Sue).
3. Improved interpersonal relations (Tom, Sam, Pedro, Steve, Al, Jill, Sue).
5. Improved work or school performance (Tom, Sam, Fred, Pedro, Frank, Aileen, Sue).
6. Gave inner peace, or relaxation, or clearer thinking, or better concentration (Tom, Sam, Frank, Al, Jill, Sue).
7. Reduced negative emotions, or increased positive ones (Tom, Sam, Pedro, Jill, Steve, Sue).
8. Improved mental health (Tom–"schizophrenia," Sam and Frank–depression, Fred–schizo-affective disorder, Steve–general, Al–anxiety).
9. Improved physical health and youthfulness (Tom, Sam, Pedro, Jill, Steve).
10. Improved self-esteem (Pedro, Frank, Sue).

Since the interviews for the case histories were open-ended, some individuals might have mentioned other improvements (such as general well-being, self-esteem and physical health). These improvements seemed apparent in many cases to the interviewer, but were not much explicitly mentioned by the interviewees.

The improvements listed fall into the categories of "increased positive traits" and "reduced problems, stress, etc.," which were well-represented response categories in a survey by Aron and Aron

(1983) in which TM meditators were requested to indicate their TM-related reasons for giving up substance abuse. It is apparent from our case histories that the individuals interviewed found that their lives were improving spontaneously in a wide variety of ways, including actual efficacy of mental, emotional, and physical performance. These changes were global and appeared to cross all the categories of theory for successful treatment of substance abuse, as reviewed by Aron and Aron (1980), namely, "situations, social influences, emotions, cognitions"; by Gelderloos et al. (1991), namely, self-actualization, self-esteem, well-being, sense of meaning in life, and rebelliousness" and "coping resources"; and by Alexander et al. (this volume), namely "environmental/social, physiological, psychological, and spiritual."

All the reviews advance as a major explanation for the global changes observed in meditating former substance abusers the equally global improvements in neurophysiological functioning indicated by extensive physiological research on TM. Aron and Aron (1980) cite physiological EEG research indicating that during TM meditators experience a heightened EEG coherence, corresponding to subjective experience of TC, or transcendental consciousness, in which ordinary, active states of thought are transcended and one experiences a field of pure silence and bliss. Experience of TC is said to increase the integration and balance of the nervous system, thereby improving performance in practical life. Thus the tendency to abuse substances for the sake of a short-term sense of relief from stress, is gradually replaced through TM practice by longer-term satisfying experiences during and outside of TM that derive from regular meditation. Substance abuse, often occurring in response to stress, produces an abnormal "high" that is followed by further physiological imbalance. Gelderloos et al. (1991) review literature indicating that natural healing occurring during TM restores balance to neurotransmitter systems (see also Walton and Levitsky; and Sharma, Dillbeck, and Dillbeck, both in this volume) that have been depleted by substance abuse.

Our meditators themselves, all staunch Twelve Step adherents, suggest another global theory by embracing TM as a particularly effective way to improve their spiritual lives and improve their relationship with God, a point also considered by Alexander et al.

and O'Connell (in this volume). If, as Maharishi (1963) asserts, mind is the basis of body and behavior, and spirit ("Being" or "pure consciousness" or "creative intelligence") is the basis of mind, then as he has always claimed, the holistic improvements that accumulate in the lives of TM meditators are due to the mind's settling down during TM to contact pure (transcendental) consciousness, whose intelligence underlies the whole of life.

It is the contact of the mind with pure consciousness, the ultimate reality of life, that allows first the mind, and therefore the body, to experience a deep, settled state, and thereby to throw off the "stresses," or abnormalities accumulated through wrong living, including chemical abuse. As the mind begins to function more and more normally, meditators begin to experience a sense of peace, energy, and happiness that is increasingly independent of outer circumstances (see Maharishi Mahesh Yogi, 1967). They thus find within themselves the strength and creativity to respond favorably and effectively to difficulties which formerly overwhelmed them and dragged them down into inebriety. Simultaneously, they begin to enjoy and appreciate positive events and situations more and more fully. The experiences of developing compassion, clarity of mind, harmony, bliss, and love reported by Tom, Sam, Pedro, Jill, and Sue exemplify these changes. According to Maharishi's Vedic Psychology, upon reaching the goal of TM, the full development of human potential referred to as enlightenment, all traces of damage due to past chemical dependency, and all tendency to abuse chemicals in the present and future, is completely eliminated. Moreover, the sense of inner peace, joy, and well-being initially sought inappropriately in alcohol and drugs would be developed to its fulfillment in unbounded inner contentment and outer effectiveness and creativity. Such a felicitous state would be worth any alcoholic's time to develop.

REFERENCES

Alcoholics Anonymous World Services, Inc. (1976). *Alcoholics Anonymous: The story of how many thousands of men and women have recovered from alcoholism* (3rd ed.). New York: Author.

Alcoholics Anonymous World Services, Inc. (1981). *Twelve steps and twelve traditions.* New York: Author.

Alexander, C. N. (1982). *Ego development, personality and behavioral change in inmates practicing the Transcendental Meditation technique or participating in other programs: A cross-sectional and longitudinal study.* Unpublished doctoral dissertation, Harvard University, Cambridge.

Alexander, C. N., Langer, E. J., Newman, R. I., Chandler, H. M., & Davies, J. L. (1989). Transcendental Meditation, mindfulness, and longevity: An experimental study with the elderly. *Journal of Personality and Social Psychology, 57,* 950-964.

Alexander, C. N., Robinson, P., & Rainforth, M. (this volume). Treating alcohol, nicotine, and drug abuse through Transcendental Meditation: A review and statistical meta-analysis. *Alcoholism Treatment Quarterly.*

Anklesaria, F. (1988). *New horizons in criminology and penetentiary science: Maharishi unified field based integrated system of rehabilitation in Senegalese prisons* (Trans.). Vlodrop, The Netherlands: Maharishi Vedic University Press.

Aron, A., & Aron, E. N. (1980). The Transcendental Meditation program's effect on addictive behavior. *Addictive Behaviors. 5,* 3-12.

Aron, E. N., & Aron, A. (1983). The patterns of reduction of drug and alcohol use among Transcendental Meditation participants. *Bulletin of the Society of Psychologists in Addictive Behaviors.* 2(1), 28-33.

Bleick, C. R., & Abrams, A. I. (1987). The Transcendental Meditation program and criminal recidivism in California. *Journal of Criminal Justice. 15,* 211-230.

Bloomfield, H. H., Cain, M. P., Jaffe, D. T., & Kory, R. B. (1975). *TM: Discovering inner energy and overcoming stress.* New York: Delacorte Press.

Bloomfield, H. H., & Kory, R. B. (1976). *Happiness: The TM program, psychiatry, and enlightenment.* New York: Simon and Schuster.

Childs, J. P. (1977). The use of the Transcendental Meditation program as a therapy with juvenile offenders. In D. W. Orme-Johnson, & J. T. Farrow (Eds.), *Scientific research on the Transcendental Meditation program: Collected papers, Vol. 1* (pp. 577-584). Livingston Manor, New York: Maharishi European Research University Press.

Gelderloos, P., Walton, K. G., Orme-Johnson, D. W., & Alexander, C. N. (1991). Effectiveness of the Transcendental Meditation program in preventing and treating substance misuse: A review. *International Journal of the Addictions. 26,* 293-325.

Maharishi Mahesh Yogi. (1963). *Science of being and art of living.* New York: Signet.

Maharishi Mahesh Yogi. (1967). *On the Bhagavad-Gita.* New York: Arkana.

Monahan, R. J. (1977). Secondary prevention of drug dependence through the Transcendental Meditation program in metropolitan Philadelphia. *The International Journal of the Addictions. 12,* 729-754.

O'Connell, D. F. (1991). The use of TM in relapse prevention counseling. *Alcoholism Treatment Quarterly.* 8(1), 53-67.

O'Connell, D. F. (this volume). Possessing the Self: The technologies of Maharishi Ayur-Veda and the process of recovery from addictive diseases. *Alcoholism Treatment Quarterly.*

Schneider, R. H., Alexander, C. N., & Wallace, R. K. (1992). In search of an optimal behavioral treatment for hypertension: A review and focus on Transcendental Meditation. In E. H. Johnson, W. D. Gentry, & S. Julius (Eds.), *Personality, elevated blood pressure, and essential hypertension* (pp. 291-312). Washington, DC: Hemisphere Publishing Corporation.

Shafii, M., Lavely, R. A., & Jaffe, R. (1975). Meditation and the prevention of alcohol abuse. *American Journal of Psychiatry. 132,* 942-945.

Sharma, H. M., Dillbeck, M. C., & Dillbeck, S. L. (this volume). Implementation of Transcendental Meditation program and Maharishi Ayur-Veda to prevent alcohol and drug abuse among juveniles at risk. *Alcoholism Treatment Quarterly.*

Taub, E., Solomon, S. S., Smith, R. B., Weingarten, E., Alexander, C. N. & Walton, K. G. (this volume). Effectiveness of broad spectrum approaches to relapse prevention: A long-term, randomized, controlled trial comparing Transcendental Meditation, muscle relaxation, and electronic neurotherapy in severe alcoholism. *Alcoholism Treatment Quarterly.*

Walton, K. G., & Levitsky, D. (this volume). Role of Transcendental Meditation in reducing drug use and addictions: Neurochemical evidence and a theory. *Alcoholism Treatment Quarterly.*

Removing the Motivator: A Holistic Solution to Substance Abuse

George A. Ellis, PhD
Pat Corum

People want love, respect, health, happiness, inner peace, and freedom from stress. If any of these fundamentals is missing from a person's life, that person becomes vulnerable to many types of disease–including substance abuse. This vulnerability is similar to weakness in the immune system, which leaves the body susceptible to outside influences that can cause myriad health problems.

George A. Ellis is the author of *Inside Folsom Prison: Unified Field Based Rehabilitation*. Dr. Ellis has over 22 years of experience in working with emotionally disturbed children and adults, prisoners in a number of state and federal corrections systems, terminally ill children and adults, and people with substance abuse problems. Dr. Ellis has conducted over 25 rehabilitation projects for the Institute for Social Rehabilitation, a non-profit educational organization. An international consultant and program director for the Institute, Dr. Ellis has conducted projects for the California Youth Authority and California Adult Authority, California state prisons (including San Quentin and Folsom prisons), Vermont Department of Corrections, and prison systems in Central America. Currently, Dr. Ellis continues to serve as a consultant to the Institute for Social Rehabilitation. Dr. Ellis also is the founder and president of Agro International Inc./Geotropical S.A. (Guatemala/Costa Rica). These companies are import/export firms headquartered in Miami, Florida. Pat Corum is a former inmate of San Quentin and Folsom prisons in California. He is currently paroled, and recently graduated from California State University's Attorney Assistant Program. Mr. Corum now operates his own business, providing support services for criminal attorneys.

[Haworth co-indexing entry note]: "Removing the Motivator: A Holistic Solution to Substance Abuse." Ellis, George A. and Pat Corum. Co-published simultaneously in the *Alcoholism Treatment Quarterly* (The Haworth Press, Inc.) Vol. 11, No. 3/4, 1994, pp. 271-296; and: *Self-Recovery: Treating Addictions Using Transcendental Meditation and Maharishi Ayur-Veda* (ed: David F. O'Connell and Charles N. Alexander) The Haworth Press, Inc., 1994, pp. 271-296. Multiple copies of this article/chapter may be purchased from The Haworth Document Delivery Center [1-800-3-HAWORTH; 9:00 a.m. - 5:00 p.m. (EST)].

I have been implementing human development programs for over twenty years, working in almost every area of social rehabilitation. My experience includes programs for emotionally disturbed children, community-centered drug programs, and programs administered in a wide range of correctional environments. This includes programs administered in county jails, maximum security prisons, and "death row."

All of that experience has led me to one basic conclusion: If deep-rooted physiological stress is removed, the behavioral symptoms of that stress disappear. These "symptoms" include alcohol and drug abuse, addictions, and all other forms of deviant or criminal behavior. The underlying motivator for all of these behaviors is stress. Remove the motivator, the underlying stress, and the undesirable behavior disappears.

When I use the term "stress," I am not referring merely to minor surface-level problems or the strain and fatigue accumulated in day-to-day living. My definition of stress also includes the deep-rooted psychological and physiological influence of mental illness, addiction, dysfunctional family life, the absence of adequate parenting, or physical, emotional, and sexual abuse suffered early in a person's life. Counselors and mental health professionals generally agree that most forms of mental illness and deviant or criminal behavior can be traced to these deep-rooted physiological and psychological stresses.

There is a simple, powerful, easily-learned technique for removing deep-rooted stress: the Transcendental Meditation (TM) program. I have used this program to successfully help hard-core criminals, addicts, emotionally disturbed children, and many other "problem" individuals in a wide variety of high-stress correctional environments. My purpose here is to explain how and why the TM program has proven so successful when applied to substance abuse, violent behavior, and the innumerable other problems that arise in correctional environments. Quite simply, TM removes the motivator.

I will not take the time here to scientifically justify the benefits of the TM program. That has been done many times over. During the past twenty years, over 500 scientific studies on the TM program have been published in a wide range of prestigious scientific journals (Chalmers, Clements, Schenkluhn, & Weinless, 1989a,b,c; 1990; Orme-Johnson & Farrow, 1976; Wallace, Orme-Johnson, & Dillbeck, 1977) Gelderloos, Walton, Orme-Johnson, and Alexander (1991) reviewed 24 studies done on the TM program and substance abuse, and found TM to be a very effective drug rehabilitation program.

The experiences I wish to discuss here are human experiences. I feel that the simple, everyday experiences of case workers, counselors, and substance abuse specialists tell more about the effects and benefits of a program than any statistical analysis or psychiatric overview. Common sense and observation are the best ways to determine that a program is working and that a person who is involved in a program has changed for the better.

I once asked an emotionally disturbed child how he felt after practicing his TM technique. He said, "The trees are prettier." This, in my opinion, was a more significant statement about the power of positive transformation than any scientific study. It is a totally subjective statement of an inner, subjective experience. "The trees are prettier" was a simple reflection of a powerful change that had taken place in that child's mind and heart. Those kinds of changes are the goal of every person who works with the disadvantaged, the addicted, or the incarcerated.

The programs I have implemented in correctional settings over the past twenty years have been for custodians and counselors as well as inmates and patients. The power of this approach is described in *Inside Folsom Prison: Unified Field Based Rehabilitation* (Ellis, 1983), the book I wrote after compiling reports, testimonials and numerous research studies from participants and observers of the TM program at Folsom State Prison in California.

The TM program has proven to be a tremendous gift to the underpaid people who deal with the human consequences of crime and substance abuse. I say "underpaid" because the price that counselors, custodians, therapists, and mental health professionals pay, in terms of the impact on their health, psychology, and lifespan, cannot be compensated by any amount of money.

Any counselor can tell you: a confrontation with a highly-stressed patient or inmate is like having hot mud thrown on you. You can actually feel the heat of it. You feel like you need a shower afterwards. The TM technique is like taking a shower inside, where it is needed the most. After twenty minutes of TM, one feels deeply rested, as after a good night's sleep, without the dullness associated with sleep. The cumulative benefits are even more important: Wallace (1986) has shown that regular practice of the TM technique provides a wide range of health improvements and actually reverses the aging process.

It doesn't matter whether the institution is a mental health hospital, a prison, or a residential treatment facility–the TM program provides better health, increased self-respect, freedom from stress, and inner happiness for all who learn the technique and practice it regularly. When the TM technique is practiced regularly and supplemented by educational programs that explain the physiological, emotional, and behavioral changes that are taking place, the benefits are dramatic and tangible. (Follow-up is a normal part of TM instruction, but in special cases, such as in prison environments, a more extensive follow-up program is recommended because of the need for support and a structure that supports their continuing practice and reentry into society.)

CASE HISTORIES

1. Pat Corum (Folsom and San Quentin Prison)

Pat Corum was one of the most intelligent and toughest men I had ever met in prison. At the time we first met, in California's maximum-security Folsom State Prison, Pat had a string of convictions for kidnapping, robbery, assaults, escape attempts, smuggling, drug trafficking, and murder. During a previous term of more than seven years in the California prison system, Pat had seen twenty-two psychiatrists, psychologists, and counselors, spending hundreds of hours in group counseling, group therapy, and individual counseling. Following all of that treatment, he had been released. Within six months, Pat Corum was back in prison again, with convictions for robbery and first-degree murder.

Here is Pat Corum's story in his own words.

> By the time I was fifteen, I had reached the conclusion that normal people did not think the way I did, and that normal

people did not act the way I did. Therefore, I decided that I was totally crazy for thinking and acting the way I did.

My feelings of isolation and loneliness were so overwhelming that I started looking outside of myself for something, anything, that would stop those feelings and the pain associated with them. I found drugs.

Drugs made me feel good. For the first time in my life, I felt like I was accepted by a group of people. They thought like I did, felt like I did, and we were all doing the same or similar activities–whatever it took to get more drugs and stay loaded. For a long time, I did not think I had a drug problem. I thought I had a money problem. I felt that if I had enough money, I could get all the drugs I needed and I could feel good.

Being accepted was a big part of this process of trying to feel good. I wanted to be accepted by my family, my peers, and society in general. I guess I thought that if I had all of the outward appearances of success, i.e., nice clothes, rings, watches, a new and expensive car, lots of money, etc., that everyone would not only like me, but they would want me to be around them.

By the time I was seventeen, I had learned that I could get more of what I wanted with a gun and a smile than I could with a smile. Even then, the "control" issues were starting to surface for me. I knew what fear felt like, and through that knowledge I quickly developed skills in intimidation, coercion, and inflicting massive amounts of pain on others through physical violence and the use of weapons. As my need to look good and feel good continued to grow, my level of anger went out of control. It was like I was in a state of rage during all my waking hours. All the things that I thought would fix me, all the things that I thought would make me whole, were not working. Everything that I thought was true was a lie. There was no longer any foundation for sanity or reason. I still recall telling my best friend at the time, "I'm going to do what I want to do, when I want to do it. If people don't like it, they can kill me before I kill them." By the time I was twenty-two, I had done time in two different states, and in a mental institution. In February of 1963, I assaulted three San Leandro police officers when they attempted to arrest me for a supermarket robbery. Shortly thereafter, I shot and wounded the Chief of Police in Hollister, California.

My last encounter with the police was in Fresno, California. I had just made an "unauthorized withdrawal" from a local bank, and when the police tried to arrest me, I shot and wounded a motorcycle cop. When the dust finally cleared, I had emptied a .38 snub-nosed revolver and two clips from a 9mm automatic pistol. And the police had put five .38 slugs into me.

After two operations and a plea bargain, I was transferred to San Mateo County. There, I was charged with a capital crime and advised that the people of California would ask for the death penalty. In exchange for a plea of guilty, I was allowed to receive a sentence of life imprisonment.

I was transported to the maximum security section of San Quentin State Prison, where I stayed until 1967. Because of my continued drug usage, association with prison gangs, and being involved in the introduction of a .38 pistol with 71 rounds of ammunition into the prison, I was transferred to the maximum-security section of the most maximum-security prison in California: Folsom State Prison.

I continued my association with the prison gangs at Folsom. Because of this, in 1970 I was charged with and convicted of the execution-style slaying of a lieutenant in a rival prison gang. This time, there was no offer of a plea bargain. The jury voted 7 to 5 to execute me. The only thing that changed about me, as a result of that experience, was that my anger about betrayal and treachery from other human beings was off the scale. Otherwise, my thinking had not changed at all. I was still convinced that all I needed was enough money to buy enough drugs to feel good.

In 1974, the Folsom prison staff started a college program. I enrolled, because I could receive G.I. bill benefits. In order to receive those benefits, however, I needed to maintain good grades. That was a problem, because I did not want to study. So, I teamed up with five other life-term inmates (between us, we had twenty-three homicide convictions). Our strategy was to make our instructors aware of our backgrounds, then impress upon them the need to give us good grades.

This worked really well until we ran into an instructor by the name of George Ellis. Initially, we thought it would be easy to intimidate him, because we were so much bigger than he was. And we thought he was on drugs, because he was so relaxed and mellow all the time. So, we "drove" on him. He just looked at us, smiled, and laughed. This was the last reaction we'd expected, and we had to fall back and regroup. Not only was this guy not intimidated by us, but he had shown no fear on any level.

After that episode, I really got to watching George. I began to notice that he wasn't just "laid back," but he also had a lot of energy, and a clarity of mind that I'd never seen in anyone else.

One afternoon after class, I went up to George and asked him what kind of drug he was taking, since he had such high energy and mental clarity, but no visible signs of stress. George then gave me my first introductory lecture about Transcendental Meditation.

George didn't just practice TM, he was also a TM teacher. For the next year, he had me read every book that had been published about TM up to that time. Then, in June of 1975, after paying my own instruction fee, I was taught the simple technique of Transcendental Meditation.

I would like to say that I stopped using drugs after the first time I meditated, but that would not be true. After using alcohol and hard drugs for over twenty years, I didn't stop immediately. However, most of my friends *did* stop using drugs as soon as they learned TM.

In my case, I just continued to meditate regularly, twice a day. I quickly reached a point where using drugs seriously interfered with how good I felt after meditation. Drugs were no longer a way to feel good, they were getting in the way of feeling good.

That was when I quit using drugs. Initially, the most dramatic and visible change was in my college work. I went from grades of B or C, with an occasional A, to straight A. I stopped getting disciplinary write-ups, and I put on twenty pounds. The process of positive change had begun. This positive change began from the inside. It had nothing to do with barbed wire or armed guards, or any other external controls. And it wasn't "peer pressure," either. My peers, the people I had been drawn to all my life for support and acceptance, were not thinking or acting or feeling the way I was. They had not changed. Instead, I was in the process of change, and part of that was getting out of the insanity that had become such an integral part of my life.

One day, after I'd been doing TM for about six months, I found myself in a difficult situation with another prisoner. A year earlier, I would have moved instinctively to injure the person. But instead of just reacting to the situation, I found myself feeling calm and relaxed. I had the clarity of mind to look at the various options I had for responding. I chose the best one: I just smiled and laughed.

As George Ellis had done with me and my friends, I did not react to someone else's drama. I didn't buy into the other person's drama, and I didn't support the drama by reacting.

This was a really beautiful experience for me. I acted in a highly responsible manner for the first time in my adult life. Looking back at all the other times I had experienced a rough time in my life, I realized that the issue had always been the same. I'd reacted to the situation without thinking. Looking even closer, I realized that in every instance I'd been stressed out, angry, hostile, tired, fatigued, and detoxifying from the effects of one or more drugs. The time, place, and person were different from one incident to the next, but the common denominator was my inability to think and respond in a socially acceptable manner.

Another thing I began to notice was that I was no longer actively creating roughness in the lives of other people. I just didn't feel like doing that anymore.

There is a big difference between reacting to life and being able to live life innocently. Life, I discovered, was neither fair nor unfair. Life was what I made of it. Life did not change from being ugly and nasty, I changed from being ugly and nasty.

After completing my A.A. degree with a 3.65 GPA in 1976, I was transferred to San Quentin State Prison so I could continue working on an advanced degree. For the first time in my life, I started getting involved in the positive aspects of prison life, especially the self-help groups. SQUIRES, a youth counseling program, was my favorite. I also became actively involved in the Alcoholics Anonymous Twelve Step program and other programs that help develop the behaviors and attitudes of a positive, responsible human being.

In 1979 I was transferred to a medium-security institution, C.C.I. Tehachapi. I continued my regular meditations, although I was housed in a dormitory with 200 other men. In fact, I discovered that I could even meditate while on a prison bus, chained to the max. I met a lot of new people and made a lot of new friends, both prisoners and staff members.

I got to know one young lady quite well during those years at Tehachapi. In 1983, we got married. She was the first woman in my life who loved me for what I was, rather than because of what I could do for her. Obviously, I couldn't take her out on a date or buy her presents. My surface-level "flash" consisted of wearing prison blues.

This lady has been a part of my life for thirteen years, and we've been married for nine years. During that time, I have never raised my voice in anger to her. We have never had an argument. We have agreed to disagree on two issues, religion and abortion. The meanest thing she has ever said to me was, "When was the last time you meditated?" In November of 1986, I was released from prison. The great adventure that I call life has become even more exciting and meaningful. I now live in a four-bedroom home that was built twenty years ago. My wife drives a car that's almost new. I drive a pickup that's a little older, I own a motorcycle, and I have a garage full of power tools that I refer to as "my toys."

I can't say that life has been easy since my release, but it sure has been enjoyable, at least for the most part. Last year, five members of my family passed away, and I was able to be there and provide support each time. I was able to experience all the feelings that come with the loss of a loved one, and

> never feel the need to resort to alcohol or drugs. I was also able to be there when two members of my family were married. And I was at the hospital when my second granddaughter was born. Due to a motorcycle accident, I've undergone surgery three times in the past two years: once to have a steel plate and six screws put in my leg, once to remove the plate and screws, and once for back surgery. Each time, I allowed the doctors to put me out with gas. However, because of my regular meditation, I did not find it necessary to use any kind of pre-operative or post-operative medication. Both of the surgeons were totally amazed at the fact that I took no medication and that I healed very fast. While I was off work from the accident, I enrolled in school again. I completed the Attorney Assistant Program at California State University and, in December 1991, I started my own business. I now provide support services for criminal attorneys. What life is like for me today can best be described by a recent experience. I drove up to my son's house, and when I got out of the car my 2 1/2-year-old granddaughter saw me. She immediately started running towards me with her little arms outstretched, yelling "Grandpa, Grandpa." I dropped to my knees and she ran up to me, put her arms around my neck, gave me a giant hug and a kiss on the cheek, and whispered in my ear, "I love you, Grandpa."

Pat Corum's experience is not unique. It is an example of what has occurred a thousand times and more in correctional settings throughout the world. At San Quentin and Folsom State Prison, for example, hundreds of inmates and staff members have learned the TM technique. The positive benefits have been documented extensively (Abrams & Siegel, 1978; Bleick & Abrams, 1987; Ellis, 1983). Pat Corum believes that the TM program should be integrated into every correctional facility in the United States, and throughout the world.

2. Central America

In 1984, I became involved in a comprehensive rehabilitation project for male and female prisoners in Guatemala and Honduras. This project also included a program that we structured for the native Mayan Indian populations. The prison project was a three-year pilot program that has been concluded, but the program for the Mayan Indians continued and is still in progress today.

At the time our rehabilitation project began, Guatemala and Honduras were in the grip of civil war, military dictatorships, and terrible poverty. Prison life under these circumstances was almost incomprehensible to Americans–there were up to twenty-five people in one cell; a typical security housing unit consisted of a hole dug underneath the prison; a normal lunch was a spoonful of black beans slapped on a tortilla, with the beans served from a filthy container that looked like a thrown-away, rusted-out old oil can.

Among the Mayan Indians, poverty was so entrenched that some families had boiled water for dinner. And everyone lived in constant fear of guerrillas who would kidnap family members or fellow villagers. Once abducted, many of the kidnap victims were never seen again.

Even in the poverty of Central America, substance abuse was widespread, especially among the Mayan Indian population. These people would try anything to get even temporary relief from their horrible living conditions.

The Prisons

We introduced the TM program into the prisons and taught thousands of prisoners and staff members how to practice TM. Creating an effective follow-up program was a challenge, because the inmates' sense of time usually meant arriving 30 to 90 minutes late for a meeting. However, we eventually were able to get meditating residents to meetings on time.

After six weeks, the research portion of the project was completed. About 50% of the prisoners continued to attend regular follow-up meetings, an amazing number when one considers the low level of support–frequently, there weren't even enough chairs to allow all the participants to sit and meditate.

The prison project was structured as an educational program for one year, for both men and women. The men's program reduced institutional violence significantly. The guards were practicing TM along with the inmates, and the guards often remarked about reduced anxiety. In Guatemala, the results were even more impressive. In Guatemalan prisons, many of the inmates were given clubs and made guards inside the deeper regions of the prison. Many of these guards began practicing TM, and reported that the incidence of beatings dropped substantially.

The extent of drug use in these settings was hard to determine. But meditating inmates reported that they often had their families learn TM too, and as a result, families tended to bring fewer drugs into the prisons. This was significant because the prisons of Guatemala were totally chaotic during visiting hours, with very little supervision.

The programs for women were much better organized. For women, the stress of prison life is more emotional. We provided the TM program along with a work program that gave the participants a sense of accomplishment. This experimental enterprise taught the women how to manufacture executive-quality scarves, sweaters, etc., for export to New York's garment district. The women received a percentage of the profits. This proved to be a highly effective project–it reinforced participation in the TM program, and the proceeds helped make an ongoing TM program possible. In many cases, the women continued to participate in activities at local TM centers after their release from prison.

The Mayan Indians

The Mayan Indians account for 45% of the population in Honduras and Guatemala. Most of these people live in abject poverty. Alcoholism is very prevalent. In fact, it is almost accepted as part of their native tradition today.

Just as we were preparing to offer the TM program to the Mayan Indians, we were told that these people couldn't possibly learn to meditate. We responded by introducing an integrated program that taught them the TM technique along with specialized agricultural training.

Over 1,200 Mayan Indians learned the TM technique. The results were consistent to the point of being unanimous: participants felt much happier and more peaceful. We also trained village leaders to conduct weekly TM educational meetings for their people. The village leaders reported a noticeable reduction in alcohol indulgence by many of the villagers.

The agricultural programs that we offered taught the Mayans how to grow better food on their land. Also, many of these people began to realize that it was better to allow their children to continue with school, rather than take them out at age 15 to work in the fields.

The program with the Mayan Indians is important because it provides an expanded vision of "rehabilitation." The program we offered did more than merely alleviate substance abuse, although that in itself was an impressive accomplishment. These are simple, poorly educated people living in deep poverty. But, like everyone else, they wanted greater dignity and a better life. We did not change their economic conditions by providing outside aid. We simply provided a program that helped them feel happier inside, along with some additional knowledge for agricultural self-sufficiency. The increased inner happiness led them to seek better ways to improve their lives.

Central America taught me an important lesson: If the TM program could be that successful in the prisons and among the Mayan people, in the midst of grinding poverty and extremely difficult circumstances, then the TM program can certainly be used to reduce substance abuse in any environment, anywhere in the world.

3. Vermont

The Vermont Department of Corrections presented some special challenges for substance abuse and rehabilitation programs. Drugs and alcohol are a serious problem in all correctional systems, but the prison population in Vermont was mostly from rural areas. We found that this, coupled with the long Vermont winters, produced a high incidence of alcoholism and crimes related to substance abuse in Vermont prisons.

The good news about Vermont was that we were able to structure a comprehensive program for both prison staff and inmates. All six prisons in the Vermont system participated, with 25% of the staff and 40% of the resident inmates learning to practice the TM technique. The positive results in these institutions were the same as those reported by Abrams and Siegel (1978), Dillbeck and Abrams (1987), and Bleick and Abrams (1987) when reviewing other TM programs in prisons.

The unique feature of the Vermont program was an integrated pre-release and post-release program. This program allowed us to observe how meditating inmates dealt with their substance abuse problems in prison, during temporary (pre-release) periods outside of prison, and after release.

For most prisoners, re-entry to the less-structured life outside prison walls is dramatic, if not traumatic. The TM program has been shown to aid this transition measurably, as indicated by Bleick and Abrams (1987) in their study of reduced recidivism among meditating ex-prisoners.

With Vermont parolees, we found that when the person stayed involved with the TM program through a local TM center, they took about three months to readjust to society and feel stable and comfortable. These people remained drug- and alcohol-free. They also were able to find and hold meaningful employment.

In some cases, when the paroled prisoner went back to an old environment and did not continue contact with a local TM center, problems arose. Parolees in these situations found themselves unable to resist negative influences. Again, the most vulnerable period seemed to be the first few months after release.

The Vermont project demonstrated the post-release value of the TM program for keeping parolees drug-free and out of prison. We have found that the importance of post-release follow-up varies, usually depending upon how well the prisoner has established a routine of daily TM practice during incarceration. But the value and importance of social and intellectual support for continuing the TM program after release is clear.

4. The California Youth Authority

In 1971, we introduced the TM program to approximately 200 wards of the California Youth Authority's Community-Centered Drug Program in Stockton, California. This was done at the request of a social worker who worked with the CYA in Stockton.

The CYA is a difficult environment, because the population is so volatile. We were working with younger people (age range 11-21), a restless group that was more interested in entertaining themselves than in taking care of their personal development. Nonetheless, with a program that included the TM technique and regular follow-up meetings as described earlier, the results were very positive.

One thing that was remarkable was the absence of racial tensions during the TM follow-up meetings. When individuals practice the TM technique in a group, there is a shared experience of silence and calmness that is unique. In the CYA programs, the group meditations had a tendency to make the participants feel unified, regardless of ethnic background.

One young man's experience succinctly summarizes the value of the TM program for the CYA. A great deal of institutional violence is related to drug transactions, and Jeffrey was an unhappy illustration of this fact. Jeffrey had been involved in seventeen assaults in the two-month period prior to his instruction in the TM technique. In the month following his instruction, Jeffrey was involved in only one assault incident–and he told me later that this was the result of one of his previous assaults on someone else. He had defended himself, without aggravating the situation. And after learning TM, he had ceased to perpetrate such incidents from his side.

It would be naive to state that substance abuse simply vanished in institutions where we taught TM, or among the group of 200 wards who learned TM. In such settings, peer pressure is just too much. To put a total halt to substance abuse, all the inmates and the entire staff would have to be practicing TM (the ideal situation, but one we were unable to create). However, the majority of the 200 wards who learned TM reported that their desire to take drugs had dropped off–and they added that when they did take drugs it no longer felt good.

This experience explains the reason for the TM program's effectiveness in treating substance abuse. People only do drugs when there's a payoff, either in personal experience or social acceptance. Give them something better, something that replaces the emptiness and heartache creating the addiction, and the motivation to do drugs is gone.

On the level of personal experience, the wards often described TM as "a natural high." They found that TM results in more refined sensory perception and sensitivity. Thus, they became more sensitive to destructive influences on the body and nervous system. Drugs became something that removed the natural good feeling they were experiencing as a result of meditation (Kimble, 1975). They had replaced the "good" feeling that they got from drugs with something better.

On the level of social acceptance, many of the wards who learned TM found that they had the courage and strength to disregard peer pressure and begin to get free of drugs while still incarcerated. The educational meetings that went along with the TM technique were vital in this regard. These meetings gave the wards an understanding of their own potential, and an appreciation for the value of the results they were getting from practicing TM regularly.

Social pressure to do drugs is a problem when a person's self-respect and self-confidence are lacking. The wards who practiced the TM technique regularly, and who also attended follow-up meetings for a deeper understanding of the mechanics of stress release through TM (described below), enjoyed consistent, positive results. This proved to be a powerful antidote to the social pressure to do drugs.

5. Residential Treatment Facilities

Children's receiving homes are found throughout the United States. These institutions serve as transition facilities for children who are innocent victims of poor parental judgment–i.e., the parents are abusing the child, or else the parents have been imprisoned or done something that leaves the child parentless.

Residential treatment facilities are essentially "minimum security" facilities. Substance abuse is not as much of a problem here as it is in other correctional settings, because of close supervision by adults. But the ongoing tension, and the uncertainty that the children feel about where they are and where they ultimately will end up, can create the basis for a lifetime of personal problems–including substance abuse.

Ironically, substance abuse is a danger for counselors and other staff members in these treatment facilities. The daily stress in such environments is quite high, leading to burnout and alcohol or drug abuse. Stress is like a poison in these settings. It can grow day after day, until the difference between the house counselor and the resident gets lost.

The TM program was introduced into a number of residential

treatment facilities in California. Once again, we designed a program for both residents and counselors.

In one facility in Sacramento, California, we taught the TM technique to five children. One child was classified as autistic, two others were classified as retarded, and the other two children had no special classification (aside from being parentless). Several staff members also received instruction in the TM technique.

The special impact of the TM program became crystal-clear in this situation. The house counselors had breaks during which they could practice their TM technique. After twenty minutes of TM, they were visibly happier, calmer, and more in command of their environment. They reported much softer interactions with the children. The discipline and structure of the facility were maintained, but overreaction to stressful encounters with the children dropped significantly.

This facility was based on the Tennessee Re-Education Model. This was a behavior modification system accompanied by daily group therapy meetings with the residents. The autistic child also had some special educational programs. When first admitted to the facility, the autistic child would scream when he wanted something. Through behavior modification techniques and charting, we taught the child to point to certain items or use certain words instead of screaming. We also were able to help this child gain better control of his behavior by involving him in group therapy meetings with the other children.

These behavior modification approaches helped the children gain some control, but they did nothing to alleviate the inner anxiety that often resulted in emotional explosions. One of the children, Tim, had been chained to a bed and beaten by his mother when he was two years old. As a result, he would have violent physical tantrums (lasting as long as seven hours) whenever confronted with authority.

For the children under age 10, we taught them the children's TM technique, which the child practices while in activity. The results of this technique have been documented extensively (Nidich & Nidich, 1990). Children who learn and practice this technique typically report more inner happiness and clarity of mind. Performance in school improves, and physical confrontations decrease. We reinforced the children in their practice by giving them games in which they were verbally praised from time to time, being told how well they were practicing the technique.

The results were impressive. The children were generating happiness from within themselves, and their behavior began to change rapidly. Positive changes were observed in weeks, changes that usually require years of behavior modification and therapy.

In Tim's case, after practicing the TM technique for a week, he found himself in a confrontation with authority. He promptly fell into his pattern of explosive behavior and tantrums. He was taken to the facility's "quiet room." This was supposed to be a place where a child or young adult was separated from the group to get himself back together, but it often became a place where Tim just broke the doors and injured himself by bouncing off the walls.

This time, it became very quiet shortly after Tim was put into the "quiet room." Tim had closed his eyes and had started to meditate. The tantrum, which normally would have gone on for hours, was over in twenty minutes. Tim explained that as soon as he began to meditate, his anger just left him, and he felt happier. This pattern continued. Tim's tantrums went from daily, seven-hour-long outbreaks to once- or twice-weekly occurrences that lasted less than half an hour. One month of practicing TM delivered better results for Tim than anything else he'd done in the previous eight years.

One evening, the director of the facility came by. He was astonished at the harmony in the house and the obedient behavior of the children–and all without the customary "behavior chip" that was used at other facilities to keep control in the environment. Even the autistic child had learned to function better, because of reduced tension in the house and a less threatening environment.

In all of these facilities, the idea was to create a home-like environment. But it was difficult to do this, even though the intentions were good. There were many diagnostic and treatment intrusions, such as required group therapy, required use of behavior-modifying drugs, and interviews with social workers. And frequently, other children would go out of control and be dragged off to jail for violent behavior.

My experience with this facility and others has led me to conclude that the TM technique, provided with love and structure, is the key to permanent, natural behavior change for the better.

THE NEED FOR A NEW PERSPECTIVE ON CRIME PREVENTION AND REHABILITATION

Our society's entire model for rehabilitation–whether for criminal behavior or substance abuse–is antiquated. It needs fundamental revision. We must learn that building more prisons, hiring more police, and reinstating the death penalty are not the answers to substance abuse or criminal behavior.

Arthur Anderson, former director of the Criminal Justice Division for the Arkansas Attorney General, explains it this way (Ellis, 1983):

> Our nation has recently re-embraced capital punishment. Our legislators are enacting more criminal laws and devising tougher penalties and tighter procedures. Bus drivers and service station attendants require exact change from us for public transportation or to buy gas after dark. Off-duty policemen guard our stores and apartment complexes. The provision of crime insurance and the production of deadbolt locks, commercial Mace, and burglar alarms have become lucrative businesses. As our crime problem continues to grow, we simply expand its container by building bigger police forces, bigger courthouses, bigger prisons, and bigger probation and parole systems. We are not so unlike the fat man who combats obesity by spending more and more money buying bigger and better suits to put around himself. He is simply shrouding, not solving, a growing problem.
>
> . . . The accumulation of stress in the nervous system causes fatigue and produces physiological and psychological disorders. In fact, it is estimated that at least 80 percent of all disease involves stress-related symptoms, which commonly take the form of anxiety, tension, depression, irritability, worry, high blood pressure, insomnia, headache, indigestion, confusion, and difficulty in solving problems. As stress

> mounts, the individual's emotions become unstable and the mind loses clarity. The likelihood of mistakes and maladaptive behavior thereby increases and inevitably leads to failure and frustration, which, in turn, reinforce his previously accumulated stresses, lower his self-esteem, and leave him weakened and more susceptible to future stresses. Hence, a stress cycle is generated in which mistakes and maladaptive behavior become unavoidable. Eventually, a collapse occurs. In some, it takes the form of a nervous breakdown or heart attack; in others, it may take the form of crime. This cycle–indeed, this downward spiral–describes the "physiology of crime" and provides a wholly new perspective on crime prevention and rehabilitation.

In the light of these disturbing trends, it is more important than ever to develop a new perspective on crime prevention and rehabilitation. We must begin to acknowledge and implement programs that address substance abuse and crime at their basis.

Mr. Anderson also succinctly describes (Ellis, 1983) how the TM program relates to a new, more holistic perspective on crime prevention and rehabilitation:

> Since stress is now medically understood as a major contributor to disease, it should also be legally recognized as a major factor in crime. And, just as many prominent physicians and psychiatrists are now prescribing the TM technique for both remedial and preventive purposes, those of us responsible for the administration of criminal justice should promptly implement it in our rehabilitation and crime prevention programs. It is a natural, and even necessary, ingredient to such endeavors. The TM technique provides what is perhaps the most expeditious, and certainly the safest, method for the nervous system to automatically release and rid itself of stress: profoundly deep rest.
>
> Scientific investigation shows that during the TM technique heart and respiratory rate significantly decrease, while overall cardiovascular efficiency increases. The system does less but

> accomplishes more. Measurements of skin resistance and blood chemistry also indicate a deep state of this efficient rest.
>
> Because the TM technique triggers a deep state of physiological rest and thereby disposes the nervous system to immediately begin ridding itself of deeply and tightly rooted stresses, the practitioner quickly experiences increased autonomic stability, more effective interaction with his environment, decreased dependence on drugs, alcohol, and tobacco, and increased inner control and self-actualization. These responses are exactly the opposite to criminal patterns of behavior. Wholeness and balance are restored to the individual (p. xvii-xxi).

NOTES ON OTHER APPROACHES

In structuring the TM program for a correctional facility, we provide a program for removing the stress. We do not analyze the innumerable sources of stress and anxiety in order to remove them. Where there is darkness, we don't curse the darkness, analyze the darkness, or counsel accommodation to the darkness. We just turn on the light, or, rather, show individuals how to turn on the light for themselves by learning and practicing the TM program.

1. Behavior Modification

Behavior modification was the basis for operations at most of the residential care facilities in California. While there was always an effort at creating a caring environment, I observed that all too often the counselors applied behavior modification techniques rather mechanically. As a result, many of the children learned how to control their behavior as if they were monkeys being rewarded with a banana. They just learned through repetition that if they didn't follow instructions, they wouldn't get the banana.

The fundamental pleasure of living and enjoying life was sadly absent in these behavior modification environments. What a contrast to the results of the TM technique, with changes in behavior coming from the inside out, from a basis of happiness and self-esteem that the children were enlivening within themselves!

2. Controlling Behavior with Prescribed Drugs

Psychotropic drugs are often used to control the behavior of people in correctional environments, especially if the ward or prisoner has a substance abuse problem. These drugs may help control undesirable behavior, but they do damage at the same time. The negative side effects of most prescribed drugs are well known, but professionals continue to administer these behavior-modifying drugs anyway, often for lack of a better solution.

The Transcendental Meditation program is a non-chemical option for improving behavior. It has been tested in a wide variety of environments, including the "worst-case scenarios" of correctional institutions. The use of drugs for behavior modification, when an alternative like TM is available, is tragic. The traditional psychotherapeutic approach, which often includes the use of drugs, does not refine the physiology and free it from the stress causing the problem. TM does refine the physiology and free it from underlying stress. More than 90% of behavior problems are stress-related. Drugs are not needed to solve the problem. At the very least, the introduction of the TM program into existing therapies can lead to lower dosages of these drugs for the patient, fewer side effects, and less time needed for the use of a particular drug.

3. The TM Program Compared to "Similar" Programs

Transcendental Meditation has been shown to be significantly more effective than other forms of meditation and relaxation in reducing anxiety and promoting psychological health (Eppley, Abrams & Shear, 1989). An extensive meta-analysis of 146 meditation and relaxation studies on trait anxiety showed that the TM technique was statistically significantly more effective in reducing trait anxiety when compared to other meditation techniques, progressive muscle relaxation, and other relaxation techniques. "Trait" anxiety refers to the general tendency to be anxious, as distinguished from "state" anxiety, the degree of anxiety at a particular moment.

Participants in the TM program have also experienced about three times the growth toward self-actualization and psychological health as participants in other programs that are popularly considered to be "similar" to the TM technique (Alexander, Rainforth & Gelderloos, 1991).

IMPLEMENTING THE TM PROGRAM IN CORRECTIONAL INSTITUTIONS

The Institute of Social Rehabilitation and Maharishi Consultants International are two organizations that focus on developing TM programs to address the problems created by crime and substance abuse. Maharishi Consultants International, for example, recently proposed to bring the TM program to the entire United States corrections system (Anklesaria, 1991). This proposal reviewed the current state of the U.S. corrections system, summarized the scientific research on the TM program and criminal rehabilitation, and offered to bring the TM program to over 802,000 inmates in the state and federal corrections systems. Participation would be voluntary, with programs for prison staff specially designed around the needs of each institution.

The proposal also provided a cost-benefit analysis. Not including the incalculable savings enjoyed by society at large through reduced police costs, court costs, victim costs, probation costs, etc., the proposal shows that a one-year TM program in federal and state prisons would save taxpayers more than $8 billion. This proposal has been introduced to officials in many states. Several officials have said that if they had more money, they would like to give the program a try.

THE CHALLENGE

When I was a child, I saw my older brother get directly involved with the criminal justice system. What was it that caused him to respond to authority in such a way? Stress. Stress got him into the situation in the first place, and stress kept him from seeing a way out.

If a person's mental and emotional state is clouded and confused by stress, that person's ability to make good decisions and stay out of trouble is limited. When the stress builds up to a certain point, substance abuse and criminal behavior are not only likely, they are almost inevitable.

The TM program develops an individual's mental and physical potential in a progressive, evolutionary direction. This creates an inner value system that spontaneously leads to action that is life-supporting and evolutionary.

Life will always offer us choices. I believe that the choice to take drugs is a choice that cannot be made by a person who has an inner value system that appreciates the dignity of life. And this is a value system that is not merely an intellectual concept or a "good idea"; it is a value system rooted in the person's physiology, in the person's nervous system and the entire body. Such a person will not accept or entertain anything that is destructive to continued growth and well-being. This is why I see the TM program as a fundamental approach for dealing with substance abuse and all of its horrible effects.

A program is now available for removing the motivator that drives people to substance abuse. This program, the Transcendental Meditation technique and the educational programs that are taught along with it, is a simple yet powerful solution to the tremendous problems posed by substance abuse and the criminal behavior related to it. My experience in some "worst case" settings, and the dramatic transformations created by a properly-administered TM program in those settings, indicates that this is more than fanciful thinking. The true fantasy is that we are trying to solve a very complex problem on our hands, with no simple solutions in sight.

As a society, we have spent many decades and billions of dollars to analyze and label the problems born of human stress. We have created thousands of institutions to study the problem, given multi-millions in grants for more studies, and seen endless Ph.D. theses on the problem. But all of this has done little to solve the problems of substance abuse and crime, problems that continue to devastate human life.

The statements I am making here may provoke some corrections and rehabilitation experts. But the ones who really care about their responsibility to society know that the conventional approaches to substance abuse and crime aren't working. These are the experts who are most likely to listen to a message that has been verified repeatedly over the past twenty-five years.

The government is always slow to respond to new ideas and change. It is usually a visionary person, or the private sector, that pushes social change forward. I feel that philanthropists of good will need to come together and create an endowment fund for making the TM program available to underprivileged peoples throughout the world.

I have not the slightest doubt that if the TM program is introduced and taught properly, funded fully, and studied impartially in any of the settings I have discussed here, the truth of what I have said will be found to be irrefutable.

It is time for us to quit playing politics, avoiding the truth, and ignoring the realities of substance abuse and crime. It is time for us to embrace and implement a program that can remove the motivator, bringing an end to these problems once and for all.

REFERENCES

Abrams, A. & Siegel, L. (1978). The Transcendental Meditation program and rehabilitation at Folsom State Prison: A cross-validation study. *Criminal Justice and Behavior* 5, 3-20.

Alexander, C., Rainforth, M. & Gelderloos, P. (1991). Transcendental Meditation, self-actualization, and psychological health: An overview and statistical meta-analysis. *Journal of Social Behavior and Personality 6*, 5, 189-247.

Anklesaria, F. (1991). *Introducing the TM program to the United States corrections system.* Fairfield, IA: Maharishi Consultants International, Inc.

Bleick, C. & Abrams, A. (1987). The Transcendental Meditation program and criminal recidivism in California. *Journal of Criminal Justice 15*, 211-230.

Chalmers, R., Clements, G., Schenklun, H., & Weinless, M. (Eds.) (1989a). *Scientific research on Maharishi's Transcendental Meditation and TM-Sidhi program: Collected papers, Vol. 2.* Vlodrop, the Netherlands: MVU Press.

Chalmers, R., Clements, G., Schenkluhn, H., & Weinless, M. (Eds.) (1989b). *Scientific research on Maharishi's Transcendental Meditation and TM-Sidhi program: Collected papers, Vol. 3.* Vlodrop, the Netherlands: MVU Press.

Chalmers, R., Clements, G., Schenkluhn, H., & Weinless, M. (Eds.) (1989c). *Scientific research on Maharishi's Transcendental Meditation and TM-Sidhi program: Collected papers, Vol. 4.* Vlodrop, the Netherlands: MVU Press.

Dillbeck, M. & Abrams, A. (1987). The application of the Transcendental Meditation program to corrections. *International Journal of Comparative Applied Criminal Justice* 11, 111-132.

Ellis, G. (1983). *Inside Folsom Prison: Unified Field Based Rehabilitation*. Burlington, VT: Accord Publications.

Eppley, K., Abrams, A. & Shear, J. (1989). Differential effects of relaxation techniques on trait anxiety: A meta-analysis. *Journal of Clinical Psychology 45*, 6, 957-974.

Gelderloos, P., Walton, K., Orme-Johnson, D., & Alexander, C. (1991). Transcendental Meditation and substance misuse: An overview. *International Journal of the Addictions 26*, 3, 239-325.

Kimble, C. J. (1975). Transcendental Meditation in the youth authority. *California Youth Authority Quarterly 28*, 1.

Nidich, S. & Nidich, R. (1990). *Growing Up Enlightened*. Fairfield, IA: Maharishi International University Press.

Orme-Johnson, D. & Farrow, J. (Eds.) (1977). *Scientific Research on the Transcendental Meditation: Collected Papers, Vol. 1*. Livingston Manor, NY: Maharishi International University Press.

Wallace, R. (1986). *The neurophysiology of enlightenment*. Fairfield, IA: MIU Press.

Wallace, R. K., Orme-Johnson, D. W., & Dillbeck, M. C. (Eds.) (1990). *Scientific research on Maharishi's Transcendental Meditation and TM-Sidhi program: Collected papers, Vol. 5*. Fairfiled, IA: MIU Press.

Importance of Reducing Stress and Strengthening the Host in Drug Detoxification: The Potential Offered by Transcendental Meditation

Frank Staggers, Jr., MD
Charles N. Alexander, PhD
Kenneth G. Walton, PhD

INTRODUCTION

Popular press now cites experts as agreeing that the best hope for success in the war against drugs is to turn from interdiction to prevention and treatment (Zuckerman, 1993). This agreement has come at least in part because more than $100 billion spent attempting to reduce the availability of illegal drugs since 1981 has

---

Frank Staggers, Jr. is affiliated with the Haight-Ashbury Free Clinic, Drug Detoxification, Rehabilitation, and Aftercare Program in San Francisco, CA. Charles N. Alexander is affiliated with the Department of Psychology and Kenneth G. Walton is affiliated with the Departments of Chemistry and Physiology at Maharishi International University in Fairfield, IA.

Correspondence should be addressed to Frank Staggers, Jr. at 75 Anair Way, Oakland, CA 94605.

[Haworth co-indexing entry note]: "Importance of Reducing Stress and Strengthening the Host in Drug Detoxification: The Potential Offered by Transcendental Meditation." Staggers, Frank Jr., Charles N. Alexander, and Kenneth G. Walton. Co-published simultaneously in the *Alcoholism Treatment Quarterly* (The Haworth Press, Inc.) Vol. 11, No. 3/4, 1994, pp. 297-331; and: *Self-Recovery: Treating Addictions Using Transcendental Meditation and Maharishi Ayur-Veda* (ed: David F. O'Connell and Charles N. Alexander) The Haworth Press, Inc., 1994, pp. 297-331. Multiple copies of this article/chapter may be purchased from The Haworth Document Delivery Center [1-800-3-HAWORTH; 9:00 a.m. - 5:00 p.m. (EST)].

not significantly reduced either their availability or their use. In turning to prevention and treatment, however, governments and private organizations are looking more carefully than ever for those approaches that are most effective, safest, and least costly to administer. This article focuses on the early withdrawal phase of treatment, outlining the special problems encountered at this phase and summarizing research suggesting that the Transcendental Meditation program is an unusually promising technology currently underutilized during drug detoxification.

For many persons attempting to break a drug or alcohol addiction, the early withdrawal or detoxification phase can be the most difficult. This is because detoxification involves major psychological and physiological stress reactions. Acute stress is associated with a constellation of neuroendocrine changes termed the "fight-or-flight" response, first characterized by Cannon (1929) in the early part of this century. An intense discharge of the sympathetic nervous system is a major component of the stress response and is a key symptom of drug withdrawal. Therefore, reducing outflow of the sympathetic nervous system is often a primary objective in contemporary approaches to drug detoxification. Although in the past Western medicine has relied heavily on medications to accomplish this goal, meditation, acupuncture, and other non-pharmaceutical means of relaxing the nervous system are gaining increasing acceptance.

The Transcendental Meditation (TM) technique is a potent non-pharmaceutical approach to eliminating stress and normalizing sympathetic nervous system activity. For this reason alone, TM is expected to be a powerful aid in drug detoxification. However, another promising advantage of this technique is its holistic effect on physical and mental health. Its wide range of benefits may be especially relevant to complicated drug detoxification cases such as in pregnancy, multiple addictions, addictions with underlying mental illness, or addictions with superimposed debilitating physical diseases. Although TM has not been investigated in detoxification specifically, studies have shown the technique to effectively reduce drug and alcohol consumption, even in severely addicted individuals (Alexander, Robinson, & Rainforth, this volume;

Gelderloos, Walton, Orme-Johnson, & Alexander, 1991; Taub, Steiner, Smith, Weingarten, & Walton, this volume).

One comprehensive way of understanding the role of TM in preventing or treating drug abuse is in the context of the public health model of disease prevention (Mausner & Bahn, 1974; Strantz, 1988). The three components of this model, as applied to physical disease, are: the *causal agent* (e.g., virus or bacterium), the *host* (e.g., human being who contracts the disease), and the *environment* (e.g., air, water and food supply). Addiction also has been considered in the context of the public health model (Miller & Hester, 1989). Application of the model to addiction is the same as for disease except the agent is the drug, and the most pertinent environmental factors may be sociological (e.g., peer pressure or psychosocial stress). In its beneficial effect in reducing physical disease and drug abuse, TM appears to act by strengthening the host. (See the last section for a more complete elaboration of this perspective.) Numerous studies of disease reduction through Transcendental Meditation suggest that TM makes the host more resistant to disease and more able to recover quickly if already afflicted (Alexander, Langer, Newman, Chandler, & Davies, 1989; Herron, 1993; Orme-Johnson, 1987; Schneider, Alexander, & Wallace, 1992; Schneider, Staggers, Alexander, Sheppard, Gaylord et al., 1991; Walton, Pugh, Gelderloos, & Macrae, submitted). The present essay focuses on the deleterious effects of stress in drug detoxification and discusses evidence that Transcendental Meditation strengthens the health of the host, reducing the perceived need for drugs and the tendency to use drugs. [See also a discussion by others in this volume on the potential of TM for modifying environmental factors: Orme-Johnson (this volume).]

MAJOR GOALS OF DETOXIFICATION, AND THE RELEVANCE OF TM

The principal goal in drug detoxification can be said to be maintaining the physical and mental stability of clients while they adjust to a drug-free state. To accomplish this goal, immediate and delayed symptoms associated with drug withdrawal must be alleviated. If these symptoms are not alleviated, relapse, severe morbidity, and even mortality may result.

Drug detoxification can take anywhere from a few days to many weeks, depending on the potency, elimination half-life, and neurohormonal effects of the specific drug involved, the length of time that a specific drug was abused, and the physical and mental state of the person being detoxified. However, except for cases involving potent benzodiazepines, long-acting opiates, or high doses of nicotine, the symptoms associated with withdrawal from most drugs can usually be managed in one month or less. Although regimens and durations vary, the main therapeutic objective of most drug detoxification treatments remains the same: counter the destabilizing effects of stress.

The Western medical model of the body's acute response to stress, which is largely based on Cannon's early studies (1929), provides a framework for understanding the physical withdrawal symptoms seen with most addicting drugs. This is because, once physical dependency has been established, withdrawal from addicting drugs is associated in varying degrees with the emotional and physical changes seen in the full-blown stress or fight-or-flight response. The importance of acute stress may not have been fully recognized in the past in part because the wide variety of beneficial treatments were not seen to have one effect in common–countering the acute response to stress. As will be discussed more completely below, medications that block activity of the sympathetic nervous system, as well as acupuncture, exercise, various relaxation techniques of clinical origin, "stress" vitamins, and herbs, all of which are currently in use in detoxification, are effective in varying degrees at blocking the acute response to stress. Thus, both pharmaceutical and non-pharmaceutical techniques that help counter the body's response to stress play a crucial role in alleviating withdrawal symptoms. Furthermore, any treatment that might offer improved performance in this area would be a candidate for use in drug detoxification.

In this context, the Transcendental Meditation technique has properties which make it an excellent prospect for a primary or adjunctive drug detoxification treatment. One of its most important attributes is its distinctively effective ability to calm the nervous system and counter psychological stress (Dillbeck & Orme-Johnson, 1987; Eppley, Abrams, & Shear, 1989). Non-pharmaceutical stress-reduction techniques with some similarities to TM, but which may be less effective at reducing stress (Eppley et al., 1989) are already widely used in drug detoxification. Although the usefulness of some of these techniques in addiction treatment has been questioned (Klajner, Hartman, & Sobell, 1984), a few have already become commonplace in detoxification programs in many institutions (see below). Before further discussing the potential of TM and other non-pharmacological approaches, however, it is important to more fully understand the stress response and its implications for both health and drug detoxification.

REVIEW OF THE STRESS RESPONSE AND ITS IMPLICATIONS FOR HEALTH AND DRUG DETOXIFICATION

In his classic book, *Bodily Changes in Pain, Hunger, Fear, and Rage,* Harvard physiologist Walter B. Cannon (1929) elaborated the changes precipitated by stressful situations. Such bodily changes include increased adrenaline release and marked activation of the sympathetic nervous system. These are the principal components of what he named the "fight-or-flight response," signifying the organism's automatic response to threat. Subsequent scientists in the field, particularly Hans Selye, broadened the model of the stress response, investigating long-term changes in physiological function and in susceptibility to disease which result from prolonged exposure to stress (e.g., Selye & Tuchweber, 1976).

Activation of the fight-or-flight response is the initial reaction to almost any stressful or threatening event, including drug withdrawal. In this sense, drug withdrawal falls in the same general class of threatening events as confrontation by a dangerous adversary, experience of acute blood loss, or experience of an insulin overdose. The autonomic nervous system mediates a major part of the involuntary psychophysiological reaction to a stress-provoking situation. The sympathetic branch of the autonomic nervous system prepares the body for vigorous activity, and also for confronting severely demanding or life-threatening situations. For example, the sympathetic nervous system precipitates release of adrenaline and related neurotransmitters, raises the blood pressure, increases the heart rate and force of contraction, increases blood sugar, dilates the pupils, and reinforces the brain's state of arousal. It is the sympathetic nervous system that is mainly provoked during intense drug detoxifications and other stressful situations. In contrast, the parasympathetic branch of the autonomic nervous system prepares the body to digest food and to refurbish tissues. When the body is in a state of peaceful rest and rejuvenation, it is the parasympathetic nervous system that tends to be more involved.

The sympathetic and parasympathetic nervous systems complement each other like the right hand complements the left hand or like the right cerebral hemisphere the left cerebral hemisphere. Thus, in a healthy person these two systems operate in balanced fashion. However, in a person exposed to chronic or frequent intermittent challenges (stressors), the sympathetic system tends to become overactive, throwing off this balance. Since the parasympathetic system principally promotes rest and rejuvenation, it is easy to see why diseases resulting from excessive activity of this branch are few in number. On the other hand, the types of activities promoted by the sympathetic system (e.g., increased blood pressure and state of arousal) make disorders resulting from its hyperactivity far more numerous. A detailed discussion of stress-related neuroendocrine factors contributing to excessive activity of the sympathetic nervous system, and how these tend to promote drug abuse and relapse, is given elsewhere (Walton & Levitsky, this volume).

Although some (e.g., Burchfield, 1979) have argued that psychological distress is a necessary component of true stress, the stress response is generally envisioned to arise from exposure to either psychological stressors or physiological stressors. Psychological stressors are primarily learned cues or signals perceived as overwhelming or dangerous, such as pressures arising from a job, finances or interpersonal relations. Moreover, psychological stressors can include conditioned cues, for example, experiences previously associated with drug use (Childress et al., 1988; O'Brien et al., 1988). In comparison, stressors identified as physiological are usually chemical changes or imbalances within the body's own internal organ systems, such as rapid changes in blood glucose, oxygen, and neurotransmitter levels. Drug withdrawal involves both physiological and psychological stressors.

If these two categories of stressors are in fact distinct, they clearly are not mutually exclusive. For example, a heroin addict who is running low on his supply of heroin may experience a stress response due to the anticipation of drug withdrawal. His worries and fears may precipitate the discharge of the sympathetic nervous system long before his body has physically begun to withdraw from the heroin. The discharge of the sympathetic nervous system will be further elevated once that person actually runs out of heroin and starts physically experiencing heroin withdrawal. Thus, in this case of the heroin addict, the psychological stressor actually preceded, and then overlapped with, the physiological stressor.

The combined physiological and psychological stress experienced during drug withdrawal can be severe and can cause a very large increase in sympathetic nervous system activity (Sytinsky, Galebskaya, & Jantunen, 1981). For example, abrupt withdrawal from sedative drugs such as the barbiturates and benzodiazepines can be so stressful as to be fatal. The reason for this added stress is that sedatives actually suppress activity of parts of the nervous system. The nervous system attempts to counter this chemical suppression by increasing its outflow, much like an engine charges up in order to pull a large weight. Therefore, when the sedative is abruptly discontinued, the highly charged nervous system suddenly finds itself unopposed by the sedative and rebounds like a loaded spring. It is generally the sympathetic nervous system that becomes excessively active and plays a key role in withdrawal from most addicting drugs, but other parts of the nervous system, as well as the hormonal system, are also involved. For example, withdrawal from opiate addiction can produce imbalances of the parasympathetic nervous system as well as the sympathetic, and withdrawal from any drug may affect activity of the adrenal cortex (Chrousos & Gold, 1992).

In addition to the episodes of acute stress occurring during withdrawal, chronic (i.e., prolonged or frequent intermittent) stress also produces effects relevant to withdrawal. Recent studies have revealed mechanisms linking prolonged or chronic stress with drug abuse (Walton & Levitsky, this volume) and with disease and aging

(Eliot, 1979; Sapolsky, 1992; Sapolsky, Krey, & McEwen, 1986). In particular, recent work has suggested that chronic elevations of adrenal steroids such as cortisol and aldosterone, and reductions in other important factors such as dehydroepiandrosterone and serotonin, during or as a result of stress, may underlie a wide variety of deleterious effects of stress on health (MacLean et al., 1992; Walton & Levitsky, this volume; Walton et al., submitted). These effects appear to include increasing the propensity to consume alcohol or to use drugs as an attempt to reduce the discomfort of acute stress (Walton & Levitsky, this volume). Also, there now appear to be experiments demonstrating how reduction or elimination of stress through interventions such as the TM technique can reduce the propensity for both drug abuse (e.g., Alexander et al., this volume; Taub et al., this volume; Walton & Levitsky, this volume) and disease (Alexander et al., 1989; Orme-Johnson, 1987; Schneider et al., 1991; 1992; Walton et al., submitted).

Thus, while the stress response can be vital to survival under many circumstances (e.g., insulin overdose), it also takes its toll on the physiology, often leading to mental and physical disease and accelerated aging (Sapolsky, 1992). Chronic stress distorts the regulatory machinery maintaining balance in the physiology. The resulting prolonged imbalances may be the source not only of physical and mental diseases but also of addictive behaviors. Use of addicting drugs may in part reflect a maladaptive attempt to correct psychophysiological imbalances that have arisen from chronic stress (Walton & Levitsky, this volume). Given that the period of early withdrawal from drugs is extremely stressful, even potentially lethal, it is critical that treatments used in drug detoxification minimize the negative effects of the stress response. This is, in fact, the key objective of most detoxification treatments.

COMPLICATING FACTORS IN DRUG DETOXIFICATION

Since the stress incurred during drug withdrawal can be severe, it is easy to see that treatment can be compounded by factors such as pregnancy, underlying mental illness, debilitating physical diseases, poly-drug addiction, and persistent exposure to cues associated with past drug use. To insure that the proposed treatment is both safe and effective, these additional factors must be addressed whenever a drug detoxification is being planned.

Pregnancy is associated with profound physiological changes in the mother, many of which are negatively impacted by drug abuse, thereby placing addicted women in the category of high-risk pregnancies. Moreover, many medications that are normally given during drug detoxification (e.g., benzodiazepines) either cannot be given, or must be given in smaller doses, to avoid damaging the fetus. Similarly, popular sympathetic nervous system drugs often cannot be used during pregnancy because they can cause severe drops in blood pressure as well as placental insufficiency and abortion.

Underlying mental diseases complicate drug withdrawal because they reflect additional severe biochemical imbalances which often become manifested as the client withdraws from the addicting drug. The health care provider who is trying to manage the mentally ill addicted person often finds himself having to manage both the drug withdrawal symptoms and the exacerbated mental illness. Thus, the mentally ill addict presents one of the greatest management challenges seen in medical practice, and usually requires a team effort involving mental health experts as well as drug recovery experts.

Debilitating physical diseases like AIDS, epilepsy, heart disease, hypertension, chronic pain, and diabetes often are exacerbated by the stress of drug withdrawal. This is mainly because the seizure threshold is altered, blood pressure is increased, blood glucose is elevated, the immune system is depressed, and other organ systems are strained. Furthermore, pre-existing pain conditions often become worse during drug detoxification, which itself can be highly painful, forcing the health care provider to manage intractable pain of separate origins at the same time. Also, certain medicines given to prevent withdrawal symptoms can be dangerous if combined with others that a client may be taking for pre-existing medical conditions. Therefore, due to the possibility of complex drug interactions, any addicted client with a debilitating disease should be followed by his primary care physician during detoxification, as well as by his drug recovery expert.

Drug withdrawal in poly-drug addiction presents another complex, clinical picture for which treatment is difficult. As an illustration, in the Drug Detoxification Program at the Haight-Ashbury Free Clinic (under the direction of one of us, F.S.) it is common to find clients who inject "speedballs" (a mixture of heroin and cocaine) and then use benzodiazepines and alcohol to balance their body's reactions. If this confounding situation is further complicated by the fact that some of the addicting drugs may have been mixed or "cut" with unknown substances and that none of the drug doses may be known for certain, then even the best neuropharmacist or neurophysiologist will have difficulty predicting how the poly-drug addict's nervous system will react once the withdrawal process starts.

When external cues (such as syringes and drug pipes), or internal cues (such as negative mood states and flashbacks) have been repeatedly paired with past drug abuse, then these cues alone may begin to trigger either withdrawal symptoms, intoxication-like symptoms, drug compensatory symptoms, craving, or various combinations of the above (Childress et al., 1988; Childress, McLellan, Natale, & O'Brien, 1987; O'Brien, Childress, McLellan, & Ehrman, 1990; Rohsenow, Niaura, Childress, Abrams, & Monti, 1990-1991). Thus, cues associated with past drug abuse have been implicated in both persistent drug abuse and relapse back to drug abuse after various periods of abstinence (Childress et al., 1988; O'Brien et al., 1988; O'Brien et al., 1990; Rohsenow et al., 1990-1991; Washton & Stone-Washton, 1990; Weiss & Cheung, 1987). These cues can be so powerful that even weeks or months after completion of detoxification, when there is no further evidence of physical dependency, they can still trigger potent withdrawal symptoms and other reactions. Therefore, because of this type of conditioning, exposure to such cues during detoxification can often prevent or disrupt successful treatment.

PHARMACOLOGICAL AND PHYSICAL METHODS FOR STRESS REDUCTION IN DRUG DETOXIFICATION

Due to the fact that drug withdrawal can be extremely stressful, any methods useful in combating stress are also, as a general rule, helpful in treating drug withdrawal. This includes psychological approaches such as counseling, psychotherapy, support groups and health education, as well as physiological approaches such as exercise, proper diet, relaxation training, acupuncture, and sedative medication. Most contemporary drug detoxification programs use any or all of the above measures.

For example, the Haight-Ashbury Free Clinic provides a comprehensive treatment package for detoxification, consisting of psychiatric care, acute medical care, life-style modification programs and special services to AIDS patients who abuse drugs, pregnant abusers, poly-addicted abusers, and abusers with severe psychiatric disorders such as schizophrenia and manic-depressive illness. Even though this program offers a wide range of medicines, it also employs physical exercise regimens, dietary supplements, acupuncture, and psychological relaxation techniques as an integral part of its therapeutic protocol. These different treatment modalities appear to complement each other in countering the stress associated with drug withdrawal. This section focuses mainly on pharmacological and physical ways of alleviating the stress associated with drug withdrawal.

Starting about 30 years ago, general sedatives like phenobarbital and Valium, which are capable of relaxing various segments of the nervous system, became the cornerstone of drug detoxification programs (Smith & Wesson, 1971; Victor, 1966). However, during the last 15 years, drugs which specifically block segments of the sympathetic nervous system (e.g., clonidine and propranolol) have moved to the forefront (Baumgartner & Rowen, 1987; Glassman, Stenter, Walsh, & Raizman, 1988; Gold, Pottash, Sweeney, & Kleber, 1980; Gottlieb, 1988; Horwitz, Gottlieb, & Kraus, 1989; Walinder, Bokstrom, & Karlsson, 1981). The drugs used in detoxification have different mechanisms of action, represent different drug categories and may treat different types of withdrawal, but virtually all are known to produce a relaxing effect, especially on the sympathetic nervous system. It should also be mentioned that since drug withdrawal may critically involve more aspects of the nervous system than the sympathetic branch, drugs that specifically inhibit the sympathetic branch are usually used in conjunction with other medications. This added coverage prevents breakthrough seizures and other withdrawal symptoms not controlled by sympathetic blockers.

The pharmaceutical approach has many advantages in detoxification. For instance, the medicines usually have a rapid onset and are quite potent. Moreover, they can be administered even to persons who are confused, incoherent, or psychotic during drug withdrawal. Also, if detoxification medications are used carefully, they can prevent the pregnant addict from experiencing withdrawal symptoms that endanger either her or the fetus. In many cases these medicines can be used to control craving and non-life-threatening withdrawal symptoms so that the client is less likely to relapse.

Besides these advantages, however, there are some drawbacks. For instance, detoxification medicines may have serious side-effects, including respiratory depression, drops in blood pressure, headaches, nausea, pulse irregularities, confusion, and the like. Some of these medications may cause an allergic reaction, or they may interact unfavorably with other medications that the person must take. Some of the medications are exceptionally potent, increasing the risk of overdosing, and certain detoxification medicines, like barbiturates or benzodiazepines, have the potential for abuse or addiction themselves. Furthermore, as mentioned above, some of these medicines may be dangerous if given to people with compromising conditions such as heart disease, low blood pressure, liver or kidney disease, malabsorption syndromes, asthma, diabetes, or pregnancy.

In addition to, or in place of, pharmaceutical approaches to detoxification, non-pharmaceutical, physical approaches such as acupuncture can be useful. This is true whether or not medications appear indicated, and is especially so in cases complicated by additional factors such as those mentioned above. As with proper diet and exercise, one advantage of these non-pharmaceutical techniques is that they can be used concurrently with virtually any medication. Most have a good safety profile, with few side effects, and are safe in pregnancy.

Evidence that the ancient technique of acupuncture is useful in reducing the symptoms of drug withdrawal shows that non-pharmaceutical modalities can have an important place in modern drug treatment protocols. Acupuncture is the portion of traditional Chinese medicine that involves insertion of needles into specific control points in the skin to regulate, according to ancient theory, the flow of life-sustaining energy through various bodily organs.

Western medicine cannot fully explain how acupuncture works; however, the commonly accepted belief is that nerve endings and neurosensory receptors are stimulated, various neurotransmitters and neuromodulators are released, and the pituitary gland, hypothalamus, and multiple aspects of the autonomic nervous system are activated (Chen, 1987; Smith & Khan, 1988; Stux & Pomeranz, 1987). Approximately 50% of the principal acupuncture points have major nerve trunks directly underneath them, and the rest of the points are within 0.5 cm of nerve trunks (Chen, 1987). In addition, naloxone, a potent opiate blocking agent, is known to prevent some of the analgesic effects of acupuncture (Stux & Pomeranz, 1987). This implies that the body's own intrinsic opiates, endorphins and enkephalins, may help mediate the effects of acupuncture. Furthermore, stress hormones like adrenocorticotropic hormone and cortisol appear to be reduced in detoxifying drug addicts treated with acupuncture (Wen et al., 1978; Wen & Cheung, 1973). The effectiveness of acupuncture in treating addictions is now thought to lie in the ability of stimulation of specific acupuncture points to normalize activity of the autonomic nervous system (Sytinsky et al., 1981). The same set of points has been found useful regardless of the type of drug involved. Furthermore, these points appear to have been useful in treating other disorders related to severe stress and pain (Smith & Khan, 1988).

The lack of a complete understanding of how acupuncture works has not prevented it from gaining wide acceptance as a therapeutic modality for a variety of medical disorders, including drug addiction (Bullock, Culliton, & Olander, 1989; Chen, 1987; Smith, 1989; Smith et al., 1982; Sytinsky et al., 1981). For example, the Haight-Ashbury Free Clinic has used acupuncture in detoxification since 1981, when clinical experience suggested it may be as effective as methadone and other medications, yet only half as costly. Pregnant crack cocaine addicts have been safely detoxified with acupuncture (Smith, 1989; Smith & Khan, 1988), and acupuncture seems to help poly-drug addicts regardless of the types of drugs involved in the addiction (Smith, 1979; Smith & Khan, 1988). Acupuncture also may relieve psychiatric symptoms such as depression, agitation, and anxiety (Smith, 1989; Stux & Pomeranz, 1987).

Traditional Chinese medicine, of which acupuncture is one

modality, is estimated to be more than 3,000 years old (Leung, 1977; Stux & Pomeranz, 1987). The Ayurvedic system of medicine, drawn from the ancient Vedic tradition of India, is credited with an even earlier origin (Schneider et al., 1990; Sharma, Triguna, & Chopra, 1991; Thatte & Dahanukar, 1986). Ayurvedic medicine involves some of the same points as acupuncture and appears to rest on a related understanding of vital channels or "shrotas" whose equivalent has not yet been clearly identified in Western science. Descriptions of these channels found in the ancient literature appear to be applicable to known information-carrying pathways in the neuroendocrine systems maintaining homeostasis in the body. An example is the hypothalamic-pituitary-adrenal axis regulating cortisol levels. The hormone cortisol is critical to survival of stressful experiences, and proper function of this axis appears disturbed in addictions (see Walton & Levitsky, this volume).

Since most of the procedures used in the Ayurvedic system are specifically intended to remove impurities which block the shrotas, it is not surprising that several aspects of Ayurvedic medicine, at least of the recently restored version known as "Maharishi Ayur-Veda," have been found useful in treatment of addictions of all varieties (Glaser, this volume; Sands, this volume; Sharma, Dillbeck, & Dillbeck, this volume). This ability to restore the effective role of the shrotas in maintaining optimal balance or homeostasis of the physiology (Schneider et al., 1990) should make Maharishi Ayur-Veda useful in drug detoxification as well. Moreover, the Ayurvedic system has extensive knowledge of combinations of plants and herbs which have a number of effects that could be beneficial in detoxification. For example, some of these mixtures are extremely potent at reducing free radicals, poisonous chemical species generated in excess by the body when it is experiencing stress (see Sharma et al., this volume).

PSYCHOLOGICAL METHODS FOR STRESS REDUCTION IN DRUG DETOXIFICATION

Aside from the purely pharmacological and physical approaches to reducing the stress associated with drug detoxification, some strictly psychological approaches are also in use. These have largely focused on the response to drug-associated cues. As mentioned previously, internal and external cues (e.g., negative mood states, syringes, a physical environment where the person previously took drugs, etc.) that have been repeatedly associated with drug use can, by themselves, evoke powerful psychological and physiological responses. These cues can often lead to relapse or drug-seeking behavior that complicates drug withdrawal. A comprehensive program for systematically extinguishing responses to drug-oriented cues has been developed at the University of Pennsylvania (Childress, Hole, & DePhilipps, 1991; Childress et al., 1988; Childress et al., 1987; O'Brien et al., 1988; O'Brien et al., 1990). The first step is to identify these drug-oriented cues. Then the client is given a wide array of relapse prevention techniques for combating the conditioned drug-using or withdrawal-symptom responses to these cues. One of the key techniques that can be used for desensitizing a person to learned cues is relaxation therapy. Generally clients receive personal or videotaped instruction on relaxation, but in practice are allowed to use virtually any relaxation technique they choose (Childress et al., 1991). Visualization, deep breathing and muscle relaxation are common. This desensitizing type of program focuses on the client's experience *during* exposure to such cues, and therefore the therapy is used primarily at the time the cue is experienced, to aid the extinction process.

Note, however, that this procedure has seldom been studied at the acute detoxification stage. In most cases, patients have already completed detoxification and are in subsequent stages of recovery (Childress et al., 1988; O'Brien et al., 1990). Nevertheless, because of the similarities between symptoms experienced during early withdrawal and symptoms triggered by drug-oriented cues later in the recovery process, the effectiveness of such relaxation techniques in relapse prevention may have implications for their use during acute detoxification as well.

In general, self-directed psychological techniques for stress-reduction have been more widely embraced by programs for smoking cessation than by programs for withdrawal from drugs and alcohol. Prior to Surgeon General Koop's highly acclaimed emphasis on preventive medicine in the 1980's (Surgeon General, 1988), a large segment of American society was reluctant to view tobacco smoking as an addictive disease. However, when Koop publicly emphasized that nicotine was as addicting as heroin and cocaine, the standard views about tobacco products began to change. Since tobacco smoking was previously perceived as either a "bad habit" or a cardiopulmonary risk factor, smoking cessation programs evolved along a different path than the classic drug and alcohol detoxification programs. Consequently, programs for smoking cessation often freely adopted principles from health disciplines outside the traditional chemical detoxification arena.

The strong emphasis on relaxation and stress reduction in smoking cessation was largely fueled by studies which suggested that smoking serves as a way of coping with stress, and that smoking relapses are most commonly triggered by stress (Leventhal & Cleary, 1980). The American Lung Association (1991) produced a smoking cessation audio tape which provides instruction on muscle relaxation and deep breathing techniques. This tape is widely used, and is even distributed as a part of a smoking cessation package by an international pharmaceutical company that makes transdermal, nicotine detoxification patches (Ciba-Geigy Corporation, 1992). Today, most smoking cessation programs, whether pharmacologically based or non-pharmacologically based, incorporate some type of relaxation technique.

THE TRANSCENDENTAL MEDITATION TECHNIQUE

Distinct from the desensitizing type of self-directed methods for reducing stress are the traditional techniques of meditation, and the recently-devised clinical relaxation procedures which have attempted to incorporate salient features of traditional meditation techniques. Among these methods, Transcendental Meditation has been most intensively investigated. Transcendental Meditation is a self-directed mental technique derived from Rik Veda, the oldest and most central treatise in the ancient Vedic tradition of knowledge in India (Maharishi Mahesh Yogi, 1963; 1969). The technique was first made available in its present form when Maharishi Mahesh Yogi brought it from the Himalayas in 1957. TM differs from most other forms of meditation in that it involves neither concentration nor contemplation. In the practice of TM, one effortlessly uses a specially selected "mantra," or meaningless sound, known from tradition to promote a natural shift of the awareness from the surface thinking level to progressively more refined levels, ultimately transcending the thinking process altogether. The resulting state of restful alertness, without thoughts or emotions, is called "transcendental consciousness" or "pure consciousness" (Alexander & Sands, 1993; Maharishi Mahesh Yogi, 1963; 1969), and is thought to be the feature of TM most responsible for the wide variety of benefits that have been observed (Alexander et al., 1990; Alexander, Rainforth, & Gelderloos, 1991).

As TM became more popular, Maharishi realized he could not personally instruct everyone who wanted to learn (Denniston, 1986; Frew, 1977). Thus, he instituted courses to train others as teachers, and encouraged the establishment of educational organizations in every country to teach this technique. "Transcendental Meditation" was legally established as a service mark to prevent the loss of integrity of the teaching that would likely occur if anyone not properly trained attempted to instruct others. Although TM is easily learned in a short course, the teaching of this technique is delicate, and instructors are intensively trained in a full-time course that usually runs for eight months. TM is practiced for 15-20 minutes twice daily, does not require a change of religious or philosophical beliefs, and can be practiced by almost anyone. Over four million individuals have now learned the TM technique worldwide.

From the beginning, Maharishi called for scientific research to test the effects of this practice. The first research to gain widespread attention reported on the physiological changes during TM practice, and was published in *Science* by Robert Keith Wallace, then at the University of California at Los Angeles (Wallace, 1970). This and subsequent research by Wallace and colleagues at Harvard Medical School indicated that TM directly counters many of the physiological effects of stress (Wallace & Benson, 1972; Wallace, Benson, & Wilson, 1971). Soon afterwards the number of studies increased dramatically, and TM, or other techniques modeled after it, became a key component of many stress management protocols.

It is important to note that the TM technique is not intended to be used primarily for treatment of disease or addiction. Rather, it is a procedure for developing the Self, a higher state of subjectivity than that usually denoted by the word self. As used in the West, the term "self-actualization" generally refers to development of the unique individual self. However, the Vedic tradition from which TM is drawn describes the potential for realizing a transcendental Self which is directly experienced in "higher states of consciousness." Through repetition of the experience of transcendental consciousness, one comes to know the higher self, or Self, as an unbounded field of intelligence, creativity and happiness at the basis of the individual mind. In higher states of consciousness, the Self becomes a permanent and universal fixture of daily life, underlying all experiences of objects, feelings, and ideas. Such *enlightened* individuals are said to find life totally effortless and blissful, free from stress of any kind–an ideal state which results of numerous research studies on TM support as an eventual outcome of regular practice (see for reviews, Alexander et al., 1990; 1991). The ancient adage, "Know thyself," expressed in many different creeds and philosophies, may well have originally denoted this same Self-revealing process. However, although other traditional methods for producing this experience may have existed, they appear to have been lost or largely eroded over the long course of time.

EFFECTS OF TM IN STRESS REDUCTION AND HEALTH

Thus far we have argued for the critical role of stress-reduction in drug detoxification and have presented evidence that behavioral as well as pharmacological means for reducing stress are now widely used. In particular, we explained that acupuncture, a traditional *physical* approach from oriental medicine, has gained increasing recognition in the addictions field. In the case of *mental* approaches to stress reduction and self-development, however, the medical field has continued to place emphasis on more recent clinically devised methods. These new approaches have included Childress' desensitization procedure, deep muscle relaxation, EMG biofeedback and the relaxation response. On the other hand, the following evidence suggests that Maharishi's Transcendental Meditation is distinctively effective in reducing stress and promoting psychophysiological health.

Several popular clinically devised methods of meditation and relaxation were largely derived from traditional practices, in particular from the Transcendental Mediation technique. Partly for this reason, the biomedical community has generally presumed that these derivatives would be equally beneficial but would not require instruction in those traditional practices (e.g., Druckman & Bjork, 1991; Holmes, 1984; Smith, 1976). Although it is recognized that pharmacological approaches to disease or stress reduction may vary widely in their impact and side effects, this same potential for heterogeneity of effects has not been broadly recognized in the field of mental approaches to stress and disease reduction.

Until recently, the comparative analysis of mental approaches has been either conceptual (e.g., Druckman & Bjork, 1991) or based on qualitative, narrative reviews of the literature (e.g., Holmes, 1984; Klajner et al., 1984; Smith, 1976). However, with the development and popularization of statistical meta-analysis techniques, it has become possible to precisely estimate effect sizes, controlling for differences in sample size, experimental design, and sample characteristics (Glass, McGaw, & Smith, 1981; Hunter & Schmidt, 1990). Average effect sizes associated with different techniques can then be statistically compared to determine quantitatively (as opposed to by subjective judgment) whether techniques differ in the magnitude of their effects.

Thus, the question of comparative effectiveness of different meditation/relaxation techniques was approached in a recent meta-analysis of 146 independent outcomes from 109 separate studies on trait anxiety, a measure of chronic stress, as evaluated by standardized questionnaires (Eppley et al., 1989). The effect of TM in reducing trait anxiety was found to be significantly greater than effects produced by progressive muscle relaxation, other forms of muscle relaxation, EMG biofeedback, the relaxation response or placebo meditation procedures. The effects of these clinically devised procedures were still significant compared to no-treatment controls, but only approximately half as large as those produced by TM. Whereas contemplative forms of meditation, on average, produced an effect equivalent in magnitude to the clinically devised relaxation procedures, concentration forms of meditation appeared to produce no effect. The above differences between TM and groups of other techniques were significant even when statistically controlling for such possible confounding variables as strength of experimental design, type of population, duration of treatment, experimenter bias, subject expectancy, and attrition rate. Whereas expectancy or placebo effects tend to wear off over time, the impact of TM, relative to other techniques, appeared to increase over time. Thus, while clinically devised relaxation procedures do reduce stress, they appear to do so to a lesser degree than TM.

To buffer the addict against the negative impact of detoxification and to aid later phases of recovery, it is important not only to relieve stress but also to enhance the positive sense of well being, self-worth and capacity to get along well with others. A second meta-analysis of 42 independent outcomes showed that TM produced approximately three times the effect of other forms of relaxation and meditation on standardized measures of self-actualization (Alexander et al., 1991). Self-actualization is operationalized by high composite scores on subscales measuring such qualities as self-acceptance, self-regard, and capacity for intimate contact. Again, this result was maintained when statistically adjusting for strength of experimental design and duration of intervention; the result was also found to increase with duration of practice.

A third meta-analysis of 20 studies meeting rigorous methodological criteria provides additional evidence that TM is differentially effective in reducing chronic sympathetic nervous system arousal. This study found that the effect of TM in reducing elevated levels of systolic and diastolic blood pressure was substantially larger than that produced by other forms of meditation. However, the numbers in each category type were too small to allow statistical comparisons between groups. In addition to this difference in effectiveness, TM had the highest compliance rate of the techniques investigated. The results of these meta-analyses are further supported by the findings of two recent randomized, controlled trials directly assessing the efficacy of TM compared to other relaxation techniques in reducing high blood pressure.

Perhaps the most compelling evidence that TM can effectively reduce a stress-related disorder resulted from the following study. In the first randomized, controlled trial ever conducted on the use of behavioral means to reduce mild hypertension in African-Americans, the relationship between high blood pressure and reduction of stress was assessed (Schneider et al., 1991). Approximately half of the elderly African-American hypertensive patients chose to discontinue their blood pressure medicines before participating in the study. Baseline blood pressure was obtained over a two-month period, so that blood pressure could fully normalize in those who went off medication. Since hypertension is thought to arise in part from hyperactivity of the sympathetic nervous system, many of the subjects had been taking standard sympathetic nervous system blockers such as propranolol, clonodine, and atenolol. (Incidentally, these are the medications mentioned above which are prescribed most for the symptoms of drug detoxification.) For purposes of safety, subjects with a history of stroke, ischemic heart disease, kidney damage, or critically elevated blood pressure were excluded from this study. The subjects were then randomly assigned to either a TM group, a progressive muscle relaxation (PMR) group, or a control group which received only the standard instructions on diet and exercise. In the final analysis, the control group displayed no change in blood pressure over the three-month intervention period. However, both the TM group and the PMR group showed significant reductions in blood pressure compared to the control group. Furthermore, the TM group displayed reductions in systolic and diastolic blood pressure (-11/-6 mm Hg) which were twice as large as those for the PMR group (-5/-3 mm Hg), adjusting for pretest values.

Because equal numbers of subjects remained on medication as elected to go off medication, TM's effectiveness for both conditions could be assessed. Interestingly, the largest TM effect was produced for individuals who were no longer on medication. This suggests that TM successfully replaced potent medications used in the standard treatment of hypertension. Thus, this behavioral technique could be not only a useful adjunct to standard drug treatment but also an effective first-line treatment for mild hypertension in elderly African-Americans. The authors surmised that TM was effective at reducing high blood pressure in part because of its ability to reduce the chronic elevation of sympathetic nervous system activity. These results also confirm by direct experimental comparison what was shown in the statistical meta-analyses, namely, that TM outperformed standard deep muscle relaxation, the most widely used approach to physical relaxation. The approach used in this study is currently being expanded upon in a larger trial supported by the National Institutes of Health.

The study also extends the findings of an earlier randomized, controlled trial comparing TM with other behavioral techniques in elderly residents of retirement homes. In that study the subjects who learned TM showed a similar significant reduction in systolic blood pressure (-12 mm Hg) compared to subjects assigned to either a generic mental relaxation technique, a "mindful" mental stimulation technique, or usual care. Furthermore, over a three-year period, the mortality rate from all causes for the TM group was significantly lower than for the other groups (Alexander et al., 1989).

TRANSCENDENTAL MEDITATION AND SUBSTANCE ABUSE

Because it is likely that the best predictor of the efficacy of TM in detoxification is its degree of effectiveness in later stages of recovery, it is important to review the general research on TM and substance abuse. The potential usefulness of TM in drug abuse was first reported in a technical letter to the *New England Journal of Medicine*. While following blood pressure changes in 20 young men who learned TM, 19 of whom had used either heroin, marijuana, LSD, barbiturates or amphetamines, it was found that all 19 reported no longer using drugs because the drug-induced feelings were extremely distasteful compared to the feelings they were experiencing as a result of TM (Benson, 1969). In a much larger follow-up survey from the same laboratory, questionnaires were completed by 1,862 out of approximately 1,950 people to whom they had been sent and who had practiced TM for an average of 20 months (Benson & Wallace, 1972; Benson & Wallace, 1977). After starting TM, a significant decrease in drug abuse was reported. Subjects stated that in the six-month period before starting TM, 80% used marijuana, 60% drank hard liquor, and 48% smoked tobacco cigarettes. After Transcendental Meditation had been practiced for up to three months, 46% used marijuana, 44% drank hard liquor, and 36% smoked tobacco. An even more dramatic change was apparent in the group who had practiced TM for over 21 months, where only 12% of the subjects continued to use marijuana, 25% to drink hard liquor and 16% to smoke tobacco. Similar impressive changes were seen in subjects who had abused amphetamines, barbiturates, hallucinogens, and narcotics.

This study also examined self-report data on drug selling. There was both a decrease or cessation of drug-selling activity and a shift away from advocating drug use to others. Approximately 20% of the subjects reported they sold drugs before starting TM, but in the subgroup who had practiced TM for less than three months, only 6% reported they continued to sell drugs. In the group practicing TM for up to 21 months, less than 1% reported they continued to sell drugs. In addition, 65% of the subjects reported they had either encouraged or condoned drug abuse by others before starting TM, but over 95% reported they began to discourage drug abuse soon after starting TM. Although this study had an impressive number of subjects and dramatic findings, it can be criticized because of its retrospective design and lack of a matched control group. Nevertheless, the results provided an impetus for further research on the use of TM in drug treatment.

In 35 subsequent studies, the effects of TM on substance abuse were assessed for people in the general population, for participants in inpatient and outpatient treatment programs, and for prisoners with histories of heavy use (reviewed in Alexander et al., this volume; Aron & Aron, 1980; Gelderloos et al., 1991). Although these studies varied widely in strength of research design, they consistently yielded results indicating that TM reduces drug use and addictions. Since most of these studies involved no separate detoxification program, it can be inferred that use of TM alone was generally sufficient to reduce stress to tolerable levels during the period of immediate withdrawal as well as to provide the basis for continued abstinence during later phases of recovery.

In particular, the comparative effectiveness of TM in reducing substance abuse was quantitatively assessed in a recent statistical meta-analysis. The effects of TM, in 19 studies explicitly reporting outcomes for drug consumption (with sufficient information to compute effect sizes), were compared with the effects of standard treatment programs reported in other available meta-analyses or, in cases where these were not available, in the original studies (Alexander et al., this volume). This meta-analysis controlled for strength of study design and sample size by appropriately weighting TM treatment outcomes on these factors. The results indicated that TM produced a significantly larger reduction than these other treatment and prevention programs in the use of alcohol, tobacco, and illicit drugs.

- For alcohol abuse, TM produced a significantly greater effect than: (1) education programs for drug prevention that were designed to foster resistance to peer pressure; (2) prevention education programs designed to enhance self-esteem and knowledge of drug consequences; (3) the average of a wide range of driving-under-the-influence (DUI) treatment programs (including educational programs, psychotherapy, anti-abuse programs such as Alcoholics Anonymous, and therapeutic probation programs); and (4) the average of other relaxation treatment programs (including biofeedback, muscle relaxation, stress-management training, and other forms of meditation).
- For tobacco smoking, TM produced significantly greater effects than: (1) drug prevention education programs; (2) counseling programs for smoking cessation; (3) bibliotherapy; (4) pharmacological treatments for nicotine addiction (including nicotine replacement programs and clonodine therapy); and (5) "unconventional" treatment (including acupuncture, hypnosis, sensory deprivation, etc.).
- For illicit drugs (cannabis, hallucinogens, and narcotics), TM produced significantly greater effects than: (1) preventive education programs combating peer pressure; and (2) preventive education programs fostering self-esteem and knowledge about drugs.

In this meta-analysis, the effect sizes for TM were of a magnitude generally considered large in the behavioral sciences (Cohen, 1977), and were typically several-fold greater than those of standard treatment programs. Also, secondary analyses revealed that the more rigorous, longitudinal experiments on TM, including random assignment studies, actually had a somewhat larger effect size than cross-sectional surveys; and that effects were also somewhat larger for serious compared to casual misusers of alcohol and illicit drugs. For example, in a randomized, controlled trial conducted over an 18-month period, addition of TM produced 2.6 times the abstinence rate of a standard AA plus counseling program in severe, skid-row type alcoholics (Taub et al., this volume). EMG biofeedback also produced favorable results in this study. This suggests that the positive outcomes for TM were not due to inclusion of studies with a weak design or studies focusing on casual users. Moreover, analysis of the time course of treatment influence indicates that TM's effects on smoking, drinking and use of illicit drugs tend to increase over time (up to two years), suggesting a cumulative effect of regular TM practice. In contrast, it is known that success rates for standard drug treatments fall off substantially over equivalent periods (Hunt, Barnett, & Branch, 1971). It should be noted that in this meta-analysis, TM was generally compared with classes or types of treatment (e.g., preventive education programs or relaxation training) and not to each particular treatment program. This is because there were not enough studies on each individual treatment program to allow separate comparisons. Thus, quantitative comparisons of the other specific treatments await the accumulation of more study outcomes. In summary, the results of this meta-analysis, and of the other studies described above on the effectiveness of TM in prevention and treatment of substance abuse, would lead one to predict that TM could also be distinctively effective during the early withdrawal phase.

WHERE TM FITS WITHIN THE PUBLIC HEALTH MODEL, AND ITS SPECIAL ADVANTAGES FOR DETOXIFICATION

Within the last decade, alcohol and drug departments in a number of agencies throughout California, including Alameda, Los Angeles, and San Diego counties, have adopted a modified version of the public health model as their conceptual framework for combating alcohol and drug abuse. As mentioned in the Introduction, the public health model assumes that there are three main factors that interact to create a disease process: the causative agent, the human host and the environment (Miller & Hester, 1989; Strantz,

1988). In many epidemics, the nature and roles of these factors are distinct and well-defined. However, in other epidemics, the three factors may be so tightly interwoven (especially environment and agent) that they can hardly be separated from one another.

The classic illustration of the public health model applied to combating disease involves the case of malaria. The infectious agent is the intracellular parasite; the host is the human being; the physical surrounding is the marsh; and the transmission vector is the mosquito. Based on the public health model, a strategy to stop malaria might involve vaccinating the host against the parasitic agent; developing a chemical that kills the malaria parasite directly, preferably before it enters the host; developing an insecticide to kill the mosquito that transports the parasite; or draining the marshlands of the stagnant water where the mosquito breeds.

Application of the public health model to combat substance abuse (e.g., Alameda County, 1988; Miller & Hester, 1989; Strantz, 1988), is basically as follows: the host is man; the disease-causing agent is the abused drug; the surroundings are the local socio-economic community; and the drug dealer or retailer is the vector of transmission. Thus, strategies developed to combat substance abuse may address any or all of the aforementioned variables. For example, health authorities in a given county may try to eliminate the "disease-causing agent" directly by locating and destroying such things as the marijuana plants, opium flowers, and psilocybin mushrooms. Or the county authorities may focus on eliminating the vectors of transmission by arresting all the main drug pushers and bootleggers in an area. Another approach authorities might take involves making the surrounding community less conducive to drug use. For instance, public media campaigns could be started that deglamorize the use of any drugs in the workplace, schools, streets, public transit systems, and sports arenas. Furthermore, the social environment could be uplifted and made more resistant to substance abuse by the promotion of adequate educational, vocational, and health care opportunities and cultural appreciation events.

As stated earlier, current information indicates that attempts to reduce drug availability have not been particularly successful in reducing drug use. While educational programs to uplift the social environment and the potential addict do appear to have some beneficial effect, there are other things that health authorities could do to combat substance abuse. Reinforcing the host, the individual human being, is an option that has not been seriously tested. If effective means are available, strengthening the health of the individual could be a direct and cost-effective means of reducing use of alcohol and drugs. Throughout the country, mental health clinics, community counseling agencies, schools, churches, drug prevention programs, employee assistance programs, and correctional facilities are now employing self-improvement courses in order to strengthen individuals and help them overcome the pressures or temptations which may lead to substance abuse. These self-improvement courses usually include such things as self-esteem and self-confidence enhancement, drug refusal skills, independent decision making skills, sober coping mechanisms, constructive assertiveness skills, communication skills, strategies to develop resistance to peer pressure, and stress reduction techniques.

As indicated above, Maharishi Mahesh Yogi's Transcendental Meditation program has been shown by meta-analysis to outperform such programs, which are each targeted at one area contributing to drug abuse. The reason for this unusual effectiveness appears to be associated with the natural and holistic influence of this practice (Alexander et al., this volume). TM not only directly counters the negative effects of the stress response (Walton & Levitsky, this volume), it also has been found to decrease anxiety, depression, anger, neuroticism and insomnia, and to increase well-being and self-esteem (see for review Alexander et al., 1991). Moreover, TM has been reported to enhance memory, learning ability, moral reasoning, and clarity of thinking (e.g., Dillbeck, 1982; Nidich et al., 1983), as well as to improve general physical health (Orme-Johnson, 1987). Strong physiological and psychological health are crucial in resisting the various effects of alcohol or drugs. Moreover, because individuals practicing TM appear to think more clearly, they may have a better foundation for absorbing the lessons of other self-improvement courses, such as those dealing with sober coping mechanisms or peer pressure resistance.

Another potential advantage of TM is its demonstrated benefits in treating complicating factors (mentioned earlier) that may be associated with drug detoxification. Because TM is natural and holistic in its physiological and psychological effects, this technique may be better able than most other approaches to safely and comprehensively address the multiple needs of these special cases. Specifically, prior research has indicated that TM is or could be useful in each of the following:

- reducing complications in pregnancy and childbirth (Heidelberg, 1979),
- treating serious mental illnesses, such as schizophrenia (e.g., Candelent & Candelent, 1975) and post-traumatic stress disorder (Brooks & Scarano, 1985),
- treating physical diseases, including epilepsy (e.g., Subrahmanyam & Porkodi, 1980), asthma (e.g., Wilson, Honsberger, Chiu, & Novey, 1975), hypertension (e.g., Schneider et al., 1992), hypercholesterolemia (e.g., Cooper & Aygen, 1979), and chronic pain (Mills & Farrow, 1981),
- recovering from multiple addictions (see Aron & Aron, 1980; Clements, Krenner, & Molk, 1988; Monahan, 1977),
- reducing susceptibility to stressors such as conditioned cues, as reflected in a more rapid habituation of galvanic skin response to physical and mental stressors (e.g., Orme-Johnson, 1973; Goleman & Schwartz, 1976), and growth in field independence and stable internal locus of control (e.g., Alexander et al., 1991; Hjelle, 1974; Pelletier, 1974).

Finally, there are several practical advantages of TM over many other forms of treatment for detoxification, including: ease of initial learning (TM is learned in a few hours over a period of five or six days); ease and simplicity of the practice (even a child of four can learn a modified form); no requirement for special instruments or for painful or invasive procedures; high cost-effectiveness relative to other standardized detoxification treatments (e.g., Greenstreet, 1988); positive health benefits rather than adverse side-effects; can be used in conjunction with other procedures (e.g., acupuncture, medications, Ayurvedic treatments); can be made available within treatment institutions as well as used in outpatient programs; and completion of initial instructions insures life-long follow-up membership and services in community-based centers teaching the Transcendental Meditation technique throughout the world.

For the reasons outlined above, Transcendental Meditation appears highly promising as a primary detoxification treatment or as a component of multifaceted treatment programs. No changes in beliefs, diet, or other aspects of lifestyle are required. However, improvements in attitude toward health and in assuming responsibility for one's health appear to increase spontaneously in subjects who learn TM, even after a relatively short time of practice (Schneider et al., 1992). Also, if structured follow-up is provided, as would be the case in detoxification treatment, adherence to regular practice can be very high. For example, in Schneider et al. (1992), the TM adherence rate (percentage who practiced TM "always or almost always twice a day") over a three-month follow-up was 97%. Research specifically on the use of TM in drug and alcohol detoxification programs remains to be done. However, given the critical importance of reducing stress and strengthening the host during drug detoxification, it would be unwise to overlook the promise of this distinctively effective, safe, and time-tested technique for personal development.

REFERENCES

Alameda County. (1988). *Alameda County Drug Program Services Plan*. Alameda County, CA: Alameda County Department of Alcohol and Drug Programs, State of California.

Alexander, C. N., Davies, J. L., Dixon, C. A., Dillbeck, M. C., Druker, S. M., Oetzel, R. M., Muehlman, J. M., & Orme-Johnson, D. W. (1990). Growth of higher states of consciousness: The Vedic psychology of human development. In C. N. Alexander & E. J. Langer (Eds.), *Higher stages of human development: Perspectives on adult growth* (pp. 286-340). New York: Oxford University Press.

Alexander, C. N., Langer, E. J., Newman, R. I., Chandler, H. M., & Davies, J. L. (1989). Transcendental Meditation, mindfulness, and longevity: An experimental study with the elderly. *Journal of Personality and Social Psychology, 57*, 950-964.

Alexander, C. N., Rainforth, M. V., & Gelderloos, P. (1991). Transcendental Meditation, self-actualization and psychological health: A conceptual overview and statistical meta-analysis. *Journal of Social Behavior and Personality, 6*, 189-247.

Alexander, C. N., Robinson, P., & Rainforth, M. (this volume). Treating and preventing alcohol, nicotine, and drug abuse through Transcendental Meditation: A review and statistical meta-analysis. *Alcoholism Treatment Quarterly.*

Alexander, C. N., & Sands, D. (1993). Meditation and relaxation. In S. N. McGill (Ed.), *McGill's survey of the social sciences: Psychology (pp. 1499-1504).* Pasadena, CA: Salem Press.

American Lung Association. (1991). *Stop smoking: Relaxation and motivation.* (Cassette Recording).

Aron, A., & Aron, E. N. (1980). The Transcendental Meditation program's effect on addictive behavior. *Journal of Addictive Behaviors, 5,* 3-12.

Baumgartner, G. R., & Rowen, R. C. (1987). Clonidine vs. chlordiazepoxide in the management of acute alcohol withdrawal syndrome. *Archives of Internal Medicine, 147,* 1223-1226.

Benson, H., & Wallace, R. K. (1972). Decreased drug abuse with Transcendental Meditation: A study of 1,862 subjects. In J. D. Zarafonetis (Ed.), *Drug Abuse: Proceedings of the International Conference* (pp. 369-376). Philadelphia: Lea and Febiger.

Benson, H., & Wallace, R. K. (1977). Decreased drug abuse with Transcendental Meditation: A study of 1,862 subjects. In D. W. Orme-Johnson, & J. T. Farrow, (Eds.) *Scientific research on the Transcendental Meditation program: Collected papers* (pp. 498-505). Rheinweiler, W. Germany: Maharishi European Research University Press.

Benson, H. B. (1969). Yoga and drug abuse. *New England Journal of Medicine, 281,* 1133.

Brooks, J. S., & Scarano, T. (1985). Transcendental Meditation in the treatment of post-Vietnam adjustment. *Journal of Counseling Development, 64,* 212-215.

Bullock, M. L., Culliton, P. D., & Olander, R. T. (1989). Controlled trial of acupuncture for severe recidivist alcoholism. *The Lancet,* 1435-1439.

Burchfield, S. R. (1979). The stress response: A new perspective. *Psychosomatic Medicine, 41,* 661-672.

Candelent, T., & Candelent, G. (1975). Teaching Transcendental Meditation in a psychiatric setting. *Hospital & Community Psychiatry, 26,* 156-159.

Cannon, W. B. (1929). *Bodily changes in pain, hunger, fear, and rage.* New York: Appleton.

Chen, G. S. (1987). Enkephalin, drug addiction and acupuncture. *American Journal of Chinese Medicine, 5,* 25-30.

Childress, A. R., Hole, A. V., & DePhilipps, D. (1991). *The coping with craving program: A manual of active tools for reducing the craving/arousal to drug-related cues.* Philadelphia: Addiction Research Center, University Pennsylvania School of Medicine.

Childress, A. R., McLellan, A. T., Ehrman, R., & O'Brien, C. P. (1988). Classically conditioned responses in opiod and cocaine dependence: A role in relapse? In B.A. Ray (Ed.), *Learning factors in substance abuse* (pp. 25-43). NIDA Research Monograph.

Childress, A. R., McLellan, A. T., Natale, M., & O'Brien, C. P. (1987). Mood states can elicit conditioned withdrawal and craving in opiate abuse patients. In L. S. Harris (Ed.) *Problems of drug dependence, 1986. Proceedings of the 48th annual science management committee on problems of drug dependence*, (pp. 137-144). NIDA Research Monograph.

Chrousos, G. P., & Gold, P. W. (1992). The concepts of stress and stress system disorders. *Journal of the American Medical Association, 267*, 1244-1252.

Ciba-Geigy Corporation (1992). *A patient's guide: Transdermal nicotine patient support booklet.* Ciba-Geigy Corporation.

Clements, G., Krenner, L., & Molk, W. (1988). The use of the Transcendental Meditation programme in the prevention of drug abuse and in the treatment of drug-addicted persons. *Bulletin on Narcotics, 40*, 51-56.

Cohen, J. (1977). *Statistical power analysis for the behavioral sciences.* New York: Academic Press.

Cooper, M. J., & Aygen, M. M. (1979). A relaxation technique in the management of hypercholesterolemia. *Journal of Human Stress, 5*, 24-27.

Denniston, D. (1986). *The TM book: How to enjoy the rest of your life* (New Edition). Fairfield, IA: Fairfield Press.

Dillbeck, M. C. (1982). Meditation and flexibility of visual perception and verbal problem-solving. *Journal of Memory and Cognition, 10*, 207-215.

Dillbeck, M. C., & Orme-Johnson, D. W. (1987). Physiological differences between Transcendental Meditation and rest. *American Psychology, 42*, 879-881.

Druckman, D., & Bjork, R. A. (Eds.). (1991). *In the mind's eye: Enhancing human performance.* Washington, DC: National Academy Press.

Eliot, R. S. (1979). *Stress and the major cardiovascular disorders.* Mt. Kisco, New York: Futura.

Eppley, K., Abrams, A., & Shear, J. (1989). The differential effects of relaxation techniques on trait anxiety: A meta-analysis. *Journal of Clinical Psychology, 45*, 957-974.

Frew, D. R. (1977). *Management of stress: Using TM at work.* Chicago: Nelson-Hall.

Gelderloos, P., Walton, K. G., Orme-Johnson, D. W., & Alexander, C. N. (1991). Effectiveness of the Transcendental Meditation program in preventing and treating substance misuse: A review. *International Journal of Addiction, 26*, 293-325.

Glaser, J. L. (this volume). Clinical applications of Maharishi Ayur-Veda in chemical dependency disorders. *Alcoholism Treatment Quarterly.*

Glass, G. V., McGaw, B., & Smith, M. L. (1981). *Meta-analysis in social research.* Beverly Hills, California: Sage.

Glassman, A. H., Stenter, F., Walsh, B. T., & Raizman, P. S. (1988). Heavy smokers, smoking cessation, and clonidine. *Journal of the American Medical Association, 259*, 2863-2866.

Gold, M. S., Pottash, A. C., Sweeney, D. R., & Kleber, H. D. (1980). Opiate withdrawal using clonidine: A safe, effective and rapid non-opiate treatment. *Journal of the American Medical Association, 243*, 343-346.

Goleman, D. J., & Schwartz, G. E. (1976). Meditation as an intervention in stress reactivity. *Journal of Consulting and Clinical Psychology, 44*, 456-466.

Gottlieb, L. D. (1988). The role of beta blockers in alcohol withdrawal syndrome. *Postgraduate Medicine, 169,* 169-174.

Greenstreet, R. L. (1988). *Cost-effective alternatives in alcoholism treatment.* Springfield, IL: Charles C Thomas.

Heidelberg, R. (1979). *Transzendentale Meditation in der geburtshilflichen Psychoprophylaxe.* Unpublished doctoral dissertation, Medical Faculty, Free University of Berlin.

Herron, R. E. (1993). *The impact of the Transcendental Meditation technique on medical expenditures.* Unpublished doctoral dissertation, Maharishi International University.

Hjelle, L. A. (1974). Transcendental Meditation and psychological health. *Perceptual and Motor Skills, 39,* 623-628.

Holmes, D. (1984). Meditation and somatic arousal: A review of the experimental evidence. *American Psychologist, 39,* 1-10.

Horwitz, R. I., Gottlieb, L. D., & Kraus, M. L. (1989). The efficacy of atenolol in the outpatient management of the alcohol withdrawal syndrome. *Archives of Internal Medicine, 149,* 1089-1093.

Hunt, W. A., Barnett, L. W., & Branch, L. G. (1971). Relapse rates in addiction programs. *Journal of Clinical Psychology, 27,* 455-456.

Hunter, J. E., & Schmidt, F. L. (1990). *Methods of meta-analysis.* New York: Sage.

Klajner, F., Hartman, L. M., & Sobell, M. B. (1984). Treatment of substance abuse by relaxation training: A review of its rationale, efficacy and mechanisms. *Addictive Behaviors, 9,* 41-55.

Leung, A. S. H. (1977). Acupuncture treatment of withdrawal symptoms. *American Journal of Acupuncture, 5,* 43-50.

Leventhal, H., & Cleary, P. D. (1980). The smoking problem: A review of the research and theory on behavioral risk modification. *Psychological Bulletin, 88,* 370-405.

MacLean, C. R. K., Walton, K. G., Wenneberg, S. R., Levitsky, D. K., Mandarino, J. V., Waziri, R., & Schneider, R. H. (1992). Altered cortisol response to stress after four months' practice of the Transcendental Meditation program. *Society of Neuroscience Abstracts, 18,* 1541.

Maharishi Mahesh Yogi (1963). *Science of being and art of living: Transcendental Meditation.* New York: Signet.

Maharishi Mahesh Yogi (1969). *On the Bhagavad-Gita: A translation and commentary.* Harmondsworth, Middlesex, England: Arkana (Penguin).

Mausner, J. S., & Bahn, A. K (1974). *Epidemiology: An introductory text.* Philadelphia: W. B. Saunders.

Miller, W. R., & Hester, R. K. (1989). Treating alcohol problems: Toward an informed eclecticism. In R. K. Hester, & W. R. Miller (Eds.), *Handbook of alcoholism treatment approaches: Effective alternatives* (pp. 3-13.). New York: Pergamon Press.

Mills, W. W., & Farrow, J. T. (1981). The Transcendental Meditation technique and acute experimental pain. *Psychosomatic Medicine, 43,* 157-164.

Monahan, R. J. (1977). Secondary prevention of drug dependence through the Transcendental Meditation program in metropolitan Philadelphia. *International Journal of the Addictions, 12,* 729-754.

Nidich, S. I., Ryncarz, R. A., Abrams, A. I., Orme-Johnson, D. W., & Wallace, R. K. (1983). Kohlbergian cosmic perspective responses, EEG coherence, and the Transcendental Meditation and TM-Sidhi program. *Journal of Moral Education, 12*(3), 166-173.

O'Brien, P. O., Childress, A. R., McLellan, A. T., Ehrman, R., & Ternes, J. W. (1988). Types of conditioning found in drug-dependent humans. In B.A. Ray (Ed.) *Learning factors in substance abuse* (pp. 44-61). NIDA Research Monograph.

O'Brien, P. O., Childress, A. R., McLellan, T., & Ehrman, R. (1990). Integrating systemic cue exposure with treatment in recovering drug dependent patients. *Addictive Behavior, 15,* 355-365.

Orme-Johnson, D. W. (1973). Autonomic stability and Transcendental Meditation. *Psychosomatic Medicine, 35,* 341-349.

Orme-Johnson, D. W. (1987). Medical care utilization and the Transcendental Meditation program. *Psychosomatic Medicine, 49,* 493-507.

Orme-Johnson, D. W. (this volume). Transcendental Meditation as an epidemiological approach to drug and alcohol abuse: Theory, research, and financial impact evaluation. *Alcoholism Treatment Quarterly.*

Pelletier, K. R. (1974). Influence of Transcendental Meditation upon autokinetic perception. *Perceptual and Motor Skills, 39,* 1031-1034.

Rohsenow, D. J., Niaura, R.A., Childress, A. R., Abrams, D. B., & Monti, P. M. (1990-1991). Cue reactivity in addictive behaviors: Theoretical and treatment implications. *The International Journal of the Addictions, 25,* 957-993.

Sands, D. (this volume). Introducing Maharishi Ayur-Veda into clinical practice. *Alcoholism Treatment Quarterly.*

Sapolsky, R. M. (1992). *Stress, the aging brain, and the mechanisms of neuron death.* Cambridge, MA: The MIT Press.

Sapolsky, R. M., Krey, L. C., & McEwen, B. S. (1986). The neuroendocrinology of stress and aging: The glucocorticoid cascade hypothesis. *Endocrine Review, 7,* 284-301.

Schneider, R. H., Alexander, C. N., & Wallace, R. K. (1992). In search of an optimal behavioral treatment for hypertension: A review and focus on Transcendental Meditation. In E. H. Johnson, W. D. Gentry, S. Julius (Eds.), *Personality, elevated blood pressure, and essential hypertension* (pp.291-315). Washington, DC: Hemisphere Publishing Corporation.

Schneider, R. H., Cavanaugh, K. L., Kasture, H. S., Rothenberg, S., Averbach, R., Robinson, D., & Wallace, R. K. (1990). Health promotion with a traditional system of natural health care: Maharishi Ayur-Veda. *Journal of Social Behavior and Personality, 5,* 1-27.

Schneider, R., Staggers, F., Alexander, C., Sheppard, W., Gaylord, C., Gelderloos, P., Smith, S., Kondwani, K., Rainforth, M., & Cooper, R. (1991). Stress management in elderly blacks with hypertension: A preliminary report. *Proceed-*

ings of the Second International Conference on Race, Ethnicity, and Health: Challenges in Diabetes and Hypertension (pp. 68-78). Salvador, Bahai, Brazil.

Selye, H., & Tuchweber, B. (1976). Stress in relation to aging and disease. In A. Everitt & J. Burgess (Eds.), *Hypothalamus, pituitary and aging* (pp. 557-573). Springfield, IL: Charles C Thomas.

Sharma, H., Dillbeck, M., & Dillbeck, S. (this volume). Implementation of the Transcendental Meditation program and Maharishi Ayur-Veda to prevent alcohol and drug abuse among juveniles at risk. *Alcoholism Treatment Quarterly.*

Sharma, H. M., Triguna, B. D., & Chopra, D. (1991). Maharishi Ayur-Veda: Modern insights into ancient medicine. *Journal of the American Medical Association, 265,* 2633-2637.

Smith, D. E., & Wesson, D. R. (1971). Phenobarbital technique for treatment of barbiturate dependence. *Archives of General Psychiatry, 24,* 56-60.

Smith, J. C. (1976). Psychotherapeutic effects of Transcendental Meditation with controls for expectation of relief and daily sitting. *Journal of Consulting and Clinical Psychology, 44,* 630-637.

Smith, M. O. (1979). Acupuncture and natural healing in drug detoxification. *American Journal of Acupuncture, 7.*

Smith, M. O. (1989). *The Lincoln Hospital acupuncture drug abuse program.* (Transcript of the testimony to the Select Committee on Narcotics, U.S. House of Representatives).

Smith, M. O., & Khan, I. (1988). An acupuncture programme for the treatment of drug-addicted persons. *Bulletin on Narcotics, 40,* 35-41.

Smith, M. O., Squires, R., & Aponte, J. et al. (1982). Acupuncture treatment of drug addiction and alcohol abuse. *American Journal of Acupuncture, 10,* 161-163.

Strantz, I. (1988). Use of the public health model for a statewide prevention strategy. In A. Mecca (Ed.), *Prevention 2000–A Public/Private Partnership.* California Health Resources Foundation.

Stux, G., & Pomeranz, B. (1987). *Acupuncture: Textbook and atlas.* Berlin: Springer-Verlag.

Subrahmanyam, S., & Porkodi, K. (1980). Neurohumoral correlates of Transcendental Meditation. *Journal of Biomedicine, 1,* 73-88.

Surgeon General. (1988). *The consequences of smoking: Nicotine addiction.* U.S. Department of Health and Human Services.

Sytinsky, I. A., Galebskaya, L. V., & Jantunen, A. (1981). Physiologo-biochemical bases of drug dependence treatment by electroacupuncture. *American Journal of Acupuncture, 9.*

Taub, E., Steiner, S. S., Smith, R. B., Weingarten, E., & Walton, K. G. (this volume). Effectiveness of broad spectrum approaches to relapse prevention in severe alcoholism: A long-term, randomized, controlled comparison of Transcendental Meditation, EMG biofeedback and electronic neurotherapy. *Alcoholism Treatment Quarterly.*

Thatte, U. M., & Dahanukar, S. A. (1986). Ayurveda and contemporary scientific thought. *Trends in Pharmacological Science, 7,* 247-251.

Victor, M. (1966). Treatment of alcoholic intoxication and the withdrawal syndrome. *Psychosomatic Medicine, 28,* 636-650.

Walinder, J., Bokstrom, K., & Karlsson, I. B. L. (1981). Clonidine suppression of the alcohol withdrawal syndrome. *Drug and Alcohol Dependence, 8,* 345-348.

Wallace, R. K. (1970). Physiological effects of Transcendental Meditation. *Science, 167,* 1751-1754.

Wallace, R. K., & Benson, H. (1972). The physiology of meditation. *Scientific American, 226,* 84-90.

Wallace, R. K., Benson, H., & Wilson, A. F. (1971). A wakeful hypometabolic physiologic state. *American Journal of Physiology, 221,* 795-799.

Walton, K. G., & Levitsky, D. (this volume). A neuroendocrine mechanism for the reduction of drug use and addictions by Transcendental Meditation. *Alcoholism Treatment Quarterly.*

Walton, K. G., Pugh, N., Gelderloos, P., & Macrae, P. (submitted). Mechanisms of prevention through stress reduction: Suggestive results on corticosteriods, salt excretion and negative emotions. *Journal of Hypertension.*

Washton, A. M., & Stone-Washton, N. (1990). Abstinence and relapse in outpatient cocaine addicts. *Journal of Psychoactive Drugs, 22.*

Weiss, R. D., & Cheung, S. Y. C. (1987). *Cocaine.* Washington, DC: American Psychiatric Press.

Wen, H. L., & Cheung, S. Y. C. (1973). Treatment of drug addiction by acupuncture and electrical stimulation. *American Journal of Acupuncture, 1,* 71-75.

Wen, H. L., Ho, W. K. Wong, H. K. et al. (1978). Reduction of adrenocorticotropichormone and cortisol in drug addicts treated with acupuncture and electrical stimulation. *Comparative Medicines of the East and West, 6,* 61-66.

Wilson, A. F., Honsberger, R. W., Chiu, J. T., & Novey, H. S. (1975). Transcendental Meditation and asthma. *Respiration, 32,* 74-80.

Zuckerman, M. B. (1993). Fighting the right drug war. *U.S. News & World Report,* p. 74.

SECTION IV: MAHARISHI AYUR-VEDA AND THE TREATMENT OF ALCOHOLISM AND DRUG ADDICTION

Introducing Maharishi Ayur-Veda into Clinical Practice

David Sands, MD

A new client, Joe, takes a seat in your office. He is middle-aged, but looks older than his stated age. It is obvious that he is not happy about having this consultation. After the introductions have been made and you have inquired politely about his social and vocational situations, you ask him about his appetite and the strength of his digestion. This surprises him because he was expecting you to ask about his drinking–the reason he believes this consultation was scheduled. You don't. Instead, you ask what he ate yesterday and whether this was typical for him. Then you ask him what time he went to bed last night. Again, he expresses surprise. Next, you ask how well he slept. Then, you inquire about his bowel habits. Finally, you ask him about the clarity of his thinking, his memory, and about whether he feels happy and satisfied with his life. You note how he has answered your questions: the rate of speech, the gestures and accessory movements, the quality of his voice, etc. You conclude your examination by checking his pulse.

Your client seems perplexed. You have not asked him why he is

---

Dr. Sands is a staff physician at the College of Maharishi Ayur-Veda Health Center, and Assistant Professor and Associate Chairman of Physiology at Maharishi International University, Fairfield, IA.

Address correspondence to: David Sands, MD, Physiology Department, Maharishi International University, 1000 North Fourth Street, Fairfield, IA 52557-1129.

[Haworth co-indexing entry note]: "Introducing Maharishi Ayur-Veda into Clinical Practice." Sands, David. Co-published simultaneously in the *Alcoholism Treatment Quarterly* (The Haworth Press, Inc.) Vol. 11, No. 3/4, 1994, pp. 335-365; and: *Self-Recovery: Treating Addictions Using Transcendental Meditation and Maharishi Ayur-Veda* (ed: David F. O'Connell and Charles N. Alexander) The Haworth Press, Inc., 1994, pp. 335-365. Multiple copies of this article/chapter may be purchased from The Haworth Document Delivery Center [1-800-3-HAWORTH; 9:00 a.m. - 5:00 p.m. (EST)].

seeing you, about his problems, his drinking, his use of recreational chemicals and tobacco, his criminal record, his childhood, or even his relationship with his mother. He decides that the experience in this clinic is going to be different. He is not sure what will happen next, but he is curious and he is ready to listen.

What you say next may be the most important thing he will ever hear about his rehabilitation. From what you tell him, he will gain new perspective, new insight, and new hope that will turn his life in a positive direction. It will empower him to heal himself, to change his ways, cope with his problems, and become happy and successful. What you are about to undertake is his education in the principles and procedures for creating health through the practice of Maharishi Ayur-Veda.

WHAT IS MAHARISHI AYUR-VEDA?

Maharishi Ayur-Veda is the oldest system of natural health care, brought to light by Maharishi Mahesh Yogi from the ancient Vedic tradition, working with distinguished physicians and Ayurvedic experts in India. The name denotes a "comprehensive system of knowledge of the life span" (*Charaka Samhita*, 1981). Maharishi Ayur-Veda is truly a holistic system of health care, accounting for all aspects of individuality–mind, body, and behavior–in health and in disease. Maharishi Ayur-Veda sees an inherent connection between mind and body, and emphasizes mental techniques and behavioral programs in creating health. There are more than twenty categories of treatment modalities in this system, all of which seek to restore balance by integrating consciousness, mind, and body into one happy, healthy unit. In evaluating and treating health problems, as illustrated above, Maharishi Ayur-Veda examines mental, physical, physiological, behavioral, social, and environmental factors. Practiced in this way, Maharishi Ayur-Veda is more encompassing than modern medicine. It is also simple, safe, cost-effective, easily employed, and readily accepted by people of all ages and all ethnic and religious backgrounds (Schneider, Alexander & Wallace, 1992; Haratani & Hemmi, 1990a & b).

Maharishi Ayur-Veda creates health by enlivening the natural healing mechanisms of the mind-body, particularly by strengthening the functioning of the homeostatic, immune, and repair mechanisms. It does not treat disease as such, but instead seeks to create health in the mind-body system by correcting the expression of nature's intelligence contained in the DNA of every cell. Both Maharishi Ayur-Veda and modern science see nature as being inherently intelligent, meaning that it functions in an orderly, systematic manner. This orderliness is structured by laws of nature at every level of creation. In biological systems, these laws govern the expression of the information encoded in the DNA. Furthermore, both modern science and Maharishi Ayur-Veda describe creation as ever-changing and, overall, moving in a evolutionary direction through a sequential expression of natural law. The evolutionary direction of the unfolding of natural law is structured in the unified field that physicists describe as underlying the entire universe and as the source of all creation and of all change. Indeed, physicists today regard all physical phenomena as manifestations or fluctuations of the unified field. Maharishi Ayur-Veda identifies the unified field of natural law as a self-interacting field of consciousness, a field awake to its own intelligent nature, and seeks to expand human awareness to comprehend this underlying field of natural law by creating balance in consciousness, mind, body, and environment. Thus, Ayur-Veda is understood to operate at the level of the unified field, the level that governs all physiological and psychological processes. By integrating consciousness with its material and mental expressions in human psychophysiology, Maharishi Ayur-Veda encompasses the entire span of life from its most subtle to its most expressed aspects.

Introducing Maharishi Ayur-Veda into a substance abuse rehabilitation program, or any other clinical setting, brings new possibilities for therapeutic success and new professional opportunities for the staff. This paper will describe some factors to be considered when introducing this system so that it may be easily and successfully implemented. Its essential, fundamental principles will be presented so that the reader may adequately appreciate the richness and scope of this health care system. This presentation is based on the author's clinical experience, his experience in educating health professionals, and on the experience of other health professionals as they introduced Maharishi Ayur-Veda in their private practices. In keeping with the traditional method of training, the points made here will be more illustrative than didactic.

INTRODUCING MAHARISHI AYUR-VEDA INTO CLINICAL PRACTICE

The introduction of Maharishi Ayur-Veda requires that sufficient time be allocated for the staff to absorb its new concepts, to develop the skills involved in using it, and to gain personal experience with the process of creating health. The introduction will proceed smoothly and succeed maximally when the practice of Maharishi Ayur-Veda starts with the leadership of a clinic, proceeds to the clinical staff, and then to the clients. This approach has been used in clinics (Schneider et al., 1990), prisons (Abrams & Siegel, 1978), and even businesses (Alexander, Swanson, Rainforth, Carlisle, Todd & Oates, 1993; Haratani & Hemmi, 1990 a & b). Although it has been successfully introduced to the general public, introducing Maharishi Ayur-Veda to the clients first in a clinical setting never succeeds because the staff cannot appreciate what they have not personally experienced.

Gaining experience with Maharishi Ayur-Veda is very satisfying. People commonly feel more energetic, less fatigued, mentally clearer, happier, or emotionally more stable. Blood pressure may decrease and minor somatic problems may disappear. Most people experience less stress and tension. Over time, individuals may suffer fewer colds, digestive upsets, sleepless nights, or headaches (Schneider et al., 1990; Janssen, 1989). Gradually, one recognizes that improving health–creating good health–is both possible *and* natural.

With this growth of personal experience, fascinating transformations take place in both attitude and perspective. First, a transformation occurs in perspective: people stop thinking that health is something they have until it is lost. Instead, feeling healthier over time, they realize that health occurs in degrees and that they can be healthier if they act appropriately. A positive attitude about health and living a healthy lifestyle results. Even habitual health-risk behaviors such as alcohol consumption and cigarette smoking give way to health-promoting behaviors (Brooks & Scarano, 1985; Monahan, 1977). Success with some recommendations strengthens the desire to try others and ultimately to adopt a comprehensive program for improving health.

These first transformations lead to another: a transformation of conceptual framework from that of modern medical science to that of Ayur-Veda. This change is truly a change of paradigms. The paradigm of modern scientific medicine shapes our understanding of disease and drug dependency, constrains our ability to comprehend other systems of knowledge, and causes us to overlook potential contributions from other traditions. Therefore, to understand this new paradigm, one must first understand the limitations of the prevailing medical paradigm.

THE MODERN MEDICAL PARADIGM

Today's health care is delivered from a problem-oriented perspective, a viewpoint inherent in modern biomedical science. In evaluating a client's situation or concerns, a problem is identified and labeled. We say a person has "a disease," drug dependency, for example. Giving the situation a label creates a perspective: it identifies a "thing" that we call a "disease" that someone "has." It is this "thing" that is to be treated, this "disease" that is to be cured (Sheldon, 1970). Hence, all treatments are focused on symptoms or diseases because these are the basic concerns of problem-oriented modern medical practice.

Medical treatment does not really *cure* disease. What happens is that doctors prescribe treatments that, at best, *allow* the natural healing mechanisms to operate. If the healing mechanisms function effectively, they will restore the person to the customary state of health. If they don't function effectively, a chronic condition or gradual decline in health results. For example, if a person breaks a bone, setting the fracture and stabilizing it with a cast creates conditions that allow the body to heal the fracture. If a person has a boil, giving antibiotics may control the infection, but the body's immune and repair mechanisms actually heal the wound.

The disease-oriented approach has many unfortunate consequences. For one, the disease, rather than the person who suffers from the disease, is the object of attention. For another, the scientific method itself compels medical science to utilize a normative approach to studying diseases and therapeutics, again ignoring the individuality of the patient. In clinical studies, statistical averaging (creating norms) masks subtle individual variations, called "host factors," responsible for unique responses in specific situations. This means that the normative approach inherently masks subtle variations among individuals that may reflect disturbances arising from a deeper level of the mind-body unit. Such variations might reflect alterations of the ability to respond to changes in the environment, e.g., to seasonal changes in temperature, relative humidity, and length of daylight, that might ultimately lead to disease. Even "case-control" studies, which may be specifically designed to assess subtle individual differences by controlling for the more obvious variations among individuals (age, gender, etc.), generally are limited in their ability to detect these important differences between people. This limitation applies in clinical practice as well. For example, during an epidemic of influenza, it is impossible to predict who will *not* fall ill among a cohort of elderly living in a nursing home. Similarly, it is not possible to predict in which patient a drug will *not* work, nor predict in whom it *will* produce significant side-effects. Because the factors responsible for such varied responses are virtually impossible to measure and almost nothing is known that will alter them, medical science virtually ignores them.

Such questions of efficacy and epidemiology reveal another unfortunate consequence of the modern medical paradigm. Medical science does not know how to describe the state of *health* of individuals to any significant degree. Modern medicine only knows how to describe states of ill-health, states of disease. If the reader doubts this, consider the health rating scales currently in use. In the book–mistakenly titled–*Measuring Health* (McDowell & Newell, 1987), the authors present a comprehensive collection of rating scales and questionnaires, all of which measure, not health, but disability or disease. Health rating scales conform to medicine's notion that being healthy means not having any detectable disease or measurable disability.

Does being free of apparent disease or measurable disability really mean that a person is healthy? We tend to think that people are healthy until they become sick, but apparently some people are healthier than others because they stay well when others fall ill. People who become ill are predisposed to their diseases due to weaknesses or disturbances in function. Most of these weaknesses are not detectable by physical examination or laboratory tests, for they are structured in the mechanisms that regulate the expression of DNA and become apparent only when specific responses of the DNA are required. The natural healing mechanisms of the body are exquisitely coordinated and balanced by constant referral to the intelligence in DNA. Health, in this view, means that immunity and the homeostatic and repair mechanisms controlled by DNA function optimally. This implies that the ability to express the intelligence in DNA, and perhaps the ability to repair DNA, must be maintained to preserve or promote health.

In contrast to the modern medical paradigm, the paradigm of Maharishi Ayur-Veda understands health as a continuum reflecting the degree to which the body's homeostatic, immune, and repair mechanisms function properly. Any limitation in the function of these mechanisms represents some weakness, some lack of perfect health. Such weaknesses are called "imbalances" to convey the notion that these mechanisms are not functioning in a balanced, integrated manner (*Charaka Samhita,* 1981). The goal of Ayur-Veda in creating health is to restore and maintain the function of DNA and all homeostatic, immune, and repair mechanisms. Modern medical treatment rarely operates at this fundamental level of life.

Overcoming these limitations of modern medicine requires both expansion of the ability to observe and a change in perspective that allows one to consider factors not customarily regarded as important, factors that indicate that a person, a specific individual, is not perfectly healthy while not yet apparently ill (Sheldon, 1970). This discussion reveals the compelling need for a means to identify these weaknesses and to correct them. As we are about to see, this is one of the most important contributions of Maharishi Ayur-Veda. It provides the theoretical framework and practical means for identifying underlying disturbances in health and ameliorating them before they produce identifiable diseases. Ultimately, it provides a real understanding of health and how to create it.

MAHARISHI AYUR-VEDA: A GOAL-ORIENTED APPROACH TO TREATING DRUG DEPENDENCY

There is yet another transformation that takes place with the introduction of Maharishi Ayur-Veda. This is the transformation to a goal-oriented approach. Here, the goal is real health. In the case of drug dependency, this goal is freedom from addiction to chemicals and from obsessive and compelling thoughts that produce a desire for drugs. Gradually, as one experiences that health is the normal, natural state of functioning of the mind-body, and that it can be created by appropriate behaviors and specific therapeutics, one focuses increasingly on being healthy, happy and successful. Problems are not ignored, but solutions become central to one's thinking. Creating health becomes a goal of daily life.

The traditional medical approach to addictions is problem-oriented: drug addiction is regarded as a disease–a disease that may or may not be curable. Typically, a person is taught how to deal with his disease, to resist compulsive thoughts and powerful urges, to control deleterious response patterns, and to accept weakness and unhappiness. This usually requires strong emotional support and frequent reinforcement of the client. Indeed, the client may be dependent on this support for a long time. Given the problem-oriented perspective of this approach, the client maintains the negative self-image of an addict even when drug-free.

In applying Maharishi Ayur-Veda, however, the approach is directed toward a positive goal: creating health and happiness. The practitioner of Maharishi Ayur-Veda functions primarily as a teacher. The practitioner teaches clients about their innate potential for becoming healthier. The provider begins with a vision of possibilities, a vision that gives hope, then educates the client in the principles for creating health, and finally prescribes an individualized program that will create balance and fulfill the desire for health and happiness.

It must be understood that treating drug dependency through Maharishi Ayur-Veda is not accomplished simply by adopting an attitude or a philosophy. Just telling someone that he or she has the potential to be healthy does not make him or her healthy. Neither does wishing that one is healthy make one healthy. Every drug dependent person knows from experience that wishes and hopes do not automatically get fulfilled. The process of growing healthy requires the active involvement of the client.

Maharishi Ayur-Veda goes further than just educating and involving the individual; it actually empowers the individual to take control of the process of growing healthy. Instead of trading dependencies, it develops independence and self-sufficiency. By using the individualized program prescribed, the client takes charge of the process. Becoming happier and healthier, the client gradually gives up the notion that life is a struggle, that pain and suffering are normal and that disease and addiction are inevitable. The client realizes increasingly that good health and happiness are the natural state of life.

THE PRINCIPLES OF MAHARISHI AYUR-VEDA

The Principle of Psychophysiological Individuality

Maharishi Ayur-Veda is founded on a system that takes into consideration the psychophysiological constitution of each individual. According to Maharishi Ayur-Veda, three constitutional elements govern the functioning of the mind and body uniquely in each individual. In the Sanskrit language, the language of origin of Maharishi Ayur-Veda, these three elements are known as the *doshas*: *Vata*, *Pitta*, and *Kapha*. Vata dosha is the element governing movement in the physiology. Vata dosha governs breathing, the passage of food through the digestive system, the flow of blood through the circulatory system, and the activity of the nervous system. Pitta dosha governs the heat, energy, and anabolic (synthetic) functions of the physiology. Pitta is responsible for turning food into healthy tissue and into energy to power bodily processes. Kapha dosha is responsible for strength, stamina, and for the lubrication and resilience of the structural elements of the body.

According to the principles of Maharishi Ayur-Veda, each individual's constitution is composed of a mixture of all three doshas. Persons vary in the relative proportions of the three doshas in their constitution. A person's constitution may be composed primarily of Vata, of Pitta, or of Kapha, or of some combination of any two doshas, or may be composed of all three doshas in nearly equal proportion. The unique mixture of doshas in a person's constitution confers individuality. Maharishi Ayur-Veda provides the means to assess the relative contribution of each dosha to the inherent constitution of any individual.

Each dosha contributes specific qualities to the mental, physical and physiological functioning of an individual. Vata contributes qualities of coldness, lightness, dryness, roughness, movement, quickness, minuteness. Pitta contributes the qualities of heat, sharpness, lightness, acidity, moistness, liquidity, foul smell and slight oiliness. Kapha contributes the qualities of heaviness, slowness, coldness, oiliness, steadiness, sweetness, stickiness, smoothness and softness. We will consider the expression of these qualities in the mind-body.

The fundamental qualities of Vata, Pitta and Kapha listed in Table 1 give rise to distinct psychophysiological features. Persons constituted primarily of Vata dosha, called "Vatas" since they display the innate qualities of Vata in their psychophysiological features, are the butterflies among people. Vatas are light, active and vivacious. Vatas flit from one thing to another, forget what they are supposed to be doing, and tend not to be organized. Pittas remind us of honey bees. They are hard workers who go about their business with determination. Pittas like organization and stick to schedules. If you interfere with them, you may get stung. Kaphas are the elephants in society. They are large, slow, steady, and they never forget.

Vatas and Kaphas tend to be quite opposite in their characteristics, as one would expect from comparing the fundamental qualities of these doshas. However, since Vata and Kapha dosha share the quality of coldness, Vatas and Kaphas are not fond of cold weather. Pittas tend to be intermediate between Vatas and Kaphas in a number of characteristics, including height, weight, adipose tissue and musculature. In other characteristics, Pittas are very distinct, owing to the expression of the qualities of heat and sharpness not present in Vata and Kapha doshas.

When two doshas predominate in the constitution of an individual, they both contribute to the apparent psychophysiological features. This can sometimes cause uncertainty as to the constitutional makeup because the observable features may result from a blending of traits. For example, when Vata and Pitta constitute the psychophysiology, a person may display the creativity and enthusiasm conferred by Vata dosha along with the goal-oriented drive conferred by Pitta dosha. When Pitta and Kapha dosha combine, the person may display the strength and stamina of Kapha with the motivation of Pitta. Pitta-Kaphas are naturally inclined to athletics and to leadership–they tend to have a warrior's nature. Thus, they are the type of person that people look to in a time of crisis because of their size, physical strength, stability of mind and courage.

In a small percentage of people, the three doshas constitute the psychophysiology approximately equally. These tri-doshic individuals usually display the "best" features of each dosha. They have very strong, compact bodies and the vitality, drive, and strength to excel in gymnastics, soccer, and volley ball. They also tend to be very healthy, since the doshas stabilize each other.

THE PRINCIPLE OF BALANCE AND IMBALANCE

Another fundamental principle of Maharishi Ayur-Veda is that health and disease are determined by the state of balance or imbalance of the doshas. One enjoys good health when each of the three doshas exists in a balanced state. Imbalanced doshas produce abnormal physical and mental characteristics and ultimately cause disease.

It is a general tendency of the doshas to accumulate and thus to become imbalanced. Accumulation of a dosha leads to accentuated expression of its characteristics. Thus, when Vata dosha is imbalanced, anxiety, worry, restlessness, weight loss, intolerance of cold, constipation, and rough, dry, dark skin are likely to emerge. Complications of long-standing imbalance of Vata include arthritis, hypertension, and mental illness. When Pitta dosha accumulates, a person may easily become irritated or angry. One may suffer from excess body heat and odor, or may have excessive hunger or heartburn. Long-standing imbalance of Pitta may give rise to ulcers, skin diseases or to inflammatory diseases. When Kapha dosha gets imbalanced, dullness, fatigue, excessive sleep, coldness, fluid retention, and weight gain are likely to occur. The complexion may become very pale and the digestion may become uncomfortably slow. Imbalance of Kapha dosha contributes to problems such as obesity, asthma, sinusitis, and backache. Long-standing imbalance of Kapha dosha may cause herniated intervertebral discs or depression.

TABLE 1. Qualities of the Three Doshas and Their Expression in Human Psychology

Doshas	Qualities of the Doshas	Physical Characteristics	Mental Characteristics
VATA Governs movement in all psychophysiologic process: heart beat, elimination, breathing, circulation, even thinking and activity of the nervous system.	Moving Quick Light Cold Dry Rough Minute Changing Leads Other Doshas	Slight Build Dry Skin Dark Complexion Small, Deep-Set or Protruding Eyes Very Large or Small or Crooked Teeth Joints Crack, May Be Unsteady, Loose, or Rigid Kinky, Dry Hair Oval, Plain Face	Creative Exhilarated Easily Excited Easily Frightened Talkative Good Short-Term Memory Sleeps About 6 Hours Dreams May Be Active, Fearful, With Trees or Mountains
PITTA Governs heat, energy, and metabolic functions. Responsible for turning food into healthy tissue and energy for bodily function.	Hot Sharp Acidic Light Fluid Slightly Oily Sour-Smelling	Medium Build Soft, Slightly Oily Skin Fair, Reddish Complexion Yellow, Moderate-Sized Teeth Flabby, Loose Joints Thin, Silky, Red or Blonde Hair Premature Graying or Balding Chiseled Face	Sharp, Penetrating Intellect Moderately Excitable Somewhat Easily Frightened Sleeps About 7 Hours Dreams May Be Angry & Violent with Lightning or Sun
KAPHA Responsible for strength, stamina, and natural resistance of structural elements of the body.	Heavy Oily Slow Cold Steady Sweet Sticky Soft Smooth Dull	Heavy Build Large Bones Soft, Smooth, Oily Skin Clear, White Complexion Large, Soft, Gentle Eyes Strong, White Teeth Strong, Firm Joints Thick, Wavy, Oily Hair Pleasant Face	Stable Personality Not Easily Frightened Good Long-Term Memory Sleeps 8-10 Hours Dreams of Water, Birds, Clouds, Romance

Physiologic Functioning	Qualities of Balanced Dosha	Qualities of Imbalanced Dosha
Quick Moving	Exhilaration	Anxiety, Worry
Speaks Rapidly	Clear, Alert, Creative Mind	Restlessness
Irregular Hunger	Sound Sleep	Weight Loss
Variable Strength of Digestion	Vitality, Perfect Health	Intolerance of Cold
Irregular Elimination of Stool	Strong Immunity	Rough, Dark Skin
Light, Fast Gait	Normal Bowel & Urinary Function	Constipation
		Arthritis, Hypertension
Sharp Hunger	Balanced, Brilliant Intellect	Irritability, Easy to Anger
Strong Digestion	Contentment	Excess Body Heat, Excess Perspiration
Frequent Bowel Movements, Stool Often Loose	Balanced Heat & Thirst	Intolerance of Heat
Stable, Purposeful Gait	Lustrous Complexion	Skin Diseases
Penetrating Gaze	Perfect Digestion	Excessive Hunger
	Compactness of Body	Heartburn, Ulcers, Inflammations
Moves & Speaks Slowly	Dignified, Courageous, Affectionate, Forgiving	Dullness, Depression
Low Hunger	Stable Personality, Not Easily Upset	Excessive Tiredness & Sleep
Slow Digestion	Strong, Properly Proportioned Body	Coldness
Regular Bowel Habit, Formed Stool	Stable, Strong Joints	Weight Gain, Fluid Retention
Slow, Ponderous Gait	Creamy Complexion	Pale Complexion
	Great Physical Strength	Slow Digestion
		Asthma, Backache

Systems of psychophysiological constitutional typing have been conceived in modern psychology and medicine. William Sheldon proposed a relationship between body habitus and temperament (Bischof, 1964). He suggested that thin, light, wiry persons, whom he called "ectomorphs," tended to have excitable, nervous personalities, which he called "cerebrotone." Large, heavily-built persons, called "endomorphs," tended to have stable personalities or "viscerotone," while persons of medium build, "mesomorphs," tended to be more assertive and goal-directed, termed "somatotone." These three categories correspond roughly to Vata, Kapha and Pitta respectively. Sheldon believed that these categories reflect primordial elements that structure the psychophysiology of all persons, combining in various ways to create the variety of personality and body habitus we observe, in a manner comparable to Maharishi Ayur-Veda. This system of psychophysiological classification was an impressive achievement for Sheldon because he lacked the independent means of assessment of the constitution and imbalance available in Ayur-Veda.

Association of personality type, behavior and disease has led to a somewhat useful categorization of "Type A" and "Type B" personalities (Schneider, 1991). Type A's are excessively achievement-oriented, aggressive, competitive, rigid, and impatient. They tend to be overly involved in their vocation. They work under a pressure of time, feeling great urgency and need to succeed. They are very reactive to environmental stimuli, in contrast to Type B persons (Harbin, 1989). Compared to Type A's, Type B's are more complacent, steady and much less prone to premature heart attacks than Type A's. Type A personality has been associated with heart attacks in middle-aged, white-collar males.

We can recognize the characteristics of Type A personality in the system of Maharishi Ayur-Veda as the qualities of Vata and Pitta dosha somewhat out of balance. Vata and Pitta are the most common doshas in our society, so it is not surprising that Type A personality occurs so often. A Type A person displays the vitality and enthusiasm of balanced Vata combined with a degree of worry, uncertainty, and restlessness resulting from imbalanced Vata, plus the characteristics of strong motivation and penetrating intellect typical of balanced Pitta with an aggressive, demanding, and irritable nature typical of imbalanced Pitta. Type B personality is typical of a person in whom Kapha dosha predominates.

It should be understood that any combination of doshas, balanced and imbalanced, may constitute the psychophysiology and contribute to the observed features. Thus, the innumerable variety of features observed in people can be explained by the tri-dosha theory of constitutional typing. By relating observed features to underlying, governing elements, Maharishi Ayur-Veda extends the ability of a health care provider to comprehend a client. Since imbalances in the doshas underlie and give rise to all diseases and all syndromes, diagnosing and treating in terms of the doshas allows truly comprehensive health care.

HOW THE DOSHAS BECOME IMBALANCED

Through study of the laws of nature, we gain understanding of the universe. This is the purpose of science. It is the fundamental principle of science that the universe functions in an orderly and systematic manner according to specific laws of nature. Indeed, if natural law did not govern the functioning of the universe, there would be no organization or evolution in creation, and there would be no science.

In the Ayur-Vedic understanding, the doshas, the basic organizing elements of life, gain expression through natural law. When life is lived in accord with natural law, the doshas are properly expressed and the individual enjoys good health. Imbalance in the doshas arises from violations of natural law. Poor eating habits, toxins, trauma, physical strain, overwork, insufficient sleep, pressures to meet deadlines or to excel–any such violations of natural law produce changes in the psychophysiology that result in imbalance in the doshas. Eventually, imbalance of the doshas weakens the homeostatic, immune and repair mechanisms and disease results. For simplicity, the term "imbalance" is used to describe any unhealthy state of the doshas.

In understanding how the doshas become imbalanced, Maharishi Ayur-Veda provides an interesting description of the pathogenesis of disease. The process of becoming diseased occurs in stages as the doshas become imbalanced. A dosha is said first to accumulate and then to become aggravated (imbalanced). This can happen in one or more doshas at the same time. An aggravated dosha then disseminates, moving through the body until it localizes in an organ or tissue. Localization of a dosha out of its natural place in the body initially causes minor symptoms or discomfort. At this stage, a patient may experience congestion, swollen glands, headaches, abdominal distress, nervousness, irritability, insomnia, etc. Feeling that something is wrong, a person may seek medical advice. But a physician may find nothing wrong, or only minor abnormalities may appear on physical examination or in laboratory testing. Eventually, when imbalanced doshas localize in sufficient quantity to significantly disrupt functioning of an affected tissue or organ, a recognizable disease manifests, the person becomes ill. Often the illness serves as a means for the body to dispose of the accumulated dosha. However, if the physiology cannot overcome the imbalance, the disruption produces a chronic problem such as arthritis, multiple sclerosis, or cirrhosis.

This knowledge of pathogenesis would be useless if it were not possible to detect imbalance in the doshas before disease arises, at a stage when the doshas are becoming aggravated, disseminated, or localized. By providing simple and effective means to identify and treat imbalances at these early stages, Maharishi Ayur-Veda confers the ability to practice truly preventive health care.

As we become increasingly familiar with the tri-dosha theory of constitutional typing in Maharishi Ayur-Veda, we recognize the expression of the doshas more easily. For example, we may identify individuals who are primarily Pitta in nature by their medium build, sharp intellect, and powerful personality, but who have imbalanced Vata manifesting as anxiety or insomnia. Or we may recognize a Pitta who has imbalanced Kapha creating symptoms of congestion or lassitude. All possible combinations can exist.

THE PRINCIPLE OF SIMILAR AND OPPOSITE

Treatment in Maharishi Ayur-Veda is based on the principle that the doshas are increased by contact with what is similar in quality and decreased by what is dissimilar. For example, the sun, being hot, increases Pitta while the moon, being cool, decreases Pitta. For persons of Pitta constitution or in whom Pitta dosha is increased (imbalanced), Maharishi Ayur-Veda recommends avoiding exercise in the hot, midday sun. To reduce Pitta, people are advised to walk in the moonlight or by water because these have a cooling effect. Vatas have the opposite problem. It is recommended that persons of Vata constitution or imbalance dress warmly, keep the neck covered, and avoid strong, cold, winter winds. Wind aggravates the light quality and cold aggravates the cold quality of Vata, chilling Vatas "to the bone."

This principle of similar and opposite applies to all interactions with the environment, extending our understanding of our interconnectedness with the environment. Every interaction influences our psychophysiology through our doshic constitution in predictable ways. A good example is the influence of the different times of day on an individual. Morning is a time of awakening. The early morning hours–generally speaking, the hours between 2 and 6 AM–are the time when the physiology increases activity. This appears as an increase in REM sleep and eventual awakening. According to Maharishi Ayur-Veda, this gives evidence of an increasing influence of Vata dosha. If the normal time of awakening is before sunrise, or in general, before 6 AM, then the influence of Vata is carried into the morning's activities, enlivening the psychophysiology. If one arises after 6 AM, the mind tends to be dull and slow, owing to the expression of those essential qualities of Kapha dosha. After about 10 AM, as the day begins to heat up under the influence of the sun, Pitta dosha, which has the property of being hot, tends to increase. This may be noted as a brightness of thinking and a determination to accomplish the activities planned for the morning. Then, as the hour gets closer to noon, hunger rises. One may notice that when food is taken at approximately noon, hunger and digestion are at their strongest. Later on in the afternoon, life may become more frantic or we may run out of energy–sometimes called "hypoglycemic" symptoms. These result from an influence of Vata dosha. Thus, we find an influence of Vata in both the very early morning hours and the afternoon. In the evening, between 6 and 10 PM, we find the influence of Kapha dosha apparent as we tire, move more slowly, and are inclined to rest. Indeed, according to the principles of Maharishi Ayur-Veda, going to bed before 10 PM is ideal because we gain the influence of Kapha dosha and more readily fall asleep. After 10 PM in the evening, we may find that we become more alert, are ready to do more work, and get increasingly hungry. These are signs of the influence of Pitta dosha. Thus, we observe that each dosha predominates twice in the diurnal cycle: Vata from 2 to 6 AM and PM, Kapha from 6 to 10 AM and PM and Pitta from 10 to 2 AM and PM. These times are approximate, and will vary somewhat with season and latitude.

The seasons of the year also influence our psychophysiology through our doshic constitution according to the principle of similar and opposite. The winter months tend to be very cold and dry. Having these qualities of Vata dosha, winter tends to increase and aggravate Vata dosha. The summer months, being rather hot, a quality of Pitta dosha, tend to increase Pitta. The rainy months of the year that typically occur in the spring in the United States, by virtue of being cool and damp, tend to increase Kapha dosha. We may even notice the influence of weather on our thinking and physiological functioning on a day-to-day basis. On cold damp days, we feel duller, slower, and inclined to inactivity. On warmer days, we feel energetic. On very hot days, we are inclined to go swimming, or for a walk in a shady park, or at least to stay in air conditioning. We do this automatically so as not to aggravate Pitta dosha. Being out on a cold, windy day may feel fine if Pitta dosha predominates in our constitution, but may chill a person in whom Vata or Kapha dosha predominates. People who are imbalanced in Vata may feel cold in all but the hottest months of the year. Conversely, people whose Pitta is imbalanced may go out on cold days only lightly dressed.

Just as the times of day and seasons of the year influence us according to our doshic constitution, so too the food that we eat affects us. Indeed, food produces an even greater influence on the balance of the doshas because it is out of food that the tissues are formed and the physiology is maintained. Therefore, Maharishi Ayur-Veda places a great deal of emphasis on our diet and on the quality of the digestive and metabolic processes. Certain foods, especially fresh produce, are regarded as particularly valuable in creating health. The foods that produce good health, called *sattvic* foods, include the dairy products milk, ghee (clarified butter), butter, whipped cream, and yogurt. Fresh fruits and freshly squeezed grape juice are regarded as especially nutritious. Maharishi Ayur-Veda recommends eating fresh vegetables cooked to the point of just being tender. Blanched almonds, sesame seeds, dates, figs, raisins and cold-processed honey are also included in the list of *sattvic* foods.

Other foods are regarded as especially unwholesome or as having particularly deleterious effects on the psychophysiology. These *tamasic* foods include anything that is fermented or not fresh. Thus, leftovers, aged cheese, mushrooms, vinegar, soy sauce, canned foods and bottled fruit juices are omitted from the diet as much as possible. Carbonated beverages are avoided because they increase Vata. Ice-cold beverages, including iced water, also are regarded unfavorably because they decrease the power of digestion. Maharishi Ayur-Veda recommends sipping warm water with a meal instead of iced water. Chocolate, artificial food colorings, preservatives, and pesticides should be avoided if possible because they place a burden on the body's ability to neutralize and remove harmful substances. Alcohol and other recreational chemicals are particularly harmful because they upset homeostasis and because they place an enormous strain on the mind. Intoxicants greatly aggravate Pitta and Vata doshas and produce stresses that result in poorer intellectual, emotional and, eventually, physical functioning.

The strength of digestion is also very important in Maharishi Ayur-Veda. When the digestive and metabolic processes are weak, then even good food cannot be turned into healthy tissue. Maharishi Ayur-Veda provides a number of procedures for balancing the strength of digestion. Obesity is the result of weakness in the digestive system, usually involving imbalance of all three doshas. The approach to obesity (addiction to food in some cases) in Maharishi Ayur-Veda stands in marked contrast to the approach in medicine where physicians often prescribe medicine to suppress appetite. From the point of view of Maharishi Ayur-Veda, appetite is a natural expression of physiological function, so suppression of appetite only further imbalances the psychophysiology. In the practice of Maharishi Ayur-Veda, obesity is treated by balancing the appetite and digestive strength and by increasing awareness of the messages the body is trying to send that can guide the selection of food. This approach allows people to experience satisfaction in eating instead of suffering through restrictive diets.

In assessing their influence on the doshas, foods are classified by their taste. Taste is an indication of the essential qualities contained in the food, qualities that interact with the qualities of the doshas. By selecting a specific balance of tastes, we can balance each of the doshas. According to Maharishi Ayur-Veda, there are six basic food tastes. In principle, one should include all six tastes in one's daily diet. Indeed, it is best to include all six tastes at every meal, although this is not always practical in an American diet. When we think of balancing the doshas through the selection of tastes, the principle of similar and opposite applies. In selecting foods to balance the doshas, we respect both the essential constitution of the individual and the imbalances that are present. One should include all six tastes, but shift the balance according to the doshas that need to be balanced. Thus, to balance Vata dosha, we shift the diet in the direction of the sweet, sour, and salty tastes. These tastes are very commonly present in the American diet, probably because most Americans have imbalance in Vata dosha and naturally select these foods in an attempt to balance Vata. To balance Pitta dosha, we include some sweet and starchy foods, plus a somewhat larger portion of leafy greens and beans. When balancing Pitta dosha, particular attention is paid to avoiding those foods that strongly increase Pitta. These include tomatoes and tomato products, vinegar, sour fruits, yogurt, cheese, hot peppers, and excess salt. To balance Kapha dosha, more spice, leafy greens, and beans should be included in the diet. In balancing Kapha dosha, care is taken to avoid heavy, sweet foods such as candy and ice cream and greasy foods such as French fries.

The manner in which food is eaten is also important. Food should be taken according to hunger, but one should avoid overeating. Maharishi Ayur-Veda recommends eating to only three-fourths the capacity of the stomach, leaving one-fourth of the stomach empty for churning the food. It is best to take foods at regular meal times. Making lunch the main meal of the day is an old tradition, and a wise one, since noon is the time of day when the digestive power is strongest. Eating a smaller meal in the evening is a valuable technique for people who have difficulty falling asleep. It is particularly important to eat sitting down, in a settled environment, without thinking about business or any worrisome matter. This allows one's attention to guide the selection and eating of food so one is less likely to gulp down an imbalanced meal or to overeat. Just following these simple suggestions can significantly improve one's digestion and help control weight. But the real value of these principles is that they allow nature's intelligence to guide eating. Thus, following them preserves balance in the doshas.

INFLUENCE OF THE DOSHAS ON PERSONAL RELATIONSHIPS

This review of the various interactions between the individual and the environment would be incomplete without consideration of personal relationships. The doshic makeup of individuals greatly affects relationships. Vatas, who tend to be inherently disorganized, may be very attracted to Pittas, who tend to be very precise and orderly. Pittas, who by their nature tend to be self-controlled, may be attracted to Vatas, whom they find more spontaneous and outgoing. In psychology, this is seen as balancing each other's traits. Kaphas, who tend to be slow moving and not easily excited, may be attracted to Pittas, who have lots of energy, or to Vatas who have lots of enthusiasm. Vatas, likewise, may find Kaphas attractive because they are very stable and calm by nature, serving in that way as a good counterpoint to a Vata's excitable nature.

When the doshas are out of balance, the psychophysiology functions abnormally and problems in relationships are likely to arise. For example, an imbalanced Vata living with an imbalanced Pitta can produce quite a contentious and unstable family situation. An imbalanced Pitta husband may find his Vata-imbalanced wife to be disorderly, unkempt, irrational, flighty, and excessively emotional. The wife in this situation may find her husband to be excessively demanding, controlling, easily frustrated, "distant," and angry. As another example, an imbalanced Pitta living with an imbalanced Kapha may berate the Kapha for being slovenly, lazy (a couch potato), dull, and inattentive. The Kapha in this situation may not pay much attention to anything besides the TV and may become depressed, while the imbalanced Pitta complains and fumes.

Analyzing relationships in this way suggests that balancing the doshas may do a lot to enhance a marriage, a family, or other important relationships. Physicians and psychologists have found that the approaches of Maharishi Ayur-Veda can be used along with family counseling to bring rapid improvement in family dynamics. Using Maharishi Ayur-Veda may have a unique and unexpected advantage: it is often not necessary to confront negative behaviors and attitudes in prescribing Maharishi Ayur-Veda treatments. The therapist or physician need only indicate which doshas need attention and how to balance them. In practice, providers should avoid pointing out to people how imbalanced they are–it may cause anxiety, disappointment or unhappiness. The therapeutic program is better served by providing reassurance that unhappiness or detrimental behaviors will improve when the doshas become more balanced and life is lived more in accord with natural law.

USING MAHARISHI AYUR-VEDA IN TREATING DRUG DEPENDENCY

In a typical case of drug dependency or chronic drug abuse, stresses in childhood initially imbalance and continue to imbalance the doshas. Then the drugs and the associated lifestyle further upset the mind-body and continue to imbalance the doshas. Since mental symptoms often predominate initially, we would expect that Vata is the first dosha to become imbalanced. Imbalance of Pitta dosha follows, reflecting emotional trauma and the influence of alcohol or other drugs, which greatly aggravate Pitta and Vata. In a typical situation where drugs are being abused, there is a great deal of anxiety and restlessness– typical of imbalanced Vata–plus hostility, impatience, and aggression–typical of imbalanced Pitta. Imbalance of these two doshas over many years can lead to physical disease. Diagnosis of imbalances is readily accomplished, and includes assessment of physical, psychological and physiological traits such as appetite, digestion, sleep and elimination as illustrated in the example at the beginning of this paper.

Treatment of drug dependency begins with assessment of the doshic constitution and diagnosis of imbalances. The doshas are explained to the client, making it clear that these elements govern all aspects of thinking, behavior and physiological functioning. Then recommendations are made for some simple changes in diet and daily routine. The Transcendental Meditation program (Wallace, R. K., 1970, 1986; Maharishi Mahesh Yogi, 1969) is recommended to reduce stress (Dillbeck & Orme-Johnson, 1987), create balance (Dillbeck & Bronson, 1981), improve mental health (Alexander, Rainforth & Gelderloos, 1991) and physical health (Orme-Johnson, 1987), and to increase receptivity and creativity (Travis, 1979), which foster appropriate changes in social behavior (Alexander et al., 1993) and substance abuse (Monahan, 1977; Gelderloos, Walton, Orme-Johnson & Alexander, 1991). A statistical meta-analysis comparing results from many studies suggests that Transcendental Meditation may be more efficacious than other meditation and relaxation techniques in reducing stress and fostering personal development (Eppley, Abrams, & Shear, 1989). By using just these simple recommendations of Maharishi Ayur-Veda, one can often bring striking improvement in substance abuse. Severe cases may require supportive services, medical care, or even detoxification in a hospital may be necessary, but education in Maharishi Ayur-Veda can be started as soon as the client is sober and continued through various levels of inpatient and outpatient treatment. A case history will illustrate the Maharishi Ayur-Veda approach to helping a person who abuses alcohol.

A man I will call "Bob" came to see me one summer day in 1991. He was in his late thirties but looked older. Bob was a laborer from the mid-west but lacked the stability typical of such people. He was very irritated at having had to wait for a few minutes to see me and told me so when I entered the room. He made sure that I understood that his life was not going well. Using some rather graphic, profane language, he complained of insomnia, difficulty with relationships, and restlessness. He cited family problems, work stresses, and smoking as causes but he would not admit that drinking was a contributing factor. However, his complexion and manner suggested that alcohol was involved. After carrying on for some time, he finally burst out angrily with his real concern and the reason for his visit. It seemed that he was suffering from a very uncomfortable rash. He then showed me what amounted to a truly severe case of tinea cruris.

Our understanding of the doshas allows analysis of his problems. From the point of view of Maharishi Ayur-Veda, the "real" source of his troubles was severe imbalance of Pitta and Vata doshas. The rash, uncontrolled temper and open hostility demonstrated the preeminent need for balancing Pitta dosha. I explained to Bob, who had some familiarity with Maharishi Ayur-Veda, that his rash, his chief concern, was the result of an imbalance in Pitta and that he needed to balance Pitta dosha in order for the rash to heal permanently. I recommended that he follow a strict, Pitta-pacifying diet, avoid summer heat, and abstain from alcohol as much as possible. He was educated about how Pitta dosha can be balanced without emphasizing the behaviors that produced the imbalances or even drawing attention to his anger and hostility. It was not necessary to focus on the role alcohol played in imbalancing Pitta. It was only necessary to point out that it aggravates Pitta and allow him to confirm this for himself. Written instructions were provided for a "cleansing" procedure, and for dietary and other recommendations. An herbal preparation to balance Pitta to be taken by mouth was ordered adjunctively, but I also prescribed a medicated cream to quiet the inflammation acutely. It was suggested that he return in a month for assessment of his progress.

Bob, however, was so hostile and agitated that he could hardly listen. He left the office as angry as when he had arrived. Things did not go well in the next few days. He called the Maharishi Ayur-Veda clinic several times, complaining that the rash was worse and that the itching was keeping him from sleeping. He was very abusive of the nursing staff and used a lot of vulgar language. He also indicated that he was not complying with the recommendations he had received. He was given reassurance at each phone call that improvement would come if he would follow the recommendations. After several days, he stopped calling. He did not keep the follow-up appointment. The staff was relieved by the lack of contact.

At his second visit about six months later, he was calmer and more polite. He had a new problem that concerned him greatly. He complained of having dry hands, caused, he said, by handling plaster board. Indeed, the skin of the hands was very thick, dry, and cracking. The tinea cruris rash, however, was much improved. I pointed out to him that he had made a lot of progress and I asked him how it happened. He said that the medicine I prescribed had not made much difference. Finally, he was so angry and so desperate that he followed the recommendations for balancing Pitta–but not as prescribed. He had taken two or three times the recommended doses for the cleansing procedure. The result, however, was that the rash immediately improved. After that, he was much more compliant with his program. He indicated, in passing, that he was drinking less than before, but I did not pursue this point. I only reminded him that the whole program, including the avoidance of Pitta-aggravating foods and alcohol, was designed to reduce the imbalance of Pitta dosha. It was not necessary to chastise him for his initial non-compliance. His experience had shown him what was useful and what was damaging, and his self-esteem was enhanced by his taking responsibility for his well-being. He did not need my praise to reinforce his good conduct–his improved health and increased happiness provided all the reinforcement he needed.

Analyzing the situation at the second visit, we find evidence in the reduction of the rash and of his anger that the imbalance of Pitta was much improved. The very dry hands and excessive worrying indicate significant imbalance of Vata dosha. So, at this visit, during the winter (Vata) season, the focus of treatment was shifted to balancing Vata. Dietary recommendations for balancing Vata included instructions to eat more ghee (clarified butter) and olive oil, to eat a heavier diet, and to favor hot dishes such as soups and freshly cooked vegetables. He was told to continue avoiding Pitta-aggravating foods to help maintain balance in Pitta dosha. He was instructed to massage every morning with sesame oil using a specific massage technique called abhyanga (*Charaka Samhita*, 1981). Daily oil massage pacifies Vata dosha especially, and applying the oil with his hands would soften and lubricate them, relieving the cracking.

Bob's departure from the clinic was much quieter this time. We did not see him again for another six months. At his third and last visit, he was a much calmer and happier person. His hands and his rash had healed. He explained that he had been working regularly, getting along well with his family and co-workers, and he was sleeping soundly. The hostility and abusiveness were gone. Bob recognized clearly the progress he had made and truly appreciated the role that the Maharishi Ayur-Veda program had played in his improvement. It appeared that this will motivate him to stay on his program. Only minor adjustments in his program were necessary at this last visit. I've seen him only once since–we passed on a street. He smiled and waved.

Bob's case, though somewhat dramatic, was relatively mild in terms of alcohol abuse. He reduced his alcohol consumption spontaneously as balance increased in the doshas. Most clients will require more frequent contact for education and for reinforcement of the Maharishi Ayur-Veda program. Some clients will need social work, counseling, and/or medical services during treatment to succeed in their rehabilitation.

This case history also illustrates one of the most striking insights gained in practicing Maharishi Ayur-Veda: as a natural consequence of restoring balance to the doshas, we find that not only is the physical body healthier but also mental health improves (Schneider et al., 1990). Just by balancing the doshas, we can produce significant improvements in mental health and behavior, while avoiding confrontations with the psychological defenses of clients. In practice, we just identify whatever imbalances exist in the doshas and prescribe accordingly. In this way, the system of Maharishi Ayur-Veda is both simple and profound.

GROWING HEALTHIER

When clients first hear that overcoming problems in life, including problems of substance abuse, can be easily accomplished through natural and simple procedures that enliven the intelligence of nature present everywhere, they usually experience a sudden rise of hope. This is the first step in the healing process. Then, as they become familiar with the principles of Maharishi Ayur-Veda and feel themselves becoming healthier, they experience a sense of self-reliance that provides strong motivation to continue. Still, after some time, doubts may arise or the person may experience that some initial progress seems to give way to old habits. At these times, it is necessary to give some reinforcement of the understanding from Maharishi Ayur-Veda of the fundamental role of nature's intelligence in our day-to-day lives. When a client experiences suffering, weakness, and giving in to temptation, it is all too easy to forget that nature's intelligence guides life. At such times, when the client feels that progress is not being made or is even lost, the provider must help the client identify signs of progress made in achieving health before the "rough" period. The client must be reassured that growth is occurring and will continue despite a brief period of less healthy behavior. At these times, the client may require some special procedures to calm the mind and strengthen the body in order to feel "in control" again. These procedures, currently available only at Maharishi Ayur-Veda Health Centers, include a specific massage technique using herbalized oil and a technique of rhythmically pouring warm oil over the forehead. This latter technique, called shirodara, has an immediate, and often profound calming effect that has benefited many patients with severe agitation, anxiety, or even mild degrees of mania. Many other therapeutic modalities can be prescribed by physicians and psychologists trained in Maharishi Ayur-Veda as the client's situation requires. Some of these techniques use the senses for balancing the doshas. These include the use of aromatic oils, recordings of the primordial sounds of nature's intelligence found in the Vedic literature, and of Gandharva Veda music, specific music from the Vedic tradition that represents and enlivens the expression of natural law in creation. and balance in mind and body. Any of these techniques may be recommended in individual cases according to the need and receptivity of the client.

HEALTH: A MEANINGFUL DEFINITION

What *is* health? Dorland's Illustrated Medical Dictionary (1965) defines health as: "A state of complete physical, mental, and social well-being, and not merely the absence of disease and infirmity." This would be a useful definition if "well-being" could be defined explicitly. Unfortunately, well-being is subjective; it is reportable but not measurable. Some would assert that health–the complete absence of disease–is "a state that would be biologically unreal" (McDermott, 1981), leaving modern medicine with "the absence of disease" as a working definition of health and "preservation of function" as its goal.

Maharishi Ayur-Veda, on the other hand, defines well-being in explicit terms and provides the means for measuring health by determining the unique psychophysiological constitution of an individual and the degree to which it is balanced or imbalanced. How does Maharishi Ayur-Veda define health? The ancient literature of Maharishi Ayur-Veda gives a concise definition of health. It is translated here into familiar language:

> He whose doshas are in balance, whose appetite is good, whose bodily tissues are functioning normally, whose excretory functions are balanced, and whose Self, mind and senses remain full of bliss, he is called a healthy person. (*Sushruta Sutrasthanam*, 15, 38)

This definition points to the components of a healthy psychophysiology; it defines well-being. Well-being is subjective, but has features recognizable by others. According to Maharishi Ayur-Veda (*Charaka Samhita,* 1981), vitality, youthfulness, and happiness are the hallmarks of perfect health. A truly healthy person experiences joy in all things and displays physical strength, a lustrous (glowing) complexion, and stability of mind. The body is compact, neither too hard nor too soft. Movements are graceful. The facial expression is serene and pleasant. The personality is composed, spontaneous, gracious, and charming. A truly healthy person appears to function without strain, without feeling pressure of time, accepting changes in life without upheaval, accomplishing goals without apparent effort. And, of course, a truly healthy person never suffers illness.

This, then, is the goal of Maharishi Ayur-Veda: perfect health and happiness. It is understood to mean that life is lived in accord with natural law. The expression "life in accord with natural law" describes a natural state of life free from disruption by imbalanced doshas, without stress and strain, without suffering and without disease. When life is lived in accord with natural law, daily activities proceed effortlessly and spontaneously, and happiness pervades every experience.

TRAINING TO PRACTICE MAHARISHI AYUR-VEDA

Currently, licensed physicians, nurses, psychologists and social workers can receive two weeks of training in Maharishi Ayur-Veda through courses sponsored by the Maharishi Ayur-Veda Medical Association. This training qualifies health care providers to perform psychophysiological constitutional assessment, diagnose imbalances, and to prescribe many of the therapies of Maharishi Ayur-Veda. Advanced training and continuing education are available periodically. Longer courses for training to higher levels of proficiency are expected to become available soon. For more information on these programs, contact the Office of the National Medical Directors, P.O. Box 282, Fairfield, IA 52556.

CONCLUSION

The introduction of Maharishi Ayur-Veda into clinical practice offers new possibilities for health professionals to help their clients live healthier and happier lives. Introduction involves special challenges as professionals and clients must learn new knowledge about creating better health. Health professionals need to practice the diagnostic and therapeutic approaches of Maharishi Ayur-Veda themselves in order to gain familiarity with the specific techniques, with the process of becoming healthier and with the conceptual framework (paradigm) of Maharishi Ayur-Veda. Adequate time must be allocated for this education and experience.

Practicing Maharishi Ayur-Veda involves a number of transformations on the part of practitioners and clients. First, one comes to understand that health is not an all-or-none phenomenon but rather exists as a continuum from moribund to perfectly healthy. Second, a change in attitude occurs as creating health becomes a part of everyday life. Becoming healthier is experienced as increasing vitality, youthfulness, creativity, happiness, tolerance, resistance to stress, and freedom from disease. Third, attention shifts from problems to solutions. Problems such as drug dependency are not solved on their own level in Maharishi Ayur-Veda. Instead, attention is put on creating balance, on growing healthier. This change in orientation is based on a shift of paradigms: problem-oriented modern medical science that treats diseases as entities is exchanged for solution-oriented Maharishi Ayur-Veda that appreciates the psychophysiological uniqueness of individuals. In practice, Maharishi Ayur-Veda examines host factors responsible for creating and maintaining health. It utilizes physical, behavioral, and mental techniques to strengthen and balance the individual person. These techniques are prescribed according to the unique needs of the individual. Clients practice these techniques on their own. Creating better health and happiness outside the clinic setting fosters independence and self-confidence. A case history illustrated both the approach to the client and the method of analysis within Maharishi Ayur-Veda. A definition of health and a description of a truly healthy person according to the principles of Maharishi Ayur-Veda was offered in conclusion.

REFERENCES

Abrams, A. I. & Siegel, L. M. (1978) The Transcendental Meditation program and rehabilitation at Folsom state prison: A cross-validation study. *Criminal Justice and Behavior*, *5*, 3-20.

Alexander, C. N., Swanson, G. C., Rainforth, M. V., Carlisle, T. W. & Todd, C. C., & Oates, R. (1993). A prospective study on the Transcendental Meditation program in two occupational setting: Effects on stress-reduction, health and employee development. *Anxiety, Stress and Coping: An International Journal*, *6*, 245-262.

Alexander, C. N., Rainforth, M. V. & Gelderloos, P. (1991). Transcendental Meditation, self-actualization, and psychological health: A conceptual overview and statistical meta-analysis. *Journal of Social Behavior and Personality*, *6*, 189-247.

Bischof, L. J. (1964). *Interpreting personality theories*. New York: Harper & Row.

Brooks, J. S. & Scarano, T. (1985). Transcendental Meditation in the treatment of post-Vietnam adjustment., *65*, 212-215.

Charaka Samhita (1981). Translated and edited by Dr. Ram Karan Sharma. Varanasi (India): Chowkhamba Sanskrit Office Series Office.

Dillbeck, M. C. & Orme-Johnson, D.W. (1987). Physiological differences between Transcendental Meditation and rest. *American Psychologist*, *42*, 879-881.

Dillbeck, M. C. & Bronson, E. C. (1981). Short-Term longitudinal effects of the Transcendental Meditation technique on EEG power and coherence. *International Journal of Neuroscience*, *14*, 147-151.

Dorland's Illustrated Medical Dictionary (24th Edition). (1965). Philadelphia: W. B. Saunders Company.

Eppley, K., Abrams, A. I. & Shear, J. (1989). The differential effects of relaxation techniques on trait anxiety: A meta-analysis. *Journal of Clinical Psychology*, *45*, 957-974.

Gelderloos, P., Walton, K. G., Orme-Johnson, D. W. & Alexander, C. N. (1991). Effectiveness of the Transcendental Meditation program in preventing and treating substance misuse: A review. *The International Journal of Addictions*, *26*, 293-325.

Haratani, T. & Hemmi, T. (1990a). Effects of Transcendental Meditation on mental health of industrial workers. *Japanese Journal of Industrial Health, 32*, 656.

Haratani, T. & Hemmi, T. (1990b). Effects of Transcendental Meditation on health behavior of industrial workers. *Japanese Journal of Public Health, 37*, 729.

Harbin, T. J. (1989). The relationship between Type A behavior pattern and physiological responsivity: a quantitative review. *Psychophysiology, 26*, 110-119.

Janssen, G. W. (1989). The application of Maharishi Ayur-Veda in the treatment of ten chronic diseases: A pilot study. *Nederlands Tijdschrift Voor Integrale Geneeskund, 5*, 586-594.

Maharishi Mahesh Yogi. (1969). *On the Bhagavad-Gita: A translation and commentary, chapters 1-6*. Arkana: Penguin.

McDermott, W. (1981). Absence of indicators of the influence of its physicians on a society's health. *The American Journal of Medicine, 70*, 833-843.

McDowell, I., & Newell, C. (1987). *Measuring health: A guide to rating scales and questionnaires*. New York and Oxford: Oxford University Press.

Monahan, R. J. (1977). Secondary prevention of drug dependence through the Transcendental Meditation program in metropolitan Philadelphia. *International Journal of Addictions, 12*, 729-754.

Orme-Johnson, D.W. (1987). Medical care utilization and the Transcendental Meditation program. *Psychosomatic Medicine, 49*, 493-507.

Schneider, R. H., Cavanaugh, K. L., Kasture, H. S., Rothenberg, S., Averbach, R., Robinson, D. K. & Wallace, R. K. (1990). Health promotion with a traditional system of natural health care: Maharishi Ayur-Veda. *Journal of Social Behavior and Personality, 5*, 1-27.

Schneider, R. H. (1991). Adrenergic Mechanisms in Type A Behavior. In O. Cameron (Ed.) *Adrenergic dysfunction in psychosomatic and psychiatric disorders*. Washington, DC: American Psychiatric Press.

Schneider, R. H., Alexander, C. N., & Wallace, R. K. (1992). In Search of an Optimal Behavioral Treatment for Hypertension: a Review and Focus on Transcendental Meditation. In E. H. Johnson, W. D. Gentry & S. Julius (Eds.) *Personality, elevated blood pressure, and essential hypertension* (pp. 291-316). Washington, DC: Hemisphere Publishing Corporation.

Sheldon, A. (1970). Toward a General Theory of Disease and Medical Care. In A. Sheldon, F. Baker & C. P. McLaughlin (Eds.), *Systems and medical care* (pp. 84-125). Cambridge, MA: The Massachusetts Institute of Technology.

Sushruta Samhita (1981). (Translated and edited by Kaviraj Kunjalal Bhishagratna.) Varanasi (India): Chowkhamba Sanskrit Office Series Office.

Travis, F. (1979) The TM Technique and Creativity: A Longitudinal Study of Cornell University Undergraduates. *The Journal of Creative Behavior, 13*, 169-180.

Wallace, R. K. (1986). *The Maharishi technology of the unified field: The neurophysiology of enlightenment*. Fairfield, IA: Maharishi International University Press.

Wallace, R. K. (1970). Physiological Effects of Transcendental Meditation. *Science, 167*, 1251-1254.

Clinical Applications of Maharishi Ayur-Veda in Chemical Dependency Disorders

Jay L. Glaser, MD

INTRODUCTION TO MAHARISHI AYUR-VEDA

Maharishi Ayur-Veda is the world's oldest and most comprehensive system of natural health care. It has been brought to light in recent years by Maharishi Mahesh Yogi from the classical Ayurvedic texts of ancient India. It is a complete science of health because no aspect of life falls outside its scope. Containing both subjective and objective approaches to health, it deals with consciousness, psychology, physiology, behavior, and environment. It simultaneously improves the health of the mind and body, as well as the individual and society, and views these apparently separate elements as interdependent aspects of the wholeness of life.

Maharishi Ayur-Veda focuses on refining and optimizing the individual's physiology and consciousness by using a variety of methods that promote both resistance to disease and development of the full potential of the individual. The term Ayur-Veda comes from the Sanskrit root, *ayus,* which means "life" or "life-span" and *Veda* which means "knowledge." So Ayur-Veda means the knowl-

---

Jay L. Glaser is Medical Director at the Maharishi Ayur-Veda Health Center for Behavioral Medicine and Stress Management in Lancaster, MA 01523.

[Haworth co-indexing entry note]: "Clinical Applications of Maharishi Ayur-Veda in Chemical Dependency Disorders." Glaser, Jay L. Co-published simultaneously in the *Alcoholism Treatment Quarterly* (The Haworth Press, Inc.) Vol. 11, No. 3/4, 1994, pp. 367-394; and: *Self-Recovery: Treating Addictions Using Transcendental Meditation and Maharishi Ayur-Veda* (ed: David F. O'Connell and Charles N. Alexander) The Haworth Press, Inc., 1994, pp. 367-394. Multiple copies of this article/chapter may be purchased from The Haworth Document Delivery Center [1-800-3-HAWORTH; 9:00 a.m. - 5:00 p.m. (EST)].

edge of the entire span of life. Maharishi Ayur-Veda is focused on preventing disease and promoting longevity, and includes techniques designed to reestablish and maintain equilibrium in physiological functioning.

As an effective and increasingly well-documented prevention strategy, Maharishi Ayur-Veda significantly reduces the need for remedial health procedures, while including procedures for treatment and cure of a number of specific diseases, including chronic diseases and psychosomatic disorders which are refractory to conventional therapy. The six ancient encyclopedic textbooks contain chapters on obstetrics, pediatrics, surgery, toxicology, internal medicine, pharmacognosy (knowledge of the use of medicinal plants), psychiatry and other disciplines describing hundreds of different disorders and their management. Substance abuse is dealt with extensively in these ancient texts and is obviously not only a modern phenomenon.

Over time, much of the ancient medical wisdom of Ayur-Veda had become fragmented or lost. In recent years, however, Maharishi, in conjunction with a panel of the distinguished Ayurvedic scholars of India, has promoted a restoration of Ayur-Veda to its full integrity. The most eminent Ayurvedic physicians, or *vaidyas,* who have worked with Maharishi to restore Ayur-Veda to its original purity and completeness, include Dr. V. M. Dwivedi, Dr. B. D. Triguna, Chairman of the National Academy of Ayur-Veda, India, and Dr. Balraj Maharshi, advisor on Ayur-Veda to the government of Andhra Pradesh, India.

Most fundamentally, Maharishi (1986) has reestablished the wholeness of Ayur-Veda by providing an understanding of the foundational role of development of consciousness in promoting an optimal state of health, and by restoring the technologies through which consciousness can be fully unfolded. This bringing to light of Ayur-Veda in the contemporary age is named Maharishi Ayur-Veda in honor of Maharishi's restoration of the complete, authentic value of this ancient comprehensive system of natural medicine.

Peer-reviewed medical journals devoted to Ayurvedic medicine have published thousands of scientific articles documenting Ayurvedic treatment strategies and properties of Ayurvedic herbs. This research effort has been dramatically accelerated in recent years by the emergence of interest in the completely systematic, scientifically verifiable approach of Maharishi Ayur-Veda by Western researchers (Glaser, 1988; Sharma, 1993; Wallace, 1993).

In this paper we present a new approach to the problem of substance abuse based upon this ancient holistic science of health. Clinical experience and laboratory research during the past twenty years indicate that Maharishi Ayur-Veda offers important principles and treatment modalities for the treatment of substance abuse that have profound practical applications in contemporary practice. It is our hope that discussion of this work will stimulate health care professionals and administrators to establish clinical programs using this system of recovery, and to scientifically document its effects.

PSYCHOPHYSIOLOGICAL BASIS OF CHEMICAL DEPENDENCY ACCORDING TO MAHARISHI AYUR-VEDA

Evolution: The Impulse of Life

In Maharishi's analysis (1963), the nature of life is to grow, or evolve, in the direction of more and more. All living beings and even inanimate creation are involved in this process of evolution. In human beings, this natural tendency to move in the direction of greater progress is expressed as behavior oriented toward the experience of more joy, more love, more prosperity. The Sanskrit word which describes the experience sought by this behavior is *ananda,* which is sometimes translated as "bliss," pure happiness or fulfillment.

Maharishi Ayur-Veda holds that a healthy individual has a balanced nervous system which naturally adopts behaviors conducive to the neurochemistry of fulfillment or bliss. Modern neurophysiology has located many chemicals that are responsible for this state. Mental health has been shown to be dependent on equilibrium of the serotonin-melatonin axis, the adrenergic and cholinergic axes, and the adrenocortical-pituitary axis. To a neurochemist, if the complex neuroendocrine systems of the body are balanced, the result is a state of well-being or fulfillment. When the nervous system is in disequilibrium, however, the resulting loss of fulfillment prompts the desire to restore an experience of greater well-being or happiness. Chemical dependency represents maladaptive behavior which may arise in a misguided effort to restore well-being.

One expression of the force of evolution in human life is the individual's desire to gain more knowledge and understanding of the structure of the cosmos and his or her role within it. According to quantum physics, the basic building blocks of the universe are the "matter fields" and "force fields"–the basic particles and forces of nature that give rise to and structure the concrete, manifest universe that we can see, touch, and feel. The source of all these diverse aspects of natural law, however, is a single, self-interacting field–an abstract, unmanifest field of pure intelligence which is described as the unified field of all the laws of nature. Thus the entire physical universe is seen as an expression of the unmanifest unified field (Hawking, 1988).

Although physicists have recently arrived at this understanding and have made progress in describing it mathematically, it is not new. The ancient Vedic tradition has always described the universe as comprising a manifest, relative, changing field of diversity, which is the expression of an unmanifest, unchanging, eternal field of unity. This underlying, universal field is described as a field of pure intelligence or pure consciousness (Maharishi Mahesh Yogi, 1963). Some physicists (Hagelin, 1987, 1989) have proposed that the unified field described by modern physics is identical to the field of pure intelligence described by Maharishi's Vedic Science and Technology. Maharishi (1963) describes how, just as the colorless, invisible sap deep within a rose creates, nourishes, and permeates all the diverse parts of the flower, the entire diverse universe emerges from the absolute, unchanging, unmanifest field of pure consciousness. Therefore, the concrete world of objects in which we live our daily lives has its foundation in, and is permeated by, this underlying unified field.

Based on this understanding, from the point of view of Maharishi Ayur-Veda, in order for an individual to enjoy a state of continuing fulfillment, he or she must not only progress on the outer, material level of diversity and activity. It is also necessary for one to experience and enliven within one's own awareness the field of pure consciousness–and thus to connect all the outer, material expressions of one's life with their source, so that they can draw complete nourishment from this field.

In this broader understanding of life, pure consciousness, the unbounded field of intelligence which constitutes the essential nature of the individual, is called the Self, and is distinguished from the self (with a small "s") which refers to the individual in terms of a localized, constrained personality and physiology (Maharishi Mahesh Yogi, 1969). "Self-realization" is understood as the gradual unfoldment of higher states of consciousness, in which an individual increasingly experiences the diverse aspects of his or her nature in terms of the unified wholeness of pure consciousness. One becomes aware that consciousness is the primary, moving force which gives rise to everything in manifest creation, including one's own physiology.

The Mistake of the Intellect: The Loss of Wholeness

Maharishi Ayur-Veda defines the root of disease and imbalance as *pragyaparadha,* a Sanskrit term which is translated as "the mistake of the intellect"–a condition common to almost the entire human population. Pragyaparadha is defined as the forgetting of the field of pure consciousness by its diversified expressions, the loss of memory of unity by the field of multiplicity. The intellect is that faculty which discriminates, and in the case of pragyaparadha, it has lost the memory of the silent, unmanifest field of pure consciousness underlying one's nature, and thus mistakenly interprets the world as consisting only of the field of differences and change. When one is caught in the mistake of the intellect, the relative, changing, manifest field of objects, constraints, problems, and deadlines dominates one's experience; diversity and change are the dominating feature of life. The nature of the Self as a blissful and silent field of consciousness is lost from the awareness.

The mistake of the intellect by itself is obviously not enough to create chemical dependency, since almost everyone is caught in its net, yet only a portion of the population ends up with addictive disorders. Pragyaparadha nevertheless creates the conditions for the problem to start. Maharishi Ayur-Veda holds that because pure consciousness is the field of pure intelligence which gives rise to manifest creation, it is the source of all the laws of nature that govern every aspect of life for the individual and the entire universe. In Maharishi Ayur-Veda, health is defined as living in accord with natural law; and this is seen as a by-product of the development of higher states of consciousness, in which all one's thinking and actions are based on and supported by the total potential of natural law in pure consciousness.

The mistake of the intellect prevents one's actions from being spontaneously guided in accord with the laws of nature, because one's daily experience is disconnected from its source in the underlying unified field. When the experience of pure consciousness is lost to the individual, this creates imbalances in the mind and body, and one begins to violate laws of nature: eating improper foods, staying up late, becoming fatigued and anxious, working too hard, playing too hard, becoming over-stimulated. These behaviors are the seeds of further imbalance. With fatigue and stress, individual well-being and effective functioning are soon compromised. One begins to experience, "I am tired," "I am not very sharp today," "I am bored," or "I am depressed." Having deviated from the path of well-being, one naturally wants to regain it. One result is the search for external activities and substances to restore inner balance and happiness.

Physicians trained in Maharishi Ayur-Veda regard all maladaptive behaviors (including addictions) as misguided attempts to restore physiological and psychological equilibrium, or balance, so that a sense of self-fulfillment and inner silence is reestablished. If the nervous system is too active, one may pacify it with a tranquilizer. If the nervous system is too inactive or lethargic, one may take a stimulant. If we are too "high" we take downers, if we are too low we take uppers, all in an attempt to regulate our psychophysiology. As another common example, if there is some lack of stimulation in life, one may try to counteract this boredom by intense sensory input, such as violent movies which provide strong stimulation, but may also result in insomnia. Maladaptive behaviors are thus a result of the *mistake of the intellect* which deprives one of the spontaneous balance in life that comes from living in accord with the laws of nature.

In this context, the obvious antidote to pragyaparadha and the consequent violation of the laws of nature is the direct experience of pure consciousness, which is provided through the approaches of Maharishi Ayur-Veda, particularly Maharishi's Transcendental Meditation technique (described below). This experience restores balance to body and mind by restoring the "memory" of the field of unity at the basis of all the diversity of life.

The Etiology of Chemical Dependency: The Perspective of Maharishi Ayur-Veda

Research studies have found in families predispositions to chemical dependency that arise from hereditary and environmental factors. Some scientists have taken the position that chemical dependency is genetically determined and therefore incurable. They cite studies showing, for example, that the allele (alternative gene form at a given locus) of the dopamine receptor gene (DRG2) is different in alcoholics than non-alcoholics. The theory of addiction as an incurable disease also fits the perspective of the popular Twelve Step programs which view recovery from addiction as the work of a lifetime.

Maharishi Ayur-Veda, on the other hand, adopts a different perspective. It assumes that all disorders are caused by both specific predispositions (one's nature, or *prakriti* in Sanskrit) as well as by other contributory factors. These factors often involve aspects of one's lifestyle, including improper diet and daily habits; they create imbalances in the mind and body which precipitate the expression of the predisposition. (Please refer to Sands, this volume, for an expanded discussion of *prakriti.*)

From the perspective of purely medical conditions, it is clear that genetic predispositions do not inevitably lead to disorders. Individuals with colon or breast cancer have been found to have strong genetic predispositions. For most of the individual's life, however, this tendency may not be manifested as a malignancy; it remains in a latent, unexpressed form which may manifest only when other factors in one's daily life or adverse environmental conditions (such as toxins or stress) precipitate its expression. In a large proportion of individuals with latent predispositions, the cancer is not expressed at all.

What, then, are those factors that may result in the expression of predispositions involved in chemical dependency? According to Maharishi Ayur-Veda, one of the most important factors causing disease of all kinds, including chemical dependency, is violation of the laws of nature governing human life and health. One form this may take is the inappropriate lifestyle choices (poor diet, etc.) mentioned above.

Maharishi Ayur-Veda thus locates the violation of specific laws of nature in both the external and internal environment of the individual as factors precipitating substance abuse. These might include one's attitudes, daily routine, upbringing, current life circumstances, and sensory exposure. To a great degree, the behaviors which abusers adopt are cultured by their environment. Children learn poor examples of coping mechanisms at home, for example when their father takes a drink to relax after work or when their mother takes a cigarette or coffee to relax and think more clearly. The behavior of taking something exogenously for small problems is likely to be adopted when the individual is confronted with more potent stressors.

According to Maharishi Ayur-Veda, those individuals who acquire a sense of self and identity by succumbing to peer pressure to smoke or use drugs are suffering from the mistake of the intellect. They see themselves as being only a small physical body in an enormous universe; they have lost the view of their larger Self. They regard themselves as insignificant and may seek drugs as a path to feelings of self-importance.

Since stressors demand a behavioral response from the individual to restore the disruption in homeostasis, physicians trained in Maharishi Ayur-Ved also regard stress as one of the most important precipitating factors for bringing out an addictive predisposition. When I ask my patients who have resumed using a substance after a significant period of sobriety what the circumstances were that led to taking that first drink, cigarette, or hit of cocaine, invariably the response is, "I was anxious," or "I was burned out because of a deadline at work," or "My mother was very sick and I had to drive an hour each way after work to see her in the hospital and got exhausted," and so on. These scenarios suggest that the nervous system becomes fatigued or overloaded, neurochemical balance begins to be disrupted, and the individual looks for the most familiar agent in an attempt to correct the disequilibrium.

In contrast, Maharishi Ayur-Veda, as a holistic system of medicine, attempts to give the individual the means to balance the psychophysiology in a natural way, through Transcendental Meditation and its other approaches and treatment modalities. According to Maharishi Ayur-Veda, self-dignity is automatic with the experience of one's inner nature as the field of pure consciousness during TM; the regular practice of TM releases stress from the physiology and eventually establishes the awareness permanently in pure consciousness, eliminating pragyaparadha and the basis of violation of natural law.

CLINICAL APPLICATION OF THE MAHARISHI AYUR-VEDA RECOVERY PROGRAM

In my own practice as an internist at the Maharishi Ayur-Veda Health Center for Behavioral Medicine and Stress Management in Lancaster, Massachusetts, I have had the opportunity to treat thousands of patients from around the world, many of whom are coming specifically to begin a Maharishi Ayur-Veda addictions recovery program. These patients are highly self-selected in the sense that they are motivated to do something about their chemical dependency; in addition, they are refractory to treatment with standard methods. Not only are they open-minded, but they are specifically interested in seeking out alternative approaches.

The treatment approach to addictions that I am setting forth represents a summary of my experience in applying principles of Maharishi Ayur-Veda to the clinical presentation of chemical dependency. While my colleagues and I have not performed careful clinical studies with each type of addiction, the encouraging results found in this population of chronic recidivists using methods that differ from standard treatment suggests that these approaches of Maharishi Ayur-Veda may be useful for many addicted populations. While the majority of my patients differ from these populations in that they are seeking alternative recovery approaches, the underlying pathologies involved in their addiction do not appear to be different from those of patients I have observed in the inner cities.

My clinical experience using Maharishi Ayur-Veda suggests that substance abusers have completely forgotten the experience of a natural state of well-being. If they can be given a taste of the experience of mental and physical balance they become more sensitive to any influence which disrupts this well-being and integration, including the deleterious effects of the abused substance. After a period of practicing Maharishi Ayur-Veda techniques they may tell me they feel better than they have in a long time. Invariably, however, the habitual desire to experiment with their substance of choice returns and they return to using. They frequently report, however, that their state of well-being provided a contrast to their previous imbalanced state and now instead of making them feel temporarily better, the substance makes them feel worse. This pattern is both a physical experience as well as an intellectual realization. If they continue their Maharishi Ayur-Veda practices, naturally and spontaneously they may begin to reduce the dosage or frequency of abuse, and eventually, over time, cease to abuse the substance.

Since the desire and willingness to change one's life so that one feels good without exogenous substances is often the primary predictor of success, the first goal of Maharishi Ayur-Veda recovery programs is the establishment of this orientation for recovery. The therapeutic strategies are focused on giving the individual a clear experience of well-being and balance and making this experience systematic and habitual. The following case illustrates this principle:

A 52-year-old single woman who had smoked 30 cigarettes per day for 34 years attended our Health Center for treatment of chronic fatigue, perimenopausal symptoms, and insomnia. Her lifestyle involved commuting 60 minutes each way to her job in New York City, eating only in restaurants, using benzodiazepines (lorazepam, etc.), and retiring late. After three days of rest, weaning from the benzodiazepines, Maharishi Ayur-Veda treatments including oil massage, twice-daily practice of the Transcendental Meditation technique, and long walks in the woods, she went outdoors to have her first cigarette, respecting our Center's no-smoking policy. She reported that the first puff of the cigarette tasted foul and induced nausea and coughing. She threw the cigarette and the rest of the pack away. She claimed that with the novel experience of balance and well-being, she had simply lost her taste for tobacco. Three weeks later she forced herself to have a cigarette despite the nausea it created after she was berated by her boss. She stated that tobacco was the only familiar coping mechanism that was available on the job. She continues to use cigarettes on occasion in stressful situations.

Several research studies have documented this pattern. Schenkluhn and Geisler (1977), then at the Max Planck Institute in Germany, observed a common pattern in illicit drug abusers who began regular practice of the Transcendental Meditation technique following a required 15-day period of abstinence before being instructed. During the first two to three weeks after instruction, some subjects violated their sobriety; by six weeks, however, they had reduced their level of consumption below their previous use. The authors hypothesized that this period represented the lag time for the experience of increasing autonomy and well-being to become established. Although the 15-day abstinence requirement is only for the use of illicit drugs, I have noted a similar pattern in users of cigarettes and alcohol.

A recent study by Royer (this volume) monitoring 110 smoking participants in Transcendental Meditation and 214 smoking non-meditators clearly showed that meditators were significantly more successful than non-meditators in quitting or decreasing smoking over a two-year period. When regularity of meditation was taken into account, the results were even more significant: 81% of individuals who meditated twice daily quit or decreased smoking compared to 33% of the non-meditating controls. Royer noted that it took several months for the smokers to quit, but there was little recidivism. These results are impressive considering that the TM technique is not a smoking cessation program and that the smokers who learned TM did not do so to stop smoking. However, these results are not surprising in light of the known effects of the TM technique on both the mind and body (see Alexander, Robinson, & Rainforth, this volume; Walton & Levitsky, this volume). The methodological rigor and large effect size of this study are encouraging not only for smoking cessation, but for the application of Maharishi Ayur-Veda to other addictive disorders.

THE EXPERIENCE OF INNER HAPPINESS AND WELL-BEING AS AN INCENTIVE TO CONTINUE THE MAHARISHI AYUR-VEDA PROGRAM

Factors responsible for the success of Maharishi Ayur-Veda treatments include (1) the high compliance rate due to the enjoyable nature of the therapeutic modalities and the immediate benefits they bring for body and mind; and (2) the resultant distraction from the abusing substance which this enjoyment and success create. The enjoyment is created by the effortlessness of the program and the inherent experience of balance and well-being generated by the treatments. Well-designed Maharishi Ayur-Veda programs are composed of simple and natural modalities that introduce substance abusers to both the concept and the experience of their own blissful inner nature.

Maharishi Ayur-Veda programs create balance and well-being using several different treatment avenues focusing on multiple levels of the client's life: sensory, emotional, intellectual, speech, motor processes, etc. As the client experiences the deeper values of his or her own awareness and develops greater psychological and physical balance, feelings of inner happiness begin to develop. The client also gains insight into the structure of his or her own consciousness as a field of intelligence that interacts with the body to create health. In my practice I have seen patients experience that within their very being is the source of every action, perception, thought and emotion, and that the nature of that source is bliss. This experience is consistent with Maharishi's explanation of the ancient Ayurvedic texts.

Balance in the physiology is essential to maintaining the experience of inner happiness and well-being. With the onset of treatment in an environment emphasizing increasing rest and good nutrition, integrating a regular daily routine, specialized herbal preparations, and the practice of the TM technique, balance begins to be restored. For the first time in years, the client may begin to notice physical balance, inner quiet, vitality, psychological well-being, and increasing clarity of mind. The Maharishi Ayur-Veda programs are predicated on the fact that this natural experience of increasing health is more attractive than the experience of substance abuse.

CLINICAL APPLICATION OF THE MAHARISHI AYUR-VEDA RECOVERY PROGRAM

One of the ancient Ayurvedic medical textbooks, *Charaka Samhita* (1981), is clear about the approach one should take in addictive disorders. The text says:

> *A wise person should give up by and by unwholesome practices to which he is addicted and he should correspondingly adopt ones which are wholesome . . . . By slowly and gradually giving up the unwholesome practices and by increasing the wholesome practices correspondingly the unwholesome practices are eradicated forever and the wholesome practices are fully adopted.* (*Charaka Samhita*, Sutrasthana 7:36-38)

In this passage, Charaka makes two important points. First, many behaviors can most effectively be discontinued in an incremental fashion. But more importantly, he emphasizes that negative behaviors must be replaced by positive, wholesome ones. It is not sufficient to simply discontinue one behavior while continuing life as usual. For permanent recovery many positive lifestyle changes are required to both rectify and prevent the recurrence of physiological disequilibrium which created the need for the negative behavior in the first place.

THE THERAPEUTIC APPROACHES

In Maharishi Ayur-Veda, the emphasis is on creating balance through simple, natural methods using principles that patients can apply on a daily basis within the context of their own lives. According to this system of health care, every individual is unique and maintains a unique physiological relationship with the fundamental physical qualities in nature (*doshas*). Maharishi Ayur-Veda diagnosis focuses on detecting the nature of the individual's inherent equilibrium (his or her psychophysiological "body type" or constitutional type) and any deviations from it (imbalances), as a first step in restoring balance (see Sands, this volume).

Most importantly, Maharishi Ayur-Veda emphasizes that physiological balance can be maintained, restored, or disrupted depending on the appropriateness of the diet, daily activity, speech, sensory stimuli and other environmental factors. Everything one "ingests" from the environment, including movies, television, music, and the influence of friends, as well as one's food, has an influence on the dynamic equilibrium of the many elements and qualities in the physiology. Health can be restored most efficiently by simultaneously utilizing many modalities to reverse existing imbalances. At least twenty therapeutic modalities of Maharishi Ayur-Veda are currently available (Sharma, 1993; Averbach & Rothenberg, 1989).

Following is a description of thirteen modalities of Maharishi Ayur-Veda which are most directly applicable to substance abuse therapy. All of these modalities can be provided either on an inpatient or outpatient basis. The nature and frequency of treatment can be tailored by the physician to the individual's specific problem area and Ayurvedic body type. In every case, clients receive instruction in simple techniques which they can continue to utilize on a self-sufficient basis at home.

1. Mental Techniques: Maharishi's Transcendental Meditation and Its Advanced Techniques

The Transcendental Meditation program is a primary approach to recovery in the Maharishi Ayur-Veda program. The individual receives a technique by which conscious awareness is allowed to settle into a state of deep stillness while remaining awake. In that deep silence, the conscious mind locates and experiences the field of pure consciousness, the unified field of all the laws of nature, and begins to become attuned with the laws of nature governing health and wholeness. The body also experiences a deep state of rest as a result of the profound settling of the mind. The many immediate benefits of this technique include increased mental clarity and reduction and prevention of stress, enabling the individual to better cope with pressures at home and the stress of detoxification and abstinence. The long-term results include improved psychophysiological functioning, disease prevention, reversal of the detrimental effects of aging, and development of higher states of consciousness (Alexander, Robinson, & Rainforth, this volume). As noted earlier, the experience of pure consciousness during TM is the basis for eliminating the mistake of the intellect, and establishes the foundation for life in accord with natural law.

The program is learned in seven steps, each lasting about an hour. Following the course, the client meditates independently at home for 20 minutes every morning and evening. Additionally, weekend in-residence courses allow additional time for meditation and provide lectures for further intellectual understanding of the practice.

2. Group Practice of the Transcendental Meditation Program

Over the past 15 years, a considerable body of scientific research has been accumulated demonstrating the positive influence of group practice of the TM and advanced TM-Sidhi program on the environment. These studies show beneficial effects of reduced societal conflict, crime and accidents, and enhanced quality of life in extended populations including cities and nations (Orme-Johnson, this volume).

Group practice of TM has an integrating influence on the individual, as well as culturing a sense of harmony both within the individual and within the immediate group and/or community which is participating in this group practice. The development of this quality is important for substance abusers who often experience alienation and isolation.

3. Client Education

Client education focuses on the intellectual understanding of the interrelationships between consciousness, mind, and body, and their roles in regaining and maintaining health. It is designed to help the client become self-sufficient in maintaining good health and preventing disease. Client education enables the client to begin to appreciate the unified structure of life, and thus to better appreciate the many transformations experienced during the program. These sessions include specific guidelines (for example regarding nutrition and daily and seasonal routines) which the physician prescribes based on the client's individual body type (see below).

Client education is a positive, enjoyable experience that puts attention on growth of knowledge and improving health, rather than on past experiences, poor relationships, and old habits. Some reading materials and taped lectures are included. These materials are currently available from the American Association of Ayurvedic Medicine, as well as from MAPI (see Resource section of this book).

4. Maharishi Ayur-Veda Nutritional Therapy

Ayurvedic principles for proper food selection and preparation are employed according to different psychophysiological body types, individual imbalances, and seasonal variations. According to Maharishi Ayur-Veda, food plays a major role in prevention and recovery, since everything one ingests has a specific influence on the restoration and maintenance of health. Upon entry to the program, when the client is examined by a physician, individual body type is determined according to specific diagnostic criteria. Individualized nutritional guidelines are then given.

5. Yoga Asanas (Maharishi Ayur-Veda Neuromuscular Integration Program)

This program involves specific sequences of postures (yoga stretching exercises) to be performed for ten minutes before morning and evening sessions of the TM practice. This brings about suppleness of the body, thus increasing mind-body coordination and balance.

6. Pranayama (Maharishi Ayur-Veda Neurorespiratory Integration Techniques)

Neurorespiratory integration techniques are specific breathing exercises performed twice daily for 5 to 7 minutes after with the neuromuscular integration program. These techniques are held to stimulate the rich neural connections between the autonomic nervous system and the respiratory apparatus in order to increase mind-body coordination and balance. They induce a profound state of restfulness.

7. Daily and Seasonal Routines

All influences in nature have an effect on the state of mind and body. In modern medicine, the influences of the time of day (circadian cycles), of the month (e.g., menstrual cycles) or of the year (seasonal cycles) have only recently begun to be appreciated. In Maharishi Ayur-Veda these rhythms have always been considered important for the maintenance of health. Maharishi Ayur-Veda provides techniques for changing behavior to bring internal biological rhythms in tune with environmental cycles. This treatment involves instructions about daily and seasonal routines which the client can use at home. If an individual eats, sleeps, awakes, works, plays, meditates, etc., according to a balanced routine that is in accord with both the cycles of nature and the needs of one's own body type, then no aspects of life necessary for mental and physical balance will be neglected. The value of this program in the treatment of substance abuse cannot be overstated. Once detoxification has occurred and abstinence is established, this consistent daily program to maintain the experience of well-being helps prevent mental, behavioral, and physical imbalances that precipitate relapse.

8. Development of the Emotions

Maharishi Ayur-Veda places a high priority on developing emotions to their fullest and most refined capacity. Emotions are the finest level of the personality and strongly influence the physiology; they are the crucial link between individual consciousness and the functioning of the body. Emotional nourishment is particularly important within the context of substance abuse, because substance abusers are frequently subject to unhealthy negative emotions and cold, hostile environments. Maharishi Ayur-Veda attempts to impart to the recovering substance abuser, through the various treatment modalities, the experience of inner happiness. This experience creates inner balance, thus promoting a return to emotional and physical health. If further emotional nourishment is necessary, the physician may also prescribe setting aside time each day for activities which create personal fulfillment, as well as helping clients modify negative behaviors which may damage the fine level of the emotions.

9. Maharishi Gandharva Veda (Traditional Music Therapy)

Maharishi Ayur-Veda applies ancient knowledge of specific effects of sound and melody to restore physiological balance. These melodies and rhythms, known as Maharishi Gandharva Veda, are described in Maharishi Ayur-Veda as the melodies and rhythms of nature. Maharishi Gandharva Veda includes a complete range of melodies appropriate to time of day, season, and place, because different laws of nature predominate at these different times. Thus, specific music is held to have particular therapeutic influences in creating balance in the individual's physiology and in the environment. Time is set aside daily in the client's routine for listening to Gandharva Veda music.

10. Maharishi Ayur-Veda Herbal and Mineral Preparations and Rasayana Therapy

Maharishi Ayur-Veda includes extensive knowledge of medicinal plants. This therapy involves the use of certain herbal preparations traditionally used to restore balance to mind and body. These preparations include food supplements which are designed to promote balance in specific areas of the physiology based on the individual's psychophysiological type and particular imbalances. They include a special class known as *rasayanas* (including Maharishi Amrit Kalash), which are designed to act at the most fundamental level of the physiology. Maharishi Amrit Kalash is described as creating balance from this level, establishing the basis for fully integrated functioning of the mind, body, and behavior, thus promoting higher states of consciousness.

The principle of *complementarity* in Maharishi Ayur-Veda holds that the sequence of biological information as stored in plants corresponds to the sequence of biological information in the human physiology. Maharishi explains that these preparations act like special biological "software" that supplies the essential program to reestablish balance in the source code of the system. In this way the body can automatically correct any imbalances that might lead to disease. When biological information is highly ordered and integrated, the result is physiological balance–a state in which the parts of the organism are functioning in an integrated and harmonious equilibrium.

The herbal preparations are processed according to classical Ayurvedic methods, under the strict supervision of Ayurvedic physicians skilled in botanical pharmacology. An important principle in

Maharishi Ayur-Veda which also promotes balance is the use of the whole plant, which allows a synergistic effect to take place in the body and eliminates the side effects usually found with modern pharmaceutical drugs, caused by the isolation of the "active ingredient."

Extensive scientific research on Maharishi Amrit Kalash (Sharma, 1993) suggests that it has anticarcinogenic properties, as well as producing beneficial effects on a variety of aspects of health, including reduction of free radicals, enhancement of immune function, and improvement of cardiovascular disease risk factors.

11. Maharishi Ayur-Veda Behavior Therapy

Maharishi Ayur-Veda Behavior Therapy is designed to reinforce in a natural and spontaneous manner the harmonious behavior which is most conducive to health. This program endeavors to culture a positive mental attitude, more refined speech and courteous relationships, which are described as "behavioral rasayanas"–a powerful tonic for enhancing the health of mind, body, and emotions. This also helps to promote a nourishing environment for the client, since friends and family tend to reciprocate in a mutually supportive way. Behavioral recommendations thus complement emotional development by helping to refine feelings.

12. Panchakarma Program

The Maharishi Ayur-Veda Panchakarma Program, also known as "rejuvenation therapy," consists of physiological purification procedures that remove accumulated stress from the body and accumulated metabolic residues (*ama*) from the body's channels of microcirculation (*shrotas*), thereby restoring vitality and flexibility to mind and body. Therefore, they are a natural and enjoyable approach to drug detoxification or as an aid to reestablishing psychophysiological balance once detoxification has been accomplished. Panchakarma includes combinations of Ayurvedic massage, gentle herbalized heat treatments, eliminative therapies such as enemas and treatments for toning the sinuses and naso-pharynx, as well as other purification therapies. The treatments are individualized according to body type and specific imbalances. Although the procedures are simple and pleasant, they are labor-intensive, and require specialized equipment, supplies, and skilled professional technicians. Each client is attended by two technicians during a half-day program for five to seven consecutive days. Many clients, after completing the program, have stated that they had their first true experience of well-being. Although the complete Panchakarma program may not be available to clients with limited financial means, many elements of the program can be adapted for practice at home (self-oil massage, etc.).

13. Consultation and Pulse Diagnosis by a Physician Trained in Maharishi Ayur-Veda

Hundreds of physicians and other health care workers in North America who are trained in Maharishi Ayur-Veda have not only learned how to apply the aforementioned therapies, but more importantly, have developed new diagnostic skills. The physician trained in Maharishi Ayur-Veda views the patient in a broader psychological, sociological, and behavioral context. Physical diagnosis is also approached differently, with emphasis placed on determining the patient's constitutional type and specific imbalances according to classical Ayurvedic *tridosha* theory. *Tridosha* theory describes the three *doshas*–operating principles which govern physiological function and the equilibrium which exists among them (see Sands, this volume). Examination of the radial arterial pulse helps reveal the interaction between these fundamental doshas and guides therapy. Many of the specific recommendations for the various treatment modalities described in this section, including those for the client to pursue at home, are made according to this assessment of constitutional type and doshic imbalances.

Prescriptions which maximize clinical benefit and cost effectiveness are best made by a physician who has been trained in these skills and who has experience with Ayurvedic techniques. In addition to the strategies described above, the physician may elect to use other modalities (see Averbach & Rothenberg, 1989, and Sharma, 1993 for a discussion of the approaches of Maharishi Ayur-Veda).

MAHARISHI AYUR-VEDA AND TWELVE STEP PROGRAMS

The Maharishi Ayur-Veda approach to recovery has many elements in common with Twelve Step programs. Some of the more important ones include: spiritual orientation, emphasis on taking responsibility for one's own life, lack of emphasis on psychological analysis, and emphasis on action here and now.

My patients in Twelve Step programs who have added Maharishi Ayur-Veda to their recovery program have remarked that the following Ayurvedic principles have been important, positive additions to their perspective on recovery:

1. Stress is an important factor in substance abuse.
2. The main purpose of starting a substance abuse program is evolution, moving in the direction of higher states of consciousness (see below). According to Maharishi Ayur-Veda, sobriety and recovery are side benefits of the process of refining the neurophysiology in order to experience one's Self as the unbounded field of pure consciousness, the unified field of all the laws of nature. The purpose of this process is to develop one's nervous system to the point where it can maintain the experience of bliss.
3. The incentive for continuing a substance abuse program and for maintaining abstinence is increasing progress on a path of spiritual fulfillment and inner well-being. The experience of a natural state of balance and well-being is what entices one to continue on the path, thereby making success in the program independent of will-power and motivation. The value of Maharishi Ayur-Veda in promoting spiritual development is discussed briefly below and in greater detail by others in this volume. The increasing fulfillment provided by the balanced physiological and psychological state promoted by the various therapeutic strategies of Maharishi Ayur-Veda is greater than any fulfillment the substance can bring.
4. Even if a disorder has a latent, potential, or even manifested genetic predisposition in an individual, this disorder need not be fully expressed.
5. Addictive disorders are therefore potentially curable.

6. Addictive disorders do not have a single etiology, i.e., a genetic predisposition; rather, there are multiple factors responsible for bringing out addictive behaviors. Rehabilitation programs should therefore address the multifactorial etiologies with multiple therapeutic strategies.

In my own practice I have used Maharishi Ayur-Veda as an adjunct to Twelve Step programs since the two programs may usefully complement each other.

INTRODUCING MAHARISHI AYUR-VEDA TO TWELVE STEP PROGRAM ADHERENTS

Many patients with addictive behaviors have approached me because they have studied or tried the Twelve Step model and feel that it has been useful, and yet they are eager to accelerate their rehabilitation. Some have remarked that the essence of the Twelve Step program for them is the spiritual aspect, yet they feel "stuck" on the first four or five steps and are unable to move on.

I respond that there is no need for them to delay putting their attention on the Eleventh step–they can begin immediately to implement those higher steps and still fully benefit from the Twelve Step program. I remind them of Maharishi's *principle of the highest first*: Using an analogy, Maharishi (1963) explains that an army which captures the fort automatically possesses all the treasures in the gold mines and silver mines within the territory of that fort. In the analogy, "capturing the fort" means development of our full human potential in higher states of consciousness, in which the experience of pure consciousness is never lost; with this state of wholeness comes development of every area of life.

O'Connell (this volume) and Alexander, Robinson, & Rainforth (this volume) have analyzed how TM and Maharishi Ayur-Veda promote spiritual development, and how this brings holistic growth in all aspects of the individual's life. Maharishi has explained that higher states of consciousness develop automatically as a result of the direct experience of the field of pure consciousness through TM and the stabilization of this experience through regular daily practice. This evolution of consciousness produces a natural state of well-being and physiological balance as automatic "side benefits." As this development proceeds through Maharishi Ayur-Veda programs, my patients are naturally motivated to make amends with those they have hurt and to share their experiences with others, and so on.

Patients also find that Maharishi Ayur-Veda helps them to more fully appreciate their Twelve Step program. Many people drop out of Twelve Step programs because they feel depressed by the experiences of others at the meetings. With the regular practice of Transcendental Meditation, the experience of increasing inner silence and bliss begins to persist during daily activities outside of meditation. My meditating patients tell me they can attend meetings without feeling overshadowed or drained, and they are more able to give and share with other members. I have never observed a sober person involved in a Twelve Step program who relapsed after adding Maharishi Ayur-Veda to their recovery.

INITIATING MAHARISHI AYUR-VEDA PROGRAMS FOR PATIENTS WITH SUBSTANCE ABUSE DISORDERS

Maharishi Ayur-Veda as applied in North America and Europe has been found especially helpful for management of chronic disorders. Although Staggers, Alexander, and Walton (this volume) suggest it has a role in detoxification, its use in these settings has not been widely applied nor significantly researched so far, as conventional medical methods have been found to be both safe and effective. The importance of Maharishi Ayur-Veda programs begins with the difficult stage after detoxification when the individual has developed an interest in maintaining sobriety but may have experienced limited success in the past with conventional methods.

Individuals may not be familiar either with the Transcendental Meditation technique or Maharishi Ayur-Veda. Health professionals without formal training in these programs should not attempt to instruct clients personally, but should aim at interesting them in these approaches and should refer them to Maharishi Ayur-Veda centers or physicians trained in Maharishi Ayur-Veda. TM must be learned from a qualified instructor who has received extensive training (the technique is very simple, natural, and easy to learn, but it is also a delicate practice, and individual experiences may vary). The following is a sample talk which addictions counselors and other health professionals can adapt for introducing the Maharishi Ayur-Veda program to clients.

"You have expressed your frustration that you have been able to stop abusing a number of times, only to relapse again. And we have talked about how your mind has always been the trigger for you to return to your old pattern of abuse, when you are under stress and your body has gotten out of balance. You have seen that when your body is addicted to the substance, the cravings of the body overshadow your will-power. We therefore need to get your mind and body to work together to maintain well-being.

"It is easy for you to quit for a few weeks, but the programs that you have started so far have not been enough by themselves to have a long-lasting effect in changing your body's craving. I am going to suggest something radically new for you. Only a new seed can yield a new crop. This approach will maximize the mind-body connection. It is called Maharishi Ayur-Veda.

"There are many different treatment strategies of Maharishi Ayur-Veda that will be used, and yet they all have one thing in common: even though they may act in some way on your body, they are also going to be changing the way your mind and body interact. Even though the techniques you will be learning seem different from the programs you tried before, and even though they may seem unusual to you, research has shown they may have benefits for conditions like yours. These techniques are all simple, natural, and enjoyable. I am only asking you to have an open mind and to approach this program with innocence.

"You will need to make a commitment of some time, energy, and resources. I will give you some reading and you will need to attend classes and patient education programs to get started. It would also be good for you to learn Transcendental Meditation, which is a simple mental technique practiced for 15 to 20 minutes morning and evening sitting comfortably with the eyes closed. We will arrange group meditation sessions where you can have your meditation checked as well as a consultation by a doctor trained in Maharishi Ayur-Veda who will prescribe a specific diet, natural herbal preparations and other enjoyable treatments. It will also be important for you to make a significant change in your irregular schedule. From now on you should try to live according to a routine that includes going to bed on time, getting daily exercise and fresh air, and practicing Transcendental Meditation. I think the commitment of time and energy will be very worthwhile, and the results will prove to be very rewarding right from the start. Is this something you would like to try?"

This is an appropriate point for the client to sit with a Maharishi Ayur-Veda patient educator who explains the basic principles. There are also several videotapes, audiotapes and books that give a brief introduction and explain the treatment modalities (see Resources section in this volume). These materials can be provided to the client who returns in several days to begin the program.

For success with Maharishi Ayur-Veda, it is critical to start patients on a good daily routine. Most people with substance abuse problems have lives that are disorganized and oriented around the abuse. I tell them to prioritize the activities they need to accomplish in their day and then to write up a schedule for posting on the mirror or refrigerator for frequent reference.

Consultation with a physician trained in Maharishi Ayur-Veda is often of benefit at the outset since the physician is best able to determine specific imbalances and make appropriate prescriptions for diet and herbal supplements. When a physician recommends modifications for diet, the changes should be made easily and gently, reminding the client that Ayurvedic recommendations are not strict rules, but guidelines to promote physiological balance. I always tell people that with respect to diet, Maharishi Ayur-Veda never says "never" or "only." Instead, the person selects from the foods he or she enjoys, taking more of the most beneficial ones and less of the others according to specific imbalances and body type. The most important Ayurvedic guideline is to eat what one *naturally* likes, and to not be swayed by past habits and memories. Exercises outlined during client education sessions help clients distinguish between natural desires and inappropriate cravings. Patient education materials are available describing the body-type specific diet and appropriate eating behaviors.

The most important step is instruction in the Transcendental Meditation technique, which provides the basis for overcoming the disorder from the level of consciousness. Health care professionals need only to recommend attending an introductory lecture given by a qualified TM teacher, and then follow up to see if the client has pursued this program. All teachers of TM have been trained by Maharishi to give the standardized seven-step course which enables the person to become self-sufficient in practicing Transcendental Meditation. TM teachers are also qualified to demonstrate simple programs of yoga asanas and pranayama (breathing exercises).

If the client is motivated and has sufficient financial means, an optional program is a one or two-week in-residence treatment with the Maharishi Panchakarma purification program as described above. This is ideally taken every two to three months during the first year of abstinence. At the Maharishi Ayur-Veda Health Center for Behavioral Medicine and Stress Management in Lancaster, Massachusetts we have found that Panchakarma provides a natural experience of health and well-being that may prove to be a turning point in recovery.

CONCLUSION

In this paper I have examined Maharishi Ayur-Veda as a means for substance abuse rehabilitation, either by itself, or as a complement to Twelve Step and other recovery programs. Maharishi Ayur-Veda has been observed by many practitioners to be useful in recovery because it is a complete science of health with a consistent theoretical framework that deals with all aspects of a client's life: mind, body, behavior, and environment. All of the treatment modalities are based on the underlying theoretical framework, and the substance abuse client is able to understand the rationale for the treatments, which are themselves enjoyable. This enjoyment and increasing well-being are also the motivators for continuing the treatments and maintaining sobriety. The treatment modalities are presented so the client can continue many of them in the home environment for self-sufficient health care and recovery. Prevention of disease and maintenance of health are the purpose of Maharishi Ayur-Veda programs, which automatically contribute to spiritual development whether the programs are used for recovery or for other medical conditions. The physician organizations which promote Maharishi Ayur-Veda are eager to see the programs implemented and rigorously evaluated in a variety of clinical settings. I invite all health care professionals and addictions counselors to visit Maharishi Ayur-Veda Health Centers and to be trained in these valuable modalities.

REFERENCES

Alexander, C. N., Robinson, P., Rainforth, M. (this volume). Treating alcohol, nicotine, and drug abuse using Transcendental Meditation: A review and statistical meta-analysis. *Alcoholism Treatment Quarterly.*

Averbach, R. & Rothenberg, S. (1989). Fundamentals of Maharishi Ayur-Veda: Natural health care for the mind and body. [Videotape and booklet]. Lancaster, MA: Maharishi Ayur-Veda Products International.

Glaser, J. (1988). Maharishi Ayur-Veda: An introduction to recent research. *Modern Science and Vedic Science*, *2*(1), 89-108.

Hagelin, J. S. (1987). Is consciousness the unified field? A field theorist's perspective. *Modern Science and Vedic Science*, *1*, 29-87.

Hagelin, J. S. (1989). Restructuring physics from its foundation in light of Maharishi's Vedic Science. *Modern Science and Vedic Science*, *3*, 3-72.

Hawking, S. M. (1988). *A brief history of time*. New York: Bantam.

Maharishi Mahesh Yogi. (1963). *Science of being and art of living*. New York, NY: Signet.

Maharishi Mahesh Yogi. (1969). *On the Bhagavad Gita: A translation and commentary (Chapters 1-6)*. Baltimore, MD: Penguin.

Maharishi Mahesh Yogi (1986). *Life supported by natural law.* Washington, DC: Age of Enlightenment Press.

O'Connell, D. F. (this volume). Possessing the self: Maharishi Ayur-Veda and the process of recovery from addictive diseases. *Alcoholism Treatment Quarterly.*

Orme-Johnson, D. W. (this volume). Transcendental Meditation as an epidemiological approach to drug and alcohol abuse: Theory, research and financial impact evaluation. *Alcoholism Treatment Quarterly.*

Royer, A. (this volume). The role of the Transcendental Meditation technique in promoting smoking cessation: A longitudinal study. *Alcoholism Treatment Quarterly.*

Sands, D. (this volume). Introducing Maharishi Ayur-Veda into clinical practice. *Alcoholism Treatment Quarterly.*

Schenkluhn, H. & Geisler, M. (1977). A longitudinal study of the influence of the Transcendental Meditation program on drug abuse. In D. W. Orme-Johnson & J. T. Farrow (Eds.), *Scientific research on Maharishi's Transcendental Meditation program: Collected papers*, Vol. 1, (pp. 544-555). West Germany: MERU Press.

Sharma, H. (1993). *Freedom from disease*. Toronto: Veda Publishing.

Charaka Samhita, I (1981). (P. V. Sharma, Ed. & Trans.). Delhi: Chaukhambha Orientalia.

Staggers, F., Alexander, C. N., & Walton, K.G. (this volume). Implementation of the Transcendental Meditation program and Maharishi Ayur-Veda to prevent alcohol and drug abuse among juveniles at risk. *Alcoholism Treatment Quarterly.*

Wallace, R. K. (1993). *The physiology of consciousness.* Fairfield, IA: Maharishi International University Press.

Walton, K. G., & Levitsky, D. (this volume). Role of Transcendental Meditation in reducing drug use and addictions: Neurochemical evidence and a theory. *Alcoholism Treatment Quarterly.*

The Application of Maharishi Ayur-Veda to Mental Health and Substance Abuse Treatment

Jim Brooks, MD

As a psychiatrist, I am deeply interested in the application of Maharishi Ayur-Veda to the fields of both mental and physical health, especially with reference to treatment for substance abuse. In this chapter, I would like to share my experience and perspective on Maharishi Ayur-Veda in clinical settings.

Ayur-Veda is the world's oldest system of traditional medicine, the source of which is the Vedic tradition of India. Its ancient textbooks include the Charaka (1981) and Sushruta (1981) Samhitas. These texts provide a comprehensive explanation of the etiology, pathophysiology, and natural treatment approaches for medical and psychiatric disorders, and are still used today in the training of Ayurvedic physicians in India. In addition to treatment approaches for mental and physical disorders, Ayur-Veda also em-

---

Dr. Brooks is a board certified psychiatrist and is Clinical Director of the Mental Health Institute of Mount Pleasant, Mount Pleasant, IA; he is also attending physician at the College of Maharishi Ayur-Veda Health Center, and adjunct clinical faculty at Maharishi Ayur-Ved at Maharishi International University, Fairfield, IA.

Please address correspondence to Dr. Jim Brooks, Mental Health Institute of Mount Pleasant, 1200 East Washington, Mount Pleasant, IA 52641.

[Haworth co-indexing entry note]: "The Application of Maharishi Ayur-Veda to Mental Health and Substance Abuse Treatment." Brooks, Jim. Co-published simultaneously in the *Alcoholism Treatment Quarterly* (The Haworth Press, Inc.) Vol. 11, No. 3/4, 1994, pp. 395-411; and: *Self-Recovery: Treating Addictions Using Transcendental Meditation and Maharishi Ayur-Veda* (ed: David F. O'Connell and Charles N. Alexander) The Haworth Press, Inc., 1994, pp. 395-411. Multiple copies of this article/chapter may be purchased from The Haworth Document Delivery Center [1-800-3-HAWORTH; 9:00 a.m. - 5:00 p.m. (EST)].

phasizes treatment strategies for disease prevention as well as for promotion of mental and physical health. The treatments from this system of health are holistic in that they involve a comprehensive approach that simultaneously addresses the psychological, physiological, behavioral, and environmental components of the individual.

Due to hundreds of years of foreign rule in India, much of the essential knowledge of Ayur-Veda was lost. However, since India gained its independence, there has been a resurgence of Ayurvedic medicine in India. Over 100 Ayur-Veda colleges have now been established in India, a number of which are fully supported by the Indian government. The World Health Organization has formally recognized and given support to the reestablishment of this system of health care. Over the last eight years in particular, there have been significant strides in restoring the knowledge of Ayur-Veda to its original stature. The individual most responsible for this is Maharishi Mahesh Yogi, the founder of the Transcendental Meditation program and a many academic institutions around the world, including Maharishi Vedic Universities and Maharishi Ayur-Veda Universities in many countries, the World Center of Maharishi Ayur-Veda and Maharishi Institute for Vedic Science and Technology in India, and Maharishi International University in the United States. Maharishi, working with leading Ayurvedic physicians in India, including Dr. V. M. Dwivedi, Dr. Brihaspati Dev Triguna, and Dr. Balaraj Maharshi, has not only brought to light from the Vedic literature the complete knowledge of the theoretical and practical aspects of Ayur-Veda, but has also made courses available to physicians around the world to facilitate implementation of this system of natural health care. This authentic, comprehensive, and scientific knowledge of Ayur-Veda is referred to as "Maharishi Ayur-Veda." Over one thousand medical doctors in all five continents have now taken courses in Maharishi Ayur-Veda and are integrating it with their current medical practices. There is also a growing body of published research demonstrating its clinical validity.

Maharishi Ayur-Veda includes many therapeutic modalities that had virtually become lost, including, most importantly, methods to develop higher states of human consciousness. The theoretical knowledge of Maharishi Ayur-Veda includes Maharishi's explanation that, in addition to three known states of consciousness, i.e., waking, dreaming, and sleeping, there are higher states of consciousness that sequentially develop to unfold the full potential of human life (Maharishi Mahesh Yogi, 1969). Modern scientific research on Transcendental Meditation, the main modality Maharishi Ayur-Veda, indicates that these higher states of consciousness have their own specific psychophysiological parameters (Alexander et al., 1990).

The consciousness approach of Maharishi Ayur-Veda includes mental techniques to directly experience and enliven the field of pure consciousness, described by Maharishi as the silent, unmanifest, unbounded field of pure intelligence, which is the basis of the individual mind and physiology, and also of all existence (Maharishi Mahesh Yogi, 1969, 1986). The purpose of these techniques is to infuse the mind with the lively silence–the alertness, calmness, and bliss–characteristic of the experience of this field. The result for the individual is more inner peace and contentment, and more mental alertness and clarity. The individual spontaneously feels fulfilled from within, maintaining a kind of internal gyroscope that is unshakable in the face of life's vicissitudes. According to Maharishi Ayur-Veda, the regular experience of this field, alternating with daily activity, is the primary factor in culturing the individual's growth toward higher states of consciousness. In his books *The Neurophysiology of Enlightenment* (1986) and *The Physiology of Consciousness* (1993) Wallace describes some of the physiological correlates found in individuals who are developing toward higher states of consciousness, known traditionally as "enlightenment."

According to Maharishi Ayur-Veda, the prevention and treatment of all physical and mental disorders should include practical techniques that promote the holistic development of both mind and body. The treatment is not limited to one part of the individual, such as one organ system or one chemical, because a disease is understood to affect the whole system due to the integration of all the parts of the system. For example, if a person has frequent colds, the physician trained in Maharishi Ayur-Veda would not only treat the immediate problem but would also instruct the patient in how to prevent future colds from occurring. Because all diseases, including colds, are understood to involve psychological as well as physiological factors, the doctor would provide a variety of treatments to ensure the advancement of not only physical but also psychological health. For example, the Ayurvedic physician would make certain dietary and herbal recommendations in order to reestablish balance in the physiology. The individual would also be taught how to understand his or her psychophysiological constitutional type (to be described below) so that foods eaten in the future would not contribute to the development of frequent colds. At the same time, the individual would be taught appropriate daily routines in order to maintain proper balance between his or her biological rhythms and the natural rhythms of the environment, which include daily, monthly, seasonal, and yearly effects. Colds, for example, may be aggravated during the winter and spring months; therefore, certain behavioral measures such as a daily warm oil massage, avoiding sleeping during the daytime, drinking hot water frequently during the day, using certain herbal seasonings on the food, and taking certain mixtures of herbal preparations that enhance the immune system, etc., may be extremely useful in reducing cold symptoms. In addition, the Ayurvedic physician may recommend that the individual learn one of the mental techniques of Maharishi Ayur-Veda, including the Transcendental Meditation (TM) technique. This technique has been shown to enhance immune functioning (Seiler, 1979).

Transcendental Meditation produces a profound state of rest in the physiology, which allows the body to heal itself more effectively. Also, research has shown that the TM technique enhances well-being and significantly reduces stress, which has a two-fold effect. Firstly, this reduction in stress may further enhance immune functioning. Secondly, an individual who is less stressed spontaneously feels more fulfilled and secure inside. Such a person is more likely to make healthier choices in terms of diet and behavior. On the other hand, feeling unfulfilled may result in addictive (unhealthy) behaviors, including smoking and intake of improper types and amounts of food. According to Maharishi Ayur-Veda, both smoking and improper diet are causative factors in the development of colds and other respiratory disorders. The above examples illustrate how even a seemingly purely physical disorder, such as the common cold, has both physiological and psychological causes. The treatment, therefore, should include a holistic approach in order to be most effective in terms of both prevention and treatment. This is a true "mind-body" approach.

Although there has been a great deal already written with regard to the physical health benefits of Maharishi Ayur-Veda (Sharma, 1993; Wallace, 1986, 1993; Averbach & Rothenberg, 1989), as a psychiatrist, I have taken a personal interest in examining the benefits of Maharishi Ayur-Veda in the fields of mental health and substance abuse rehabilitation. In the remainder of this chapter, I would like to share with you my perspective on this most important subject.

THE PERSPECTIVE OF MAHARISHI AYUR-VEDA ON THE CAUSE OF MENTAL ILLNESS AND ADDICTIVE BEHAVIORS

The classical textbooks of Ayur-Veda describe the etiology of mental illness from several different perspectives; in other words, the cause is usually multifactorial, but all these factors are usually intertwined. These factors can be understood to be primarily either psychological, physiological, behavioral, or environmental.

The main cause of mental illness (and of all disease), according to Maharishi Ayur-Veda, involves what is called in Sanskrit *pragyaparadha*. The English translation of this word is "mistake of the intellect." Maharishi defines pragyaparadha as the loss of memory of pure consciousness, which is the field of unity at the basis of the mind, by its diversified expressions in the mind, body, and all spheres of life.

Pure consciousness, or transcendental consciousness, is understood by Maharishi Ayur-Veda to be the essence of our nature as human beings. Maharishi (1963) explains that just as the silent ocean rises up in waves, the ocean of pure consciousness underlying our awareness rises up to form the waves, or content, of consciousness, i.e., our thoughts and feelings, which in turn form the basis of our entire personality. Subjectively, pure consciousness is experienced during Transcendental Meditation as a state in which the mind is completely quiet and calm and yet remains alert. This state of "restful alertness" has a corresponding style of physiological functioning that includes EEG coherence (Banquet, 1973), marked reduction in metabolic rate (Wallace, 1970), increased skin resistance (Orme-Johnson, 1973), low levels of cortisol (Bevan, 1980), and a constellation of other neurophysiological parameters (Wallace, 1993).

According to Maharishi Ayur-Veda, the regular experience of pure consciousness during meditation results in a dramatic and significant change in the qualitative experience of the individual. Maharishi explains that before learning to meditate, since the clear experience of pure consciousness is not dominant, the tendency of the individual is to identify with and become overly attached to sensory experience. This is referred to as "object referral," because the world outside ourselves takes on primary importance. This way of experiencing the world has its basis in the mistake of the intellect, or pragyaparadha, because one has lost sight of the unified basis of life in pure consciousness. The net effect is that one feels an inner lack that only seems to be satisfied when the senses are successful in obtaining the object that they desire. According to Ayur-Veda, however, one can never achieve complete happiness in life through sensory experience alone. Since everything around us is always changing, by definition there can be no lasting satisfaction from the material-objective world in and of itself.

Maharishi (1986) describes pure consciousness as being "self-referral," because in that state consciousness knows, or is aware of, itself alone. When this self-referral state is experienced through Transcendental Meditation, and as it gradually becomes stabilized through the regular practice of this technique, one develops a stable core of inner security and fulfillment, which is never lost, even in the midst of dynamic activity and change. One has thus made a qualitative quantum shift in daily experience to a life based on the self-referral field of pure consciousness, which Maharishi (1969) describes as the Self (capital "S"), as distinguished from the "small self," the realm of thoughts, feelings, and actions with which one has previously identified.

When the Self dominates in one's awareness, the mistake of the intellect disappears, because the diverse aspects of life have been reconnected to their source in pure consciousness. One's perception of oneself and of one's relationship to the outer environment becomes more stable and more accurate. Perception is no longer colored by underlying feelings of inner lack. Therefore one can spontaneously enjoy and appreciate all sensory experiences fully, but one is no longer dependent upon the outer world to feel happy and well.

Thus, enlivening this deeper aspect of our personality and stabilizing it in daily life promotes psychophysiological balance, and thereby eliminates the cause of many mental disorders as well as addictive behaviors. When a person's thinking and action are not established in pure consciousness, he or she becomes a slave to inconsistencies and losses, which are inevitable in the outer sphere of our life, and is at much higher risk for the experiences of fear, sadness, anger, anxiety, depression, lust, greed, and envy. The effects of TM practice significantly enhance a stable sense of inner satisfaction coupled with an increased ability to perform effectively in one's daily activity, regardless of what events might be going on externally; thus the internal, steady experience of the Self promoted by TM is seen in clinical practice to be a wonderful vaccine against a wide variety of mental imbalances and addictive behaviors.

Clinically, I have found that the application of this principle of promoting balance between mind, body, and pure consciousness (Self) is extremely useful in treating both psychiatric and addictive disorders. This can be illustrated in the case of Susan, a woman in her sixties who carried the "dual diagnosis" of substance abuse and major depression, linked with panic attacks and agoraphobia. Susan came into the hospital "a bundle of nerves." She had been unable to fully grieve the death of a close friend and had become housebound from the ensuing development of panic attacks. Her doctor had put her on sedatives, to which she had become addicted. Over time, she became increasingly despondent and dysfunctional, and at the time of hospitalization she was feeling that suicide was her only option. Since she was already on sedative and antidepressant medicines, which were not effectively eliminating her symptoms, I discussed a few "alternative" Maharishi Ayur-Veda strategies with her, which she was quite eager to learn. In addition to my training in psychiatry, I am a qualified teacher of Transcendental Meditation. I taught her the Transcendental Meditation technique, along with a few other Ayurvedic therapies such as nutritional counseling, recommendations for her daily routine (self-oil massage), and neurorespiratory/neuromuscular integration techniques (breathing techniques and yoga exercise postures). (See Averbach & Rothenberg, 1989, and Glaser, this volume, for a discussion of the various treatment approaches of Maharishi Ayur-Veda.) Within ten days of this natural, nonpharmacological approach, Susan was well enough to go home. She was no longer depressed, but was instead seen to be frequently smiling and more positive in her outlook. She was no longer experiencing panic attacks and was making progress with her agoraphobia. She had cut down on the regular use of sedatives to only periodic usage on an "as needed" basis.

What happened? How could such a dramatic transformation occur in so short a time? Basically, the TM technique enabled Susan to experience, on a regular basis, her innermost Self–pure consciousness. The other Maharishi Ayur-Veda strategies created balance in mind and body, which supported this experience. Very quickly she began to describe a welling up of inner calm and joy from within. This experience during her Ayur-Veda practice, especially during TM, resulted in a lessening of her worries and fears, and new zest for life. In other words, her newfound calmness, energy, and happiness were related to loss of object referral and the development of functioning based on the self-referral state of pure consciousness. At eight months' follow-up, she continues to show improvement in all of her symptoms.

A second factor seen by Maharishi Ayur-Veda to be causative in the development of psychiatric conditions takes more of a physiological perspective. The ancient knowledge of Ayur-Veda includes a very complete and practical understanding of human physiology. In Maharishi Ayur-Veda, there are three basic underlying metabolic principles that govern the human physiology (as well as the physiology of the animal and plant kingdoms). These three organizational principles are called *Vata, Pitta,* and *Kapha* (Averbach & Rothenberg, 1989). Vata represents the principle of movement in the physiology and is responsible for the functioning of the nervous system and the flow of the circulatory and digestive systems. Pitta is responsible for digestion and metabolism, and Kapha is responsible for the structure and fluid balance of the body. All of the modern and scientific understandings of the body's composition and function can be organized according to these three categories.

There are several advantages to categorizing the physiology according to Vata, Pitta, and Kapha. Firstly, every individual can be categorized as one of ten different psychophysiological constitutional types, based on the combination of these three elements, which are called *doshas*. Once an individual's constitutional type (determined through a comprehensive history and physical examination, including a special Ayurvedic examination of the pulse) is determined, then it is possible to determine what types of food would promote balance in that individual. Also, both mental and physical ill health are seen as arising as a consequence of imbalances among the doshas. Thus, if there is some psychological or physiological imbalance present, herbal preparations, as well as other recommendations of Maharishi Ayur-Veda, can be prescribed that will restore balance for that given individual. For example, if an individual has primarily a Vata type of constitution, then if Vata increases or becomes "aggravated" in that individual, this may produce imbalances leading to such psychological conditions as insomnia and anxiety; more severe imbalances may lead to psychiatric disorders. For such an individual, certain food types that reduce excess Vata in the system, such as warm and heavy foods having more of a sweet, sour, or salty taste, will be extremely helpful in reducing the symptoms. Also, regular mild exercise, a daily warm oil massage, regular practice of Transcendental Meditation, certain herbal preparations that are extremely effective in providing a soothing influence to the nervous system, and a variety of other behavioral recommendations will all serve to correct the anxiety and insomnia, because they treat, not the symptoms themselves, but the underlying imbalances that are causing them. Ayurvedic treatments often can be administered without having to resort to modern drugs, which may have a tendency to have harmful and unwanted side effects. This simple and yet profound system for understanding the human physiology is easy to learn, for both the physician and patient, and it gives the psychiatric or substance abusing patient a tremendous sense of control over his or her own health and destiny.

In my clinical experience, patients greatly appreciate this simple but elegant psychophysiological approach to treating their psychiatric condition because they have a sense of truly understanding what is wrong and also have the opportunity to be intimately involved in their own recovery. Many of the therapies of modern psychiatry, including psychotherapy and medication, often have the unwanted side effect of promoting dependency and a sense of lack of control over one's own healing process. The advantage of a Western-trained physician who is also trained in Maharishi Ayur-Veda is that he or she can use an integrated approach emphasizing natural treatment methods primarily; however, if necessary, he or she can add Western medical approaches in an adjunctive fashion. In this way, patients truly get "the best of both worlds."

Using these principals of Vata, Pitta, and Kapha, can be extremely practical in treating psychiatric disorders. Ed, for example, is a 45-year-old male who was presented with a diagnosis of major depression. From the Ayurvedic point of view, he had a Pitta type depression with his main complaint being extreme irritability (a sign of Pitta imbalance). Because he was against taking medications, and wanted a natural treatment approach for his depression, he was prescribed a Pitta-reducing regimen. This included a Pitta-pacifying diet (which favors sweet, bitter, and astringent foods, a reduction in salty, spicy, sour, and oily foods, an increase in milk and ghee [clarified butter]); an herbal tea; milk *shirodhara* (a Pitta-reducing procedure where a stream of milk treated with special herbs is poured across the forehead for 30 to 40 minutes); a breathing technique known in Ayur-Veda to have a "cooling effect" on the mind; and TM (which provides mental calmness and reduces irritability). At his next appointment ten days later, Ed was much more relaxed, was cheerful (less depressed), and reported a significant reduction in his anger outbursts at home and at work. In Ed's case no medication was needed. In some more resistant cases, however, a combination of antidepressant medication along with Ayurvedic recommendations might be the best approach.

Maharishi Ayur-Veda also understands the etiology of mental imbalance and addictions from a third perspective–behavior. Of course, behavioral approaches have become increasingly popular in modern psychology and psychiatry. Maharishi Ayur-Veda provides an expanded understanding of human behavior that is quite useful in both treating as well as preventing mental and emotional imbalance. In short, this angle on the etiology of disease refers to a principle known in Maharishi Ayur-Veda as *violation of natural law.* This principle basically refers to the idea that we create much of our own misery by failing to think and act in accord with the laws of nature that govern human life and the environment. In medicine, this idea is becoming not only well known but also substantiated scientifically. (For example, such disorders as lung and throat cancer, heart disease, strokes, and hypertension, as well as auto accidents, homicides, and suicides have been related to cigarette smoking and alcohol consumption. These behaviors are clearly not life-supporting and thus can be understood as being not in accord with the natural laws upholding the health of the body.) Maharishi Ayur-Veda not only recognizes this idea but also, more importantly, provides a methodology for reducing and ultimately eliminating the tendency to violate natural law. In order to behave in such a manner as to prevent harming oneself or others, Maharishi Ayur-Veda recommends procedures that help individuals to become physically and mentally well; thus, they have less of a tendency to behave in ways that may produce harm to themselves or others. In other words, behaviors which result in self-harm often are due to an inner feeling of discomfort, emptiness, or unhappiness. The individual is wanting to "feel better," at least temporarily. Thus, improper diet, too little or too much exercise, smoking, drinking, drug abuse, etc., will be significantly reduced if a person can find a healthier means to promote mental and physical well-being. This may sound simple, but having practical tools to increase one's inner sense of happiness and wellness, as well as techniques to enhance one's ability to be more successful in one's daily activities, naturally reduce the likelihood that an individual will have to rely on behaviors that temporarily enhance well-being but ultimately result in a worsening of psychological and physiological health. Each of the approaches of Maharishi Ayur-Veda serves in a natural way to greatly enhance one's sense of self, and scientific research clearly demonstrates improvements in both psychological and physiological health.

The practice of Transcendental Meditation is fundamental to this process, because it gives the direct experience of pure consciousness. Maharishi (1986) explains that the field of pure consciousness underlying human physiology and psychology is the unmanifest field of pure intelligence–the totality of natural law–which gives rise to and structures the entire physical universe. With the daily experience of this field, the individual's thinking and action are brought increasingly into accord with the evolutionary direction of natural law governing all of life, and one becomes less inclined toward non-life-supporting behaviors.

Moreover, current treatments for substance abuse help an individual to cope with the loss of his or her habit but do not provide a way to effectively "replace the high." TM promotes the experience of pure consciousness, an experience of inner bliss and fulfillment, and other techniques of Maharishi Ayur-Veda also promote a natural experience of well-being in body and mind. These experiences successfully replace those found with the substance that was being abused, which often come to be seen as inferior to those found with TM.

The fourth factor seen to be causative in mental illness and addictive behaviors is environmental influences. The environment in which we live definitely plays a role in our daily life. It is obvious, for example, that a loving, nurturing family environment does a lot more to foster normal human development than one in which parents and/or siblings are hostile, judgmental, and stressed.

Maharishi Ayur-Veda suggests that it is possible for us to improve our environment from two perspectives. The first is that although it may be difficult to change another person's behavior, we can certainly change our own. If a person is improving his or her physical and mental well-being through the technologies of Maharishi Ayur-Veda on a daily basis, then he or she can often step out of the "vicious cycle" of blame that is often seen in unhealthy relationships. If we can improve ourselves and develop more inner strength and stability, we can often begin to respond to our family and/or peers in a less defensive and more supportive and empathic manner. This often can go a long way to reverse negative trends and tendencies that we formerly viewed as unchangeable and hopeless aspects of our environment.

Secondly, Maharishi Ayur-Veda notes that even though on the surface we appear separate from one another, on the deepest level of our mind we are intimately connected with those around us. Pure consciousness, the basic field underlying all existence, lies at the deepest level of our own personality. Thus, universality is basic to our nature, and therefore we are all connected on this fundamental level of human experience. This phenomenon on the level of human experience has parallels to modern theories of quantum physics.

In quantum field theory, physicists have shown mathematically that there is an underlying unified field of nature's intelligence, which has the property of being unmanifest (silent) but nonetheless gives rise to everything that is manifest in the physical universe. This unified field is the basis and the cause of everything in nature, according to physics. Because it has the property of infinite correlation, it is the integrating factor that maintains orderliness in nature.

Some physicists (Hagelin, 1987) have arrived at the same understanding that has always been a part of the knowledge of Ayur-Veda: that the unified field of natural law is the field of pure consciousness, and that therefore humans have the unique characteristic of being able to experience the unified field. This would explain how we might be able to holistically influence not only our entire physiology, but also our surrounding environment, through the procedure of contacting and enlivening the unified field of pure consciousness deep within us. Because of this infinite correlation value of pure consciousness, if we enliven this field through both individual practice and especially through group practice of Transcendental Meditation, it is possible to influence our environment significantly in the direction of greater peacefulness and positivity. It is interesting to note that there is extensive published scientific research (e.g., Dillbeck, Landrith, & Orme-Johnson, 1981; Dillbeck, Cavanaugh, Glenn, Orme-Johnson, & Mittlefehldt, 1987; Orme-Johnson, Gelderloos, & Dillbeck, 1988) indicating that group practice of TM and the advanced TM-Sidhi program results in a reduction of crime, accidents, sickness, and suicides in society.

MAHARISHI AYUR-VEDA IN CLINICAL PRACTICE

In this section, I will be describing the clinical applications of Maharishi Ayur-Veda in the fields of both mental health and substance abuse rehabilitation. In the United States and many other countries, there are many mental health professionals who are incorporating Maharishi Ayur-Veda into their practices. I personally have been using these techniques in my clinical practice for the past ten years. I will briefly describe a number of diagnostic categories and give case examples of how Maharishi Ayur-Veda has helped patients with these disorders.

Major depression is one of the more common psychiatric conditions, with approximately 20% of the population afflicted at some point in their lifetimes. This condition is characterized by a sad or irritable mood, difficulty sleeping, poor or increased appetite, and decreased ambition. It is associated with a 15% mortality rate due to suicide. This condition is usually treated with a combination of antidepressant medication and psychotherapy. Often chronic stress is a contributing factor to this condition, along with a genetic predisposition. Due to significant side effects from medications and a high recurrence rate, the mental health profession is looking for more effective ways of treating this condition. The techniques of Maharishi Ayur-Veda help in treating this condition to a significant degree because scientific research has demonstrated that herbal medications (Sharma, 1988), purification procedures (Schneider, 1985) which include shirodhara (an ancient treatment for mental conditions that involves pouring herbalized oil and other natural substances, as described above, across the forehead), and Transcendental Meditation (Brooks & Scarano, 1986) are all helpful in treating not only depression but a number of other conditions. These treatments appear to work by virtue of physiological parameters including changes in EEG (Banquet, 1973), serum cortisol (Jevning, 1978), endogenous endorphin production (Sharma, 1988), and endogenous imipramine receptor binding (Sharma, 1988). Also, psychological factors such as stress reduction, increased inner contentment associated with enhanced self-esteem, and increased energy all contribute to the alleviation of depression.

A patient of mine, a nurse who is married with two children, presented with severe symptoms of major depression that made her unable to function at work or at home. She was extremely suicidal. She was given a trial of antidepressant medication in the hospital, but due to side effects, she was unable to tolerate an effective dose. She was prescribed Transcendental Meditation, and within a few days, she had a significant improvement in her depression to the point where she was able to leave the hospital. One interesting sideline to this case is that this patient previously was "stuck" in her therapy sessions. She was unable to look at some difficult issues related to early childhood abuse. After learning to meditate, she had more self-confidence and therefore was able to face many difficulties in her life that she had been unable to confront before. This brings out a very important point. Techniques of Maharishi Ayur-Veda, which include meditation, diet, herbal preparations, purification treatments, recommendations for daily routine, taste and aroma therapies, etc., all act in a holistic and synergistic way. These treatments serve to enhance the benefits of other more traditional treatments such as psychotherapy.

Mental health professionals who integrate Maharishi Ayur-Veda into their practice are finding similar benefits in the treatment of a variety of other conditions, including anxiety disorders, borderline and narcissistic personality disorders, psychotic disorders, and substance abuse disorders.

One last case example is that of Ralph, a 40-year-old male attorney who unfortunately suffers from a variety of addictions, including narcotics, amphetamines, and minor tranquilizers. He had been struggling unsuccessfully, off and on for years, to get off these substances. With a combination of Maharishi Ayur-Veda therapies, including herbal preparations, Transcendental Meditation, dietary recommendations according to his constitutional type, music therapy, etc., he has been able to stop using drugs altogether. He is also feeling a sense of inner happiness and strength, a feeling that he previously was able to achieve only by taking drugs. He has been gracious enough to describe his experience with Ayur-Veda as follows:

> Having been a poly-substance abuser for the last twenty years, I was nearly ready to give up and simply maintain a crippled lifestyle. I had studied TM in the 1970's, but my drug use had all but precluded its use in my daily life. After some promptings from my Maharishi Ayur-Veda-oriented physician, I began twice-daily meditation. Any attempt at describing the positive effects would be minimizing. It has been the only competing approach to altered consciousness that has been effective against the tremendous anxiety and craving produced

> by the drug withdrawal I have had to endure. After twenty minutes of meditation, I become relaxed, focused, and feel that my life has meaning. Meditation is so simple yet powerful that it seems almost impossible that its effect can be so valuable. My aftercare plan's foundation is the inclusion of this most useful tool. I would recommend its use unconditionally for those who suffer, as well as for those who are healthy but simply want to greatly improve their lives.

In summary, Maharishi Ayur-Veda has many practical applications to the field of both mental health and substance abuse rehabilitation. The theoretical underpinnings are sound and simple to understand, and the clinical application of the principles provides a significant contribution to the treatment modalities that we currently have in place in contemporary practice. I would strongly encourage my colleagues in the mental health and substance abuse-rehabilitation fields to explore some of the recent books written by Dr. Sharma, Dr. Wallace, and others (see Resources section of this book), and also to look at the rather extensive research being conducted in the clinical application of Maharishi Ayur-Veda to this branch of medicine. In addition, one-week physician training programs where one can learn to integrate Maharishi Ayur-Veda into one's daily clinical practice are also available.

REFERENCES

Alexander, C. N., Davies, J. L., Dixon, C. A., Dillbeck, M. C., Druker, S. M., Oetzel, R. M., Muehlman, J. M., & Orme-Johnson, D.W. (1990). Growth of higher stages of consciousness: Maharishi Mahesh Yogi's Vedic psychology of human development. In C. N. Alexander and E. J. Langer (Eds.), *Higher stages of human development: Perspectives on adult growth* (pp. 286-340). New York: Oxford University Press.

Averbach, R., & Rothenberg, S. (1989). *Fundamentals of Maharishi Ayur-Veda: Natural health care for the mind and body* [educational packet and videotape]. Lancaster, MA: Maharishi Ayur-Veda Products International.

Banquet, J. P. (1973). Spectral analysis of the EEG in meditation. *Electroencephalography and Clinical Neurophysiology, 35*, 143-151.

Bevan, A. W. (1980). Endocrine changes in Transcendental Meditation. *Clinical and Experimental Pharmacology and Physiology, 7*, 75-76.

Sushruta Samhita (1981). (K. L. Bhishagratna, Ed.). Varanasi, India: Chaukhamba Sanskrit Series Office.

Brooks, J., & Scarano T. (1986). Transcendental Meditation in the treatment of post-Vietnam adjustment. *Journal of Counseling and Development, 64*(3), 212-215.

Dillbeck, M. C., Cavanaugh, K. L., Glenn, T., Orme-Johnson, D. W., and Mittlefehldt, V. (1987). Consciousness as a field: The Transcendental Meditation and TM-Sidhi program and changes in social indicators. *The Journal of Mind and Behavior, 8*, 67-104.

Dillbeck, M. C., Landrith, G., & Orme-Johnson, D. W. (1981). The Transcendental Meditation program and crime rate change in a sample of 48 cities. *Journal of Crime and Justice, 4*, 25-45.

Glaser, J. L. (this volume). Clinical applications of Maharishi Ayur-Veda in chemical dependency disorders. *Alcoholism Treatment Quarterly.*

Hagelin, J. (1987). Is consciousness the unified field? A field theorist's perspective. *Modern Science and Vedic Science, 1*, 29-87.

Jevning, R. (1978). Adrenocortical activity during meditation. *Hormones and Behavior, 10*(1), 54-60.

Maharishi Mahesh Yogi. (1969). *On the Bhagavad Gita: A translation and commentary (Chapters 1-6).* Baltimore, MD: Penguin.

Maharishi Mahesh Yogi. (1986). *Life supported by natural law.* Fairfield, IA: Maharishi International University Press.

Orme-Johnson, D. W. (1973). Autonomic stability and Transcendental Meditation. *Psychosomatic Medicine, 35*, 341-349.

Orme-Johnson, D.W., Gelderloos, P., and Dillbeck, M. C. (1988). The effects of the Maharishi Technology of the Unified Field on the US quality of life (1960-1984). *Social Science Perspectives Journal,* 2(4), 127-146.

Schneider, R. H. (1985). Improvements in mental and physical health with Maharishi Ayur-Veda Panchakarma program. Paper presented at the 8th World Congress of the International College of Psychosomatic Medicine, Chicago, Illinois.

Seiler, G. (1979). The effects of Transcendental Meditation on periodontal tissue. *Journal of the American Society of Psychosomatic Dentistry and Medicine, 26* (1), 8-12.

Sharma, H. M. (1993). *Freedom from Disease*. Toronto: Veda Publishing.

Charaka Samhita, I. (1981). (P. V. Sharma, Ed. & Trans.).Delhi, India: Chaukhambha Orientalia.

Sharma, H. M. (1988). Effect of Maharishi Amrit Kalash (MAK) on brain opioid receptors. *FASEB, 2*, 4.

Wallace, R. K. (1970). Physiological effects of Transcendental Meditation, *Science, 167*, 1751-1754.

Wallace, R. K. (1972). The physiology of meditation. *Scientific American, 226*, 84-90.

Wallace, R. K. (1986). *The neurophysiology of enlightenment.* Fairfield, IA: Maharishi International University Press.

Wallace, R. K. (1993). *The physiology of consciousness.* Fairfield, IA: Maharishi International University Press.

The Family Practitioner and the Treatment of Alcoholism Through Maharishi Ayur-Veda: A Case Report

Linda Keniston-Dubocq, MD

INTRODUCTION

When I was a medical student in New York City, my impression of the alcoholic was quite literally the skid-row drunk who had lost his job, his home, his family and his health in his pursuit of bottled spirits. My clinical experience with alcoholism did not change much during my Family Practice Residency. My first Christmas as an intern was spent taking care of someone who was drunk, fell down a set of stairs, broke his neck, and almost froze to death. During my first few years of private practice in a middle class suburban neighborhood, the problem of alcoholism seemed to disappear. That changed five years ago when a patient who was also a substance abuse counselor suggested on my intake questionnaire that I ask patients about a family history of alcoholism and a personal history of substance abuse. A recovered alcoholic and addict, from a prominent New England family, she opened my eyes to a

---

Linda Keniston-Dubocq has a family practice at 151 Silver Street, Waterville, ME 04901.

[Haworth co-indexing entry note]: "The Family Practitioner and the Treatment of Alcoholism Through Maharishi Ayur-Veda: A Case Report." Keniston-Dubocq, Linda. Co-published simultaneously in the *Alcoholism Treatment Quarterly* (The Haworth Press, Inc.) Vol. 11, No. 3/4, 1994, pp. 413-428; and: *Self-Recovery: Treating Addictions Using Transcendental Meditation and Maharishi Ayur-Veda* (ed: David F. O'Connell and Charles N. Alexander) The Haworth Press, Inc., 1994, pp. 413-428. Multiple copies of this article/chapter may be purchased from The Haworth Document Delivery Center [1-800-3-HAWORTH; 9:00 a.m. - 5:00 p.m. (EST)].

different type of alcoholism, one that is very pervasive and democratic. I have since done much personal and professional work in the area of alcoholism through Twelve Step programs, workshops, and training seminars and now help to teach Family Practice residents about alcoholism.

Drug and alcohol abuse and related addictions, such as cigarette smoking, eating disorders, gambling and workaholism are extremely common. It is difficult to get accurate statistics on the exact prevalence of alcoholism, but it is estimated, depending on the diagnostic criteria used, that between 5%-10% of the population are alcoholic (Hilton 1987), and that 25% of patients in general hospitals have alcoholic problems (Moore et al., 1989). In addition to the medical problems associated with alcohol abuse, the illness can cause widespread disruption for the patient, the family and the community at large. For example, 50% of all fatal motor vehicle accidents are directly related to alcohol abuse (NIAAA, 1990 and NIDA, 1990). Most substance abuse counselors estimate up to 70% of the entire population has been affected by the abuse of alcohol and other drugs.

This presents an enormous problem for physicians in primary care, first in identifying patients with alcohol or alcohol related disorders, and secondly, in helping to orchestrate a comprehensive and effective treatment program. Alcoholism screening devices such as the CAGE questionnaire (Ewing, 1984), SMAST test (Selzer, Vinoker, & Van Rooijen, 1985) are very useful. Taking a psycho-social history, asking very specifically about issues of emotional and physical abuse, as well as a thorough medical history and exam are important (Brown, Carter, & Gordon 1987; Coulehan, Zettler-Segal, Block, McClelland & Schulberg, 1987). Also significant is a family history of alcoholism (Lanier, 1984). The etiology of alcoholism is multifactorial and may include genetic neurochemical defects, as well as environmental factors. Ultimately though, all substance abuse arises from a basic inability to fulfill the needs and desires of life satisfactorily, resulting in some physical or emotional pain that leads the suffering individual to seek relief from a substance or behavior even though the person knows that ultimately his actions are self-destructive. If a physician's job is to improve the quantity and quality of life, then this essential core of unhappiness must be treated.

Rehabilitation strategies for substance abuse have conventionally included counseling, Twelve Step programs such as Alcoholics Anonymous, alternative drug therapy, education, and in-patient treatment programs. It is the opinion of Alcoholics Anonymous (1976), the largest and most successful treatment organization, that true recovery from all addiction comes about as a result of a spiritual transformation. This process, which is never clearly defined by AA, but is fully supported by personal testimony, breaks the vicious cycle of frustration, tension, and self-destructive activity.

Transcendental Meditation (TM) greatly facilitates the effectiveness of any treatment approach. This has been documented in many studies over the past 20 years (Clements, Krenner, & Molk, 1988). Although not a rehabilitation program per se, TM is a self-development program that unlocks the individual's own creative intelligence, producing an overall and stable state of well-being that removes the craving and need for drugs.

TM is a core element of Maharishi Ayur-Veda, the ancient system of medicine of India that was introduced to the West by Maharishi Mahesh Yogi in collaboration with leading Ayurvedic physicians (Sharma, Triguna, & Chopra, 1991). Maharishi Ayur-Veda seeks to prevent disease, restore health, and promote longevity in the individual physiology by correcting imbalances in the disrupted self-regulatory homeostatic mechanisms. The individual is conceived of as a psychophysiologic unit comprising consciousness, mind, and body. Three psychophysiologic principles, called "doshas," regulate the different functions of the individual: Vata is said to underlie all processes involving motion in the body; Pitta pertains to all metabolic functions; and Kapha underlies all structural aspects of the nervous system (Sharma, 1993). Imbalances in the three doshas are responsible for all disease processes, including alcoholism (see the article by Dr. Sands in this volume for a full discussion of the doshas).

The Ayurvedic physician is trained to detect imbalances within the individual primarily through a special form of pulse diagnosis. There are more than twenty different treatment approaches in Maharishi Ayur-Veda in five main areas: consciousness, mind, body, behavior and environment. Specifically, these techniques include the use of TM, diet, exercise, herbs, panchakarma (purification techniques), aroma therapy, and music therapy, among others. For physicians involved in health maintenance and prevention, Maharishi Ayur-Veda adds new depth to the approach to a wide variety of medical problems. For those working in the area of substance abuse, Maharishi Ayur-Veda adds a powerful new dimension to the rehabilitation process. Maharishi Ayur-Veda specifically seeks to restore balance to the whole individual, in a non-pharmacological way.

To illustrate better how Ayurvedic techniques can mesh with conventional rehabilitation strategies, the following case about a young woman's recovery process is presented. This case was selected because it is representative of many of the common problems faced by alcoholics. These include a history of alcoholism within the family of origin, physical and emotional abuse, low self-esteem, dysthymia (unhappiness), anxiety, anorexia, alienation, and relationship problems. The patient was willing to try both conventional and Ayurvedic treatment modalities in her recovery process, with an excellent outcome despite many stressful environmental factors. (This case is presented with the permission of the patient. In order to ensure confidentiality, some details of her social history have been changed.)

CASE PRESENTATION

The patient was a 32-year-old white female who presented with complaints of insomnia, depression and anxiety. She was an attorney in private practice with her husband, also an attorney, and had two children less than five years of age. She had been married for six years.

The patient had been generally very well except for an overwhelming feeling of fatigue. She had no major surgeries, took no medications, and had never been hospitalized. She admitted that during college her weight dropped to 95 pounds and she had been amenorrheic during that time.

Two months prior to her consultation, her husband announced to her that he was very unhappy in the marriage and was thinking about a divorce. Since then she had experienced extreme insomnia and had been drinking two to three glasses of wine almost nightly to help her sleep, and would drink after work two to three times a week to relieve severe headaches. She also had intense bowel spasms and chronic constipation. Another doctor had prescribed Xanax as an anxiety reducer but she found that it made her too "groggy and spacey."

The patient expressed a strong desire for a non-pharmacological approach to her symptoms and was very worried about her own use of alcohol. The patient's physical exam was entirely normal except for a moderate kyphoscoliosis. Her weight was 115 pounds, BP 100/70. CBC, SMA-17, and lipid studies were also normal. In terms of Maharishi Ayur-Veda she had a marked Vata imbalance, indicating problems with anxiety, sleep and constipation; a Pitta imbalance that pointed to deeply rooted emotional conflicts; and a Kapha imbalance that indicated back pain. The pulse diagnosis also revealed that the patient's overall vitality was very suppressed.

The treatment program was comprehensive, comprising both conventional and Ayurvedic components. She was referred to a psychologist who was sensitive to issues of spirituality to help her cope with some of the severe emotional issues of the divorce. She was also referred to an osteopathic doctor for manipulation therapy for treatment of her headaches and back pain. Multiple modalities of Maharishi Ayur-Veda were also employed. In addition to her practice of the TM program, herbal supplements, including a supplement to help her sleep (MA-107), one to facilitate digestion (MA-154), and Maharishi Amrit Kalash (see below), were strongly recommended. The patient was strongly advised to be as regular as possible in terms of her daily routine, and to go to bed before 10:00 p.m. Aroma therapy and a light stretching exercise routine were suggested. The patient was also strongly encouraged to have panchakarma (physiological purification) done as soon as possible.

The issue of the patient's drinking was gently addressed during the first consultation. The patient readily admitted she was drinking and clearly wanted to stop. Both her parents were alcoholic and her father had died when she was 18 years old, of a drug overdose. She had never attended any Twelve Step programs such as Alcoholics Anonymous but was willing to go to Adult Children of Alcoholics.

At this point she did not think her drinking impaired her in any way. She thought of herself as a "potential alcoholic," especially given her family history.

The patient followed most of the recommendations. After a few sessions in therapy, the patient realized how abusive, both physically and emotionally, her husband was to her and how that was related to her having been abused as a child. When she realized that there was little hope of her husband changing, she decided to proceed with the divorce. The divorce itself was very complicated and stressful for the patient. She was followed by a private detective, was twice physically assaulted in her office by her husband, and by an unusual court order was forced to live only on alternate weeks in her own home and thus during weeks not at home was unable to see her children.

Despite these significant stressors, the patient's physical symptomatology improved. She had more energy, was sleeping better, had no constipation and far fewer headaches. She started dating again and developed a new circle of friends. She still drank on occasion, largely to help her sleep. Approximately nine months after the patient presented to therapy, she learned that her son had also been abused by her husband. She went on an all-night drinking binge and at times was suicidal. After this, she reluctantly agreed to go to a substance abuse counselor, and after much encouragement started to attend AA meetings on a regular basis. All therapists involved were actively supporting her recovery through Ayurvedic techniques and Twelve Step programs.

The next several months were very difficult for the patient. For the first time in her life, through her work in AA and strongly supported by her Ayurvedic routine, she became more in touch with her emotions. She had been denying for years how destructive her family had been. Years and years of grief and held-in anger finally began to surface. The patient came to understand how much she had abused alcohol as a drug to medicate feelings of anxiety, anger, depression, and loneliness. After she decided to stop drinking, her subjective experiences during meditation became clearer and more satisfying and, despite some very obvious stressful external forces, she started to experience greater levels of internal well-being, joy, vitality, and a sense of purpose. After nine months of sobriety she underwent a five-day course of panchakarma therapies which consisted of medicated oil massages, herbalized steam treatments, and other gentle purification techniques.

The patient also had a Maharishi Jyotish consultation and a Maharishi Yagya was recommended. Maharishi explains that Maharishi Jyotish is an approach of Maharishi Ayur-Veda that is based on the premise that all creation unfolds in a sequence that is so orderly that it is subject to calculation. Through the mathematical techniques of Jyotish, trends and tendencies of individual life can be located within the sequentially unfolding pattern of life (Morris, 1990). The practical value of this knowledge is that in advance, one can determine if some difficult period of life is coming. Therefore, action in the present can be undertaken to amend a future difficulty. Techniques to handle the future in the present are called Maharishi Yagyas (Morris, 1990). Yagyas are Vedic procedures (sometimes called Vedic engineering) which utilize the primordial sounds of nature (sounds from the Vedic Literature), and are designed, and are to restore balance between the individual and the environment. They are performed by specially trained Vedic experts. In this particular case, a Maharishi Yagya was done with the intent of settling domestic disputes. Two months later the patient received a favorable settlement in her highly contested divorce.

The patient seemed to be doing extremely well in her recovery process until she started having memories of being badly abused as a child by her father (who incidentally was a physician). The patient was still in regular psychotherapy, attending AA, and was in a group for Adult Children of Alcoholics. She did not resume drinking, but again started having severe bouts of insomnia, headaches, mood swings and muscular cramps. Because of the intense nature of her muscular spasms which were causing severe headaches and backaches, she was referred to a physical therapist who specialized in treating survivors of abuse.

Gandharva Veda music was recommended to help relieve some of the distress caused by her negative memories. The music of Gandharva Veda is explained by Maharishi to be the melodies and rhythms of nature itself, rather than the compositions of individual composers (Morris, 1990). Its purpose is to neutralize stress in the atmosphere and create a harmonizing and balancing influence for the individual. The sounds of Maharishi Ayur-Veda vary according to the time of day and the change of the season, since at these times, different laws of nature preside. When the appropriate Gandharva Veda music is played at the correct time, the physiology of the listener and his environment can be brought into balance. The patient played this music at low volume 24 hours a day in her home and over the next few months found her insomnia and mood swings greatly improved.

The patient is currently doing very well. She has been completely sober for two years and occasionally attends AA meetings. She is in a new, committed relationship and has developed a very good support system of friends within her community. Her professional practice is flourishing. Her outlook on life is cheerful and hopeful. Despite significant stresses, both past and present, she lost no time from work, suffered only minor illnesses such as colds and took no medications other than an occasional aspirin, during the three years of her recovery process. This is remarkable considering that women admitting abuse have been diagnosed with more long-term chronic illness and more lifetime surgeries than women denying abuse (Radomsky, 1992).

CASE DISCUSSION

Women who experienced childhood trauma due to abuse have symptoms that closely fit the diagnostic criteria for post-traumatic stress disorder as defined by the psychiatric criteria, the DSM-III-R (Lindberg, 1985). These symptoms include anxiety, guilt, recurring nightmares or intrusive daytime imagery. Other long-term self-destructive behavior patterns include substance abuse, feelings of worthlessness, suicide or suicide attempts, isolation and/or emotional humbling. The childhood trauma survivor, like the Vietnam veteran, has a latency period of repression, denial, and emotional avoidance following the severe trauma. This latency period, which can last up to decades, is followed by an intrusive-repetitive phase in which disquieting symptoms of nightmares, etc., recur. Just as Transcendental Meditation has been found to be effective in the treatment of post-Vietnam adjustment disorder (Brooks & Scarano, 1986), it follows that it might also be useful in the treatment of other traumatic events such as childhood abuse. TM can mitigate abreactive experience (in which prior negative experiences are remembered or relived) and allow patients maximum comfort while they are removing imbalances and creating a more integrated neurophysiological state.

This case illustrates the great power of Maharishi Ayur-Veda coupled with conventional approaches in the treatment of substance abuse. The patient had developed dysfunctional patterns of behavior, including drinking, because of deeply rooted feelings of pain and separation as a result of severe childhood trauma. Unaware of this past, she repeated the patterns of her abuse in her marriage. Her anorexia nervosa resolved innocently without intervention. Her level of alcohol addiction was mild by DSM-III-R criteria, but she was considered truly alcoholic. Although it never caused any interference with her functioning at work or any physiological problems, clearly it emotionally handicapped the patient. The use of TM helped the patient tap into her own inner resources of creative intelligence, allowing her to fully capitalize on all the other treatment modalities, making her recovery a smoother process. The Ayurvedic techniques also helped many of her physical symptoms of imbalance such as insomnia, headaches, and fatigue, which might otherwise have led to more substance abuse. Most importantly, despite bouts of depression, she never completely lost her sense of purpose in life. In fact, she felt ever-increasing feelings of joy and well-being throughout the recovery process. The patient felt that the single most important component of her recovery process was her continued practice of the TM program.

The abuse of drugs, as illustrated by this and many other cases, is strongly connected to internal psychological processes (Long & Scherl, 1984). Psychological distress, with its attendant emotional and physical disequilibrium, is very important in the problematic use of drugs. Lack of direction in life, low self-esteem, alienation, depression and meaninglessness coalesce into a feeling of helplessness on the part of the substance abuser. In addition to this lack of coping resources, a stressful environment may trigger substance abuse. This stress may include difficulties in family relations, general economic difficulties, or problems in the work or school environment. Another important factor, the depletion of neurotransmitter systems (Tennett, 1985) has been implicated in the development and continuation of substance abuse.

Ayurvedic herbal compounds called *rasayanas* are described as having the effects of increasing resistance to disease and promoting longevity. Studies done by Dr. Sharma and his colleagues (Sharma, Hanissian, Rattan, Stern, & Tejwani, 1991), suggest that one of these rasayanas, known as Maharishi Amrit Kalash (MAK), modulates the activity of brain opioid receptors in the direction of interacting selectively with molecules associated with a wide range of positive affects including well-being, contentment and happiness. He found that MAK blocked delta receptors, which may help calm the central nervous system. MAK also prevented the binding of antagonist molecules understood to be associated with negative mood opiod receptors in the brain. Finally, in depressed individuals, MAK was associated with a reduction of depression scores on the Beck Depression Inventory and the SCL-90-R.

In this particular case, the patient was experiencing chronic psychological distress for obvious reasons. Almost all individuals who have come from abusive, alcoholic, or otherwise dysfunctional homes have some elements of dysthymia, low self-esteem, and alienation. (In recovery literature this is commonly referred to as the syndrome of Adult Children of Alcoholics.) Considering the enormous stress and poor coping skills that the patients have, it is easy to speculate that they may have an alteration in their neurochemistry that may induce them to seek mood-altering drugs.

This patient was treated in a very conventional manner beginning with a careful drug and alcohol history, referral to appropriate counselors and therapists, and participation in Alcoholics Anonymous (Khantzian, 1985). Some of the Ayurvedic modalities which have been shown to be clinically effective (but not yet widely studied scientifically), were much appreciated by the patient. These included panchakarma, aroma therapy, Maharishi Jyotish, specialized herbs for specific symptoms, and recommendations about daily and seasonal routine. Two of the most powerful tools of Maharishi Ayur-Veda, TM and MAK, have been studied and show great promise in the treatment of substance abuse. A large number of studies have shown that TM reduces psychological distress (Gelderloos, Walton, Orme-Johnson, & Alexander, 1990; Geisler, 1978;

Alexander et al., 1990; Dillbeck, 1977; Dillbeck & Orme-Johnson, 1987; Ferguson & Gowan, 1976). TM has also been shown to enhance serotonin turnover (Bujatti & Riederer, 1976). TM and MAK taken together address both the main issues of psychological distress and physiologic depletion of neurotransmitters and may have been key elements in the patient's recovery.

COMMENTARY

Eric Fromm (1956) believes that the unique characteristic of being human is that "life [is] aware of itself." He points out that while this affords the opportunity for more control over life, it can also result in a sense of separation from others and the larger environment. Maharishi (1983) has explained that love is that powerful force that can unify or overcome any separations that we may experience in our lives; he states that love takes life from the pangs of separation to the bliss of eternal union. We naturally grow in our capacity for union through love throughout the course of human development. Maharishi (1983, pp. 18-19) writes:

> In its most infant state love finds an expression on the lap of mother, in the sweetness of the mother's eyes. It grows in toys and playfields, in the sweetness of friends and folks of society, it grows in the sweetness of husband and wife. With age and experience, the tree of love grows; it grows with the growth of life and evolution and finds its fulfillment in the eternal love of the omnipresent God, which fills the heart and overthrows the darkness of ignorance.

Thus, during what may be called the first phase of love during early childhood, potential feelings of separateness are simply overcome by the mother's comforting presence. As the child grows, the sense of separation is overcome through loving relationships with friends and family. The child learns to trust and enjoy life innocently.

This natural process of the development of love as described by Maharishi can become stunted and distorted in dysfunctional homes. In my clinical experience, feelings of separation, far from being overcome, are frighteningly reinforced in dysfunctional homes. Fear, distrust, anxiety, further separation, and shame can build up. Extreme degrees of self-alienation can result in dissociative states and other emotional disorders. The problem of alcoholism can often involve such a feeling of intense shame, a feeling that the individual is inherently evil merely because he exists. This kind of shame, termed "toxic shame" (Bradshaw, 1988), is caused by a basic feeling of separation of the individual from his true self.

For patients from dysfunctional homes, this lack of connection to the self leads to further dysfunctional patterns. For instance, the individual may seek attention by being an overachiever, a clown, an enabler, a delinquent. The intellect mistakenly assumes that getting approval for oneself by one's achievements, appearances, or possessions will restore this loss of self-worth. Unfortunately, when this fabricated shell crumbles because of external stressors, the individual feels more ashamed and resorts to more self-destructive methods of coping, including substance abuse.

Maharishi Ayur-Veda, especially the practice of TM, can break this cycle of disaster. TM is a simple, natural, scientific technique that reconnects the individual to his inner or "higher Self." According to Maharishi (1969, p. 339), the lower self refers to the ordinary individual self which is experienced as localized in space and time and as constantly changing in response to the environment. In contrast, the higher Self is described as that innermost aspect of the personality which never changes, the silent completely tranquil state of Being, which is the very basis of the entire field of change, including the individual self. Unfortunately, outwardly caught up in our everchanging stressful lives, we lose contact with the silent inner state of Being. When individuals are able to experience the inner Self, they are able to experience pure happiness or bliss deep within, which is the essence of their true Being. This experience of inner bliss and self-contentment dissolves feelings of toxic shame. As this experience of inner bliss grows, it begins to naturally spill out in the form of more loving feelings toward others in our environment (Maharishi, 1969, p. 307). Life is no longer a stupefying, painful experience but becomes one of continuous joy and evolution. This is the Light that overpowers the darkness.

This healing process is also the goal of Twelve Step recovery programs, although the language used is different. These programs provide the individual with much educational material in terms of literature and personal testimony about both the problem of addiction and means through which it can be overcome. More importantly, they give group support and a sense of connection to someone else trying to cope with similar problems. Perhaps most essentially, Twelve Step programs offer a hope that recovery is possible. The addition of TM would make these programs far easier and more effective. Through releasing stress from the nervous system and unfolding one's inner Self, the TM program would provide a strong inner foundation for more fully achieving all the steps of recovery–especially Steps 3 and 11 which are directly concerned with realizing one's full spiritual potential. O'Connell (this volume) provides a more detailed account of how TM can facilitate the different phases of recovery; Glaser (this volume) elaborates on how the other approaches of Maharishi Ayur-Veda may complement and enrich Twelve Step programs.

The physician can be very instrumental in the recovery process. The case presented illustrates the multifaceted nature of the illness and how the family practitioner (and other healthcare professionals) can intervene to help resolve this problem. Alcoholics may present themselves to their doctors with a variety of symptoms that may make the diagnosis of a substance abuse problem difficult. These include psychosomatic complaints and concurrent mental disorders, along with a family history of alcoholism and a personal history of trauma. There is a continuum of substance use and abuse starting from abstinence and moving to non-problematic use, misuse, abuse and dependence. Classification of the type of substance abuse is important in developing a long-term treatment plan. However, in the initial phases of diagnosis and treatment, it is perhaps most important to simply recognize that there is some type of substance abuse problem. Randomized controlled trials suggest that even brief interventions by health care providers can reduce substance use in those who are not dependent (U.S. Preventive Services Task Force, 1989).

A physician trained in Maharishi Ayur-Veda learns how to treat the patient holistically. The consciousness, mind, and body are treated as one integrated wholeness, and all complaints are considered valid and remediable. Treatment focuses on correcting basic imbalances in the psychophysiology of the patient. Pain can be eliminated at its source by a variety of modalities such as TM, Gandharva Veda music, and herbs that produce side benefits rather than deleterious side effects. Perhaps most important is the physicians' own growing sense of intuition and self-awareness that naturally arises through their personal use of the TM program and practice of sensitive Ayurvedic pulse diagnosis techniques for detecting imbalances in psychophysiological functioning (in one's own functioning as well as that of others). The healing process really starts when physicians listen with their hearts as well as their minds. When the doctor truly understands the patient's problem, love is working. When the doctor cares and trusts in the patient's own intrinsic ability to heal, the doctor is helping to place the patient back on a natural path to restoring balance. This intrinsic process of healing, gently yet powerfully nurtured through the approaches of Maharishi Ayur-Veda, allows the forces of life to once again flow spontaneously and harmoniously in accordance with the laws of nature. Through this process, full recovery and perfect health and happiness are naturally generated.

REFERENCES

Alcoholics Anonymous, 3rd edition. (1976). New York, NY: Author.

Alexander, C. N., Davies, J. L., Dixon, C. A., Dillbeck, M. C., Druker, S. M., Oetzel, R. M., Muehlman, J. M., & Orme-Johnson, D.W. (1990). Growth of higher stages of consciousness: Maharishi Mahesh Yogi's Vedic psychology of human development. In C. N. Alexander and E. J. Langer (Eds.), *Higher stages of human development: Perspectives on adult growth* (pp. 286-340). New York: Oxford University Press.

Bradshaw, J. (1988). *Healing the shame that binds you.* Deerfield Beach, FL: Florida Health Communications.

Brooks, J. & Scarano, T. (1985). Transcendental Meditation in the treatment of post-Vietnam adjustment. *Journal of Counseling and Development, 64*(3), 212-215.

Brown, R. L., Carter, W. B., Gordon, M. J. (1987). Diagnosis of alcoholism in a simulated patient encounter by primary care physicians. *Journal of Family Practice, 25*, 259-264.

Bujatti, J., & Riederer, P. (1976). Serotonin, noradrenaline, dopamine metabolites in Transcendental Meditation technique. *Journal of Neurotransmitters, 39*, 257-267.

Clements, G., Krenner, L., & Molk, W. (1988). The use of the Transcendental

Meditation program in the prevention of drug abuse and in the treatment of drug-addicted persons. *Bulletin on Narcotics, 40*(1), 51-56.

Coulehan, J. L., Zettler-Segal, M., Block, M., McClelland, M., & Schulberg, H. C. (1987). Recognition of alcoholism and substance abuse in primary care patients. *Archives of Internal Medicine, 147,* 349-352.

Diagnostic and statistical manual of mental disorders. (3rd Edition Revised). (1987). (pp. 165-169). Washington, DC: American Psychiatric Association.

Dillbeck, M. C. (1977). The effect of the Transcendental Meditation technique on anxiety level. *Journal of Clinical Psychology, 33,* 1076-1078.

Dillbeck, M. C., & Orme-Johnson, D.W. (1987). Physiological differences between Transcendental Meditation and rest. *American Psychologist, 42,* 879-881.

Ewing, J. A. (1984). Detecting alcoholism: The CAGE questionnaire. *Journal of American Medical Association, 252,* 1905-1907.

Ferguson, P. C., & Gowan, J. C. (1976). Psychological findings on Transcendental Meditation. *Journal of Humanistic Psychology, 16*(3), 51- 60.

Fromm, E. (1956). *The art of loving.* New York: Harper & Row.

Geisler, M. (1978). Therapeutische Wirkungun der Transcendentalen Meditation auf Drogenkonsumenten [Therapeutic effects of Transcendental Meditation in drug abusers]. *Zeitschrift fur Klinische Psychologie, 7,* 235-255.

Gelderloos, P., Walton, K. G., Orme-Johnson, D.W., & Alexander, C. N. (1990). The effectiveness of the Transcendental Meditation program in preventing and treating substance abuse: A review. *The International Journal of the Addictions, 26,* 293-325.

Glaser, J. L. (this volume). Clinical applications of Maharishi Ayur-Veda in chemical dependency disorders. *Alcoholism Treatment Quarterly.*

Hilton, M. E. (1987). Drinking patterns and drinking problems in 1984: Results from a general population survey. *Alcoholism, 11,* 167-175.

Khantzian, E. (1985). The injured self, addiction and our call to medicine. *Journal of American Medical Association, 254,* 249-252.

Lanier, D. K. (1984). Familial alcoholism. *The Journal of Family Practice, 18*(3), 415-422.

Lindberg, F. M. (1985). Post-traumatic stress disorders in women who experienced childhood incest. *Child Abuse and Neglect, 9,* 329-334.

Long, J.V. F. & Scherl, D. J. (1984). Developmental antecedents of compulsive drug use: A report on the literature. *Journal of Psychoactive Drugs, 16,* 169-182.

Maharishi Mahesh Yogi. (1969). *On the Bhagavad Gita: A new translation and commentary.* Baltimore, MD: Penguin.

Maharishi Mahesh Yogi. (1983). *Love and God.* USA: Age of Enlightenment Press.

Moore, R. D., Bone, L. R., Geller, G., Marrion, J. A., Stokes, J., & Levine, D. M. (1989). Prevalence, detection and treatment of alcoholism in hospitalized patients. *Journal of American Medical Association 261,* 403-407.

Morris, B. (1990). Introduction to Volume 5. In R.K. Wallace, D.W. Orme-Johnson, & M. C. Dillbeck (Eds.), *Scientific research on Maharishi's Tran-*

scendental Meditation and TM-Sidhi program: Collected papers, Vol. 5. Fairfield, IA: Maharishi International University Press.

National Institute on Alcoholism and Alcohol Abuse. (1990). *Seventh special report to US Congress on alcohol and health*. Rockville, MD: Author.

National Institute on Drug Abuse. (1990). *Third triennial report to US Congress*, Rockville, MD: NIDA.

O'Connell, D. F. (this volume). Possessing the Self: Maharishi Ayur-Veda and the process of recovery from addictive diseases. *Alcoholism Treatment Quarterly*.

Radomsky, N. (1992). The association of parental alcoholism and rigidity with chronic illness and abuse among women. *Journal of Family Practice, 35*, 54-60.

Sands, D. (this volume). Introducing Maharishi Ayur-Veda into clinical practice. *Alcoholism Treatment Quarterly*.

Selzer, M. L., Vinoker, A., & Van Rooijen, L. (1985). A self-administered short Michigan alcoholism screening test. *Journal of Studies on Alcohol, 36*(l), 117-126.

Sharma, M., Hanissian, S., Rattan, A. K., Stern, S. L., Tejwani, G. A. (1991). Effect of Maharishi Amrit Kalash on brain opioid receptors and neuropeptides. *Journal of Research Education Ind. Medicine, 10*, 1-8.

Sharma, H. M., Triguna, B. D., & Chopra, D. (1991). Maharishi Ayurveda: Modern insights into ancient medicine, *Journal of American Medical Association, 265*, 2633-2637.

Sharma, H. M. (1993). *Freedom from disease*. Toronto: Veda Publishing.

Tennett, F. S. (1985). *Primer on neurochemistry of drug dependence*. West Covina, CA: Veract.

US Preventive Services Task Force. (1989). *Guide to clinical preventive services*. Baltimore, MD: Williams & Wilkins.

Implementation of the Transcendental Meditation Program and Maharishi Ayur-Veda to Prevent Alcohol and Drug Abuse Among Juveniles at Risk

Hari M. Sharma, MD
Michael C. Dillbeck, PhD
Susan L. Dillbeck, PhD

SUMMARY. The purpose of the proposed treatment program is to provide a holistic, natural approach to prevent alcohol and drug abuse among high-risk preadolescent and adolescent children by reducing psychological distress and physiological imbalance, and by enhancing protective resources through an individual and family program. To achieve this goal, juveniles referred for alcohol and drug abuse treatment and also their families participate in a special treatment implementing the Transcendental Meditation program and aspects of a natural system of health care known as Maharishi Ayur-Veda. A large body of scientific research has demonstrated that this program reduces anxiety, depression, and hostility; increases psy-

---

Hari M. Sharma is Professor of Pathology and Director of Cancer Prevention and Natural Products Research at The Ohio State University College of Medicine, Columbus, OH. Michael C. Dillbeck is Professor of Psychology at Maharishi International University, Fairfield, IA. Susan L. Dillbeck is Professor of Education at Maharishi International University, Fairfield, IA.

[Haworth co-indexing entry note]: "Implementation of the Transcendental Meditation Program and Maharishi Ayur-Veda to Prevent Alcohol and Drug Abuse Among Juveniles At Risk." Sharma, Hari M., Michael C. Dillbeck, and Susan L. Dillbeck. Co-published simultaneously in the *Alcoholism Treatment Quarterly* (The Haworth Press, Inc.) Vol. 11, No. 3/4, 1994, pp. 429-457; and: *Self-Recovery: Treating Addictions Using Transcendental Meditation and Maharishi Ayur-Veda* (ed: David F. O'Connell and Charles N. Alexander) The Haworth Press, Inc., 1994, pp. 429-457. Multiple copies of this article/chapter may be purchased from The Haworth Document Delivery Center [1-800-3-HAWORTH; 9:00 a.m. - 5:00 p.m. (EST)].

chophysiological balance and resistance to stress; promotes more harmonious relations; and most importantly, naturally reduces dependence on alcohol, drugs, and other substances. The key components of the treatment program are the following: twice-daily practice of the Transcendental Meditation technique; twice-daily use of the herbal food supplement Maharishi Amrit Kalash; daily after-school sessions to ensure regularity and maximum benefit; a weekly treatment/class meeting for participants to understand their own experience of developing consciousness in the context of unifying principles that apply equally to their academic studies, to society, and to nature as a whole; and parental and peer participation. Structure and details of the proposed treatment program are outlined in the paper, as well as details of treatment outcome evaluation and procedures to evaluate the successful implementation of the program.

INTRODUCTION

Need for a Holistic and Positive Approach to Prevention and Treatment of Alcohol Abuse

Alcohol addiction and other addictive behaviors have multiple and interacting causes (Jones & Battjes, 1985). The environment plays an important role as either a risk or protective factor in the exposure of young people to alcohol and other addictive substances, including the influences of parents and peers as models (Baumrind, 1985; Evans, Rozelle, Berry, & Havis, 1978; Margulies, Kessler, & Kandel, 1977; Patterson, 1982). At the same time, the development of a chronic habit of dependence is strongly influenced by such internal factors as lack of coping or protective resources and the presence of risk factors such as psychological distress (Long & Scherl, 1984; Wills & Shiffman, 1985). These risk factors include depression (Paton, Kessler, & Kandel, 1977), anxiety or emotional distress (Swaim, Oetting, Edwards, & Beauvais, 1989), and antisocial behavior (Jessor & Jessor, 1978; Jones, 1968; Robins, 1978). Among the psychological resources supporting resistance to chronic alcohol and drug use are school success (Dryfoos, 1990), self-esteem (Steffenhagen, 1980; see Jessor & Jessor, 1978, for a discussion of inconclusive findings in this area), and field independence (Kalliopuska, 1982). Although there are mixed results in studies of whether field dependence is a predisposing factor or consequence of alcohol abuse, field independence is found to increase as a result of therapy (Drejer et al., 1985; Lafferty & Kahn, 1986; Tartar et al., 1986). In addition to the social and psychological influences on alcohol and drug abuse, the physiological effects of addictions, such as depletion of neurotransmitters, have also begun to come to light (Tennant, 1985). Alcohol abuse results in a greatly increased level of free radicals in the body (Fink et al., 1985), which are implicated in up to 80% of all diseases, including aging (Niwa, Kasama, Miyachi, & Kanoh, 1989; Richards & Sharma, 1991). Also, in chronic alcoholics glutathione, a free radical scavenger, is decreased (Lieber, 1988).

This paper thus assumes the following risk and protective factors for alcohol and drug abuse:

1 Risk factors: depression; anxiety and emotional distress; rebelliousness and antisocial behavior.
2. Protective factors: school success; self-esteem; field independence; mature family interaction and positive parental role modeling; peer support.

Because of the complexity of the factors influencing addiction to alcohol and drugs, the effectiveness of treatment and prevention programs has been limited. In the area of alcoholism treatment, review studies indicate very small treatment effects, and small effects of variations in treatment, such as length (Emrick, 1975; Miller & Hester, 1986).

Similar limited results are found for prevention programs for adolescents (Bangert-Drowns, 1988; Tobler, 1986). It has been proposed that comprehensive preventive interventions may be more effective than those addressed only to the individual level (Benard, 1986).

We conclude that there is a need for a comprehensive prevention program for young people at risk for alcohol and drug abuse, which addresses all levels of the individual's functioning–cognitive, emotional, physiological, and behavioral–as well as the social environment.

The Transcendental Meditation Program–A Natural Technology for Holistic Development

Maharishi's Transcendental Meditation (TM) is a simple mental technique practiced twice daily, sitting quietly with eyes closed.

The technique has been learned by four million people worldwide, including one million Americans. It is practiced by people of all cultures and religious faiths; it requires no beliefs or change in lifestyle. The technique is simple to learn and easy to practice; however, it requires systematic instruction by a qualified teacher to ensure correct practice. The technique is taught in a uniform manner worldwide. The course of instruction for the general public is given over four days, with a systematic follow-up program thereafter (Roth, 1987). When the technique is offered as part of a treatment program, on either a residential or non-residential basis, an intensive program is structured after initial instruction to provide confirmation of correct practice and intellectual understanding of the development being naturally experienced by the participants.

Transcendental Meditation is a technique for holistic personal development rather than a specific treatment program for alcohol or substance abuse. It is a systematic technology for the development of consciousness (Roth, 1987). At the same time, it has been highly successful in treatment and prevention of alcohol and substance abuse. (For an excellent review of this research, please refer to Gelderloos, Walton, Orme-Johnson, & Alexander, 1991.) The reason for this success is that the program genuinely promotes holistic personal development, and in so doing it alleviates many of the risk factors for alcohol and substance abuse and promotes many of the protective factors that naturally guard against addiction.

One way to understand the holistic effects of Transcendental Meditation is that the technique promotes advanced levels of human development that naturally extend current conceptions of developmental psychology (Alexander et al., 1990; Dillbeck & Alexander, 1989). The growth that is fostered by the technique is holistic and natural in much the same way that human development, particularly through adolescence, is holistic and natural, encompassing the physiological, cognitive, affective, and social-behavioral domains.

The Transcendental Meditation program is the most widely researched program of personal development. During the past 22 years, there have been over 500 research studies conducted in 25 countries on the effects of the technique. Many of these studies have been published in leading research journals. The first 430 research studies have been collected in five volumes (Chalmers et al., 1989a,

1989b, 1989c; Orme-Johnson & Farrow, 1977; Wallace, Orme-Johnson, & Dillbeck, 1990). This section briefly reviews categories of the research on the general effects of the Transcendental Meditation program, referring the reader to other papers in this volume that review the same findings in greater detail, and addresses the significance of these general findings for influencing the risk/protective factors for alcohol and drug abuse. It also briefly reviews research studies that specifically implement the Transcendental Meditation program in prevention and treatment for abuse of alcohol and other substances.

Physiological Changes During the Practice

During the practice of Transcendental Meditation (TM), the participant experiences a unique state of restful alertness, as indicated by physiological measurements such as reduced respiration rate and plama lactate, and increased basal skin resistence (e.g., Dillbeck & Orme-Johnson, 1987; Wallace, 1970).

One area of the physiological effects of the Transcendental Meditation program that is particularly relevant to substance abuse treatment is that of its biochemical effects. In general, biochemical research indicates that the practice normalizes biochemical functioning, leading to a more balanced state of the key neurotransmitters most directly involved in psychological functioning. (For a review of this research in the context of alleviating substance addiction, please refer to Walton and Levitsky, this volume.) The importance of this research for prevention and treatment of alcohol and drug abuse is that the Transcendental Meditation program, by promoting physiological and biochemical balance and resistance to stress, addresses a very fundamental and substantive area of the effects of alcohol and drug use that is not usually directly addressed by treatment programs.

Physiological Effects of Maharishi Amrit Kalash

Ayur-Veda is a holistic system of health care originating in the ancient Vedic times of India. With the passage of time, knowledge of this system was fragmented or lost. Maharishi Mahesh Yogi, in collaboration with prominent Ayurvedic physicians and scholars, has rejuvenated and revived this health care system in accordance with the classical texts. This comprehensive and standardized restoration of Ayurvedic therapeutic approaches is known as Maharishi Ayur-Veda (Sharma, Triguna, & Chopra, 1991).

Maharishi Ayur-Veda includes various strategies for the maintenance and promotion of health and the prevention and treatment of disease. One of these approaches is the use of special herbal food supplements known as "rasayanas." These formulations are purported to enhance general well-being, maintain homeostasis, increase immunity and promote longevity. The most prominent of the rasayanas utilized in Maharishi Ayur-Veda are two formulations collectively known as Maharishi Amrit Kalash. These formulations consist of a paste form designated Maharishi Amrit Kalash-4 (M-4) and a tablet form designated Maharishi Amrit Kalash-5 (M-5). These herbal food supplements contain a collection of various herbs; the herbal content of M-4 is different from that of M-5. On analysis, these mixtures were found to contain low molecular weight substances and multiple antioxidants, including alpha-tocopherol, ascorbate, polyphenols, catechin, beta-carotene, flavonoids, riboflavin and tannic acid (Sharma, Dwivedi, Satter, & Abou-Issa, 1991; Sharma et al., 1990). Recent research on these mixtures has confirmed their health-promoting properties, including antineoplastic (Patel, Wang, Shen, Sharma, & Brahmi, 1992; Sharma, Dwivedi, Satter, & Abou-Issa, 1991; Sharma et al., 1990), immunomodulatory (Dileepan, Patel, Sharma, & Stechschulte, 1990; Niwa, 1991), cardioprotective (Panganamala & Sharma, 1991; Sharma, Feng, & Panganamala, 1989; Sharma, Hanna, Kauffman, & Newman, 1991), neurochemical (Sharma, Hanissian, Rattan, Stern, & Tejwani, 1991) and antioxidant (Dwivedi, Sharma, Dobrowski, & Engineer, 1991; Niwa, 1991; Panganamala & Sharma, 1991; Richards & Sharma, 1991; Sharma, Hanna et al., 1991) effects. These generalized effects most likely represent the prevention of widespread damage caused by free radicals and reactive oxygen species (ROS).

Free radicals and ROS are highly reactive, unstable atoms and molecules which are by-products of metabolism. They function to protect the body from microorganisms, fungi, parasites and viruses;

however, when generated in excessive amounts they can result in widespread injury to tissues and organs, mediated by damage to lipids (lipid peroxidation), proteins, carbohydrates, DNA and cell membranes. It is estimated that 80% of all human diseases, including aging, are related to damage caused by free radicals and ROS. Excessive production of free radicals is caused by alcohol abuse, smoking, environmental pollution, excessive exposure to sunlight, radiation, certain chemotherapeutic agents, fertilizers, pesticides, etc. (Richards & Sharma, 1991). Antioxidant compounds such as those found in M-4 and M-5 are effective in scavenging excess free radicals and ROS (Niwa, 1991), thereby preventing the damage that might otherwise occur.

Alcohol is known to produce excessive free radicals, resulting in widespread damage to tissues and organs (Fink et al., 1985). This damage can be prevented and treated by scavenging the excess free radicals. Both M-4 and M-5 have been found to decrease free radicals and ROS in vitro, in both cellular and noncellular systems (Niwa, 1991). It has also been found that the antioxidant effect of M-4 and M-5 is at least 1,000 times more potent than the antioxidants vitamin C, vitamin E and probucol (an antioxidant drug), when tested in vitro in the prevention of human plasma low density lipoprotein peroxidation (Sharma, Hanna et al., 1991). This antioxidant activity of M-4 and M-5 may prove very beneficial in the prevention and treatment of alcohol abuse.

Maharishi Amrit Kalash-5 has also been found to decrease brain opioid receptor activity in vitro (Sharma, Hanissian et al., 1991), a property which could be useful in preventing substance abuse. In a study conducted on the in vitro effect of M-5 on brain opioid receptors and neuropeptides, a generalized inhibition of opioid receptor activity was seen. M-5 inhibited the activity of mu, kappa, and delta receptors. Mu receptors are specific for morphine; the inhibition of these receptors indicates M-5 may be effective in blocking the activity of exogenous opioid compounds, thereby proving useful in the prevention and treatment of drug abuse. Delta receptors bind enkephalins, natural morphine-like substances which are produced within the body; the inhibition of these receptors may indicate an ability of M-5 to decrease excessive cellular activity, thereby calming the system.

A further indication of the possible usefulness of M-5 in the prevention and treatment of substance abuse is the finding of significantly reduced Substance P levels ($p < 0.01$) in subjects who took M-5 for 3 months (Sharma, Hanissian et al., 1991). Substance P is a neurotransmitter involved in pain pathways, as well as pulmonary and gastrointestinal inflammation. The reduction of Substance P indicates M-5 may be helpful for the modulation of pain, a property which could prove useful in preventing individuals from turning to substance abuse for dealing with pain. Also, M-5 may be helpful for gastrointestinal inflammation, a condition commonly associated with alcohol abuse.

Reduction of Psychological Risk Factors

Practice of the Transcendental Meditation program reduces the psychological risk factors described below: depression, anxiety and emotional distress, and rebelliousness and antisocial behavior. Please refer to the paper by Alexander, Robinson, and Rainforth in this volume for a more extended discussion of effects on these factors.

Depression

Among the psychological effects of the Transcendental Meditation program replicated in a number of research studies is reduction of depression. For example, in a study of Vietnam veterans seeking treatment for problems of adjustment following service, veterans were randomly assigned to either an ongoing psychotherapy treatment program or to learn the Transcendental Meditation program (Brooks & Scarano, 1985). After three months, the group of TM participants showed reduced depression in contrast to controls; they also showed reduced anxiety, reduced family problems, increased employment, and reduced alcohol use.

Anxiety and Emotional Distress

A large body of research studies has repeatedly documented reduced anxiety and emotional problems among those who learn the Transcendental Meditation program. Perhaps the most important study in this area is a meta-analysis which found that the Transcendental Meditation program had approximately twice the effect size in reducing trait anxiety as did any other meditation or relaxation procedure (Eppley, Abrams, & Shear, 1989).

Rebelliousness and Antisocial Behavior

Antisocial behavior has been found to decrease among even the most hardened individuals–prison inmates–after beginning this program, as indicated by such effects as reduced recidivism (e.g., Bleick & Abrams, 1987). For an extensive review of this research, please refer to the paper by Alexander et al. in this volume.

Enhancement of Protective Factors Against Alcohol and Drug Abuse

Psychological and behavioral factors that protect against abuse of alcohol or drugs–school success, self-esteem, field independence, and mature family interaction and positive parental role modeling–have also been found to be enhanced through practice of the Transcendental Meditation program.

School Success

Research studies show that practice of the Transcendental Meditation program improves academic performance (Kember, 1985) and increases interest in continuing on to higher education (Penner, Zingle, Dyck, & Truch, 1974). The practice also enhances mental clarity, as indicated by tests of fluid intelligence (e.g., Cranson, 1989; Shecter, 1978), as well as reduces anxiety (see above), contributing to more effective academic performance.

Self-Esteem

Practice of the Transcendental Meditation program has been found to increase self-esteem among high school and college age students, including those with drug abuse problems (Geisler, 1978).

For a more extensive review of this research, please refer to Alexander et al. in this volume. A study of inner-city children who learned the Transcendental Meditation technique as part of an after-school program found that they showed improved self-concept and increased intellectual performance compared to matched controls receiving other after-school enrichment programs (Dillbeck, Clayborne, & Dillbeck, 1990).

Field Independence

Longitudinal research has demonstrated that students who learn the Transcendental Meditation program show increased field independence over a three-month period, in contrast to randomly assigned controls (Pelletier, 1974).

Mature Family Interaction and Positive Parental Role Modeling

Research on families that have learned the Transcendental Meditation program indicates that the parents show greater marital satisfaction and adjustment (Aron & Aron, 1982; Suarez, 1976), as well as increased emotional maturity, reduced anxiety, and an increase in the ability to be on the one hand sympathetic and compassionate and on the other hand objective and fair-minded (Marcus, 1977). These qualities also contribute to more effective parenting. Families that have learned Transcendental Meditation also demonstrate more healthy patterns of functioning (Chen, 1985). Research demonstrating reduction of alcohol and drug abuse among adults who learn the Transcendental Meditation program (please see below) indicates that through this program parents, other family members, or significant others will naturally become better role models for the children.

Reduction of Alcohol and Drug Abuse

There have been at least 18 studies demonstrating reduction in the use of alcohol and drugs among those who learn the Transcendental Meditation program. This research has progressed in design from retrospective surveys to prospective surveys, and also to implementation in treatment programs. Please refer to Gelderloos et al. [1991] for a detailed review of most of these studies, and to Alexander et al., in this volume, for meta-analysis of this research. For the sake of brevity, we will just note some of the treatment studies here.

In Germany, a study of 76 young people receiving crisis aid at a drug rehabilitation center (ages 15-23) assessed drug use retrospectively for the two years prior to treatment and each month after learning the TM program for one year (Schenkluhn & Geisler, 1977). Participants showed reduced usage of all types of drugs, with 75% reporting no drug use after six months. In Sweden, young drug users (ages 17-24) were randomly assigned to either group psychotherapy or participation in the Transcendental Meditation treatment program (Brautigam, 1977). After three months, TM participants showed decreased drug use and improved mental health compared to the other group. In the United States, members of a population with addiction problems at a V.A. hospital who learned the Transcendental Meditation program showed improved behavioral adjustment, as indicated by increased employment and reduced need for institutional care (Bielefeld, 1981). A study of low income chronic alcoholics in Washington, D.C. who were randomly assigned to either the Transcendental Meditation program, a standard treatment, or relaxation programs, studied participants during an initial treatment program of three months and afterward with regular field assessment for 18 months (Taub, Steiner, Smith, Weingarten, & Walton, this volume). After 18 months, 65% of the participants in the TM program were completely abstinent, compared with 25% of the patients receiving standard treatment. The muscle relaxation group also demonstrated favorable results. This study indicates that the Transcendental Meditation program is an appropriate treatment for disadvantaged and chronically addicted populations.

Summary of Effects of the Program on Risk and Protective Factors

Table 1 summarizes the effects of the Transcendental Meditation program in alleviating the risk factors for alcohol and drug abuse and in strengthening the protective factors against abuse. In order to take advantage of the potential positive influence of the family and

TABLE 1

TREATMENT	RISK/PROTECTIVE FACTORS	OUTCOME MEASURES
Maharishi Amrit Kalash	Risk factor: Physiological imbalance	Reduction of free radicals
Transcendental Meditation Program (increased psychophysiological integration)	Risk factors: Depression Anxiety and emotional distress Rebelliousness and antisocial behavior	 Reduced depression Reduced anxiety Reduced hostility Fewer school discipline problems
	Protective factors: School success	 Improved academic performance Reduced absenteesim Improved teacher ratings (school behavior, school performance)
	Self-esteem Field independence	Increased self-esteem Increased field independence
Family participation in the TM program	Mature family interaction and positive parental role modeling	Improved relationships
Group participation in the program with age peers	Peer support	
		Reduced alcohol use Fewer arrests or hospitalization associated with alcohol use

peers in the treatment approach, the program should be made available to the parents and family members of the adolescents who participate in the treatment, and group meetings with other participants of similar age can provide peer support for the individual effects of the treatment.

The table also lists the type of outcome measures used to evaluate the effects of the Transcendental Meditation program in previous research on these factors, or which may be used in subsequent research based upon this treatment program for prevention and treatment of alcohol and drug abuse.

Conclusion of Research Review

Maharishi's Transcendental Meditation program appears to fulfill the need for an approach to prevention and treatment of alcohol and drug abuse that is holistic and positive. The program is holistic, with a balancing influence on the physiological, cognitive, emotional, and behavioral levels. It is also a specific and systematic technology that the client can make use of as a positive step for self-development rather than merely focus on the lacks in his or her personal life or environment. In this regard, it is important to note that the reduction in alcohol and drug use among those who learn the Transcendental Meditation program is consistently found to be a by-product of the practice, even when it is not the reason for which the person is beginning. As a result of systematic, holistic development and an increase in psychophysiological balance, substance usage falls away in a natural and balanced way and gains are long-term as the participant continues with the practice. The use of Maharishi Ayur-Veda herbal food supplements (Maharishi Amrit Kalash) further promotes the development of psychophysiological and physiological balance by scavenging free radicals and reactive oxygen species, inhibiting lipid peroxidation, and possibly through the modulation of brain opioid receptor activity.

The Transcendental Meditation program has demonstrated effectiveness as both a preventive and treatment modality against alcohol and drug abuse. Prevention of such abuse by strengthening the individual at an early age is of greatest importance for the individual and the whole society. In the remainder of this paper, we outline a sample treatment program implementing Transcendental Meditation and Maharishi Amrit Kalash for prevention of alcohol and drug addiction among juveniles with early indications of alcohol or drug abuse. Our goal was to design an ideal treatment program, which could ensure substantial and lasting benefit to the participants and their families.

TREATMENT PROGRAM

Identifying, Recruiting, and Retaining the Participants

Subjects

The participants are juveniles with alcohol and other substance abuse problems. They can be referred to the program by the school system, by hospitals, or other treatment programs. The participants in the project should also have expressed a desire to participate fully in the proposed treatment program.

Screening

The students are first screened or assessed to be sure there is no evidence of psychosis or major illness. Then the program is described to the students. If they are willing to participate, the program is described to their parents or significant others. At least one parent or significant other must be willing to participate in the TM program with the child.

Signed Permission from Parent or Guardian

If both student and parent or guardian are interested, the parent or guardian signs a note giving permission for the child to participate in the project and committing to support the child's regular attendance in the program and their own participation (see next point below).

Commitment to Treatment

The student also will sign a commitment to attend the Transcendental Meditation and Maharishi Amrit Kalash (TM/MAK) treatment program for one year. This includes (1) instruction in Transcendental Meditation (about 9 hours total); (2) five times per week after-care treatment meetings for 20 minutes at their school during the 9 months of the school year; (3) once per week TM treatment/SCI class (for description of SCI, see Treatment section below) every month of the year; and (4) twice daily use of Maharishi Amrit Kalash herbal food supplement. (During the summer months, the students have one meeting per week–the one hour, 15 minutes treatment/class.)

The parent or significant other commits to (1) learning Transcendental Meditation before or at the same time that the child learns; (2) a meeting two times per month every month of the year (for description of meeting, see Treatment section below).

Assignment to Treatment Groups

If a research evaluation is planned for the treatment program, then the students are randomly assigned, if possible, to either the TM/MAK treatment program, or to another standard treatment program only. The TM/MAK treatment group may also participate in the standard (control) treatment program, so that a most exact assessment of the specific effects of the TM/MAK treatment program is possible. (Please refer to Evaluation section, below.)

Students will be screened and informed of the programs as soon as they are referred, throughout the period of the study. The students will join the on going after-care treatment meetings and weekly treatment/classes as soon as they receive instruction in Transcendental Meditation. Although the SCI curriculum sequentially unfolds, each lesson is self-sufficient; the students can join anytime and understand the material.

Retention of the Target Group

Because of the critical importance of twice-daily practice of TM (15 minutes per session) and use of MAK, attendance should be taken at all after-care treatment meetings and treatment/classes, and through self-report, the students' TM practice in the mornings and on weekends should be noted during each of these meetings. The parents or significant others are expected to encourage and support the morning and weekend practice, particularly by their own example.

For the students' convenience, the 20-minute after-care treatment meetings will be held near their schools directly after the last school class.

Treatment

The Transcendental Meditation and Maharishi Amrit Kalash (TM/MAK) treatment program for students over a one-year period comprises the following:

Personal Instruction in the Transcendental Meditation Program

The TM technique is learned in about 6 meetings, 9 hours total time.

Use of Maharishi Amrit Kalash

M-4 and M-5 may be taken individually, or for maximum benefit, both may be taken together. One teaspoonful of M-4 is taken twice a day, before breakfast and before bedtime, with warm milk or water or juice. One tablet of M-5 is taken twice a day with warm water, before breakfast and before bedtime. If both M-4 and M-5 are taken, it is necessary to allow 1/2 hour between taking the two formulations.

Supervised After-Care Treatment Five Times per Week During the School Year

This after-care treatment meeting, which will last approximately 20 minutes including 15 minutes of Transcendental Meditation practice, will be held near the students' schools, so that they may go directly to the meeting after the end of the school day. During the summer, the students will meet in a central location once per week for their treatment/class (please refer to description below).

Treatment/Class Held Once Per Week for One Hour Throughout the Academic Year, Once Per Week for One Hour 15 Minutes During the Summer Months

This treatment/class gives the basis for the students to appreciate their own growth of creative intelligence. Part of this treatment/class is the Science of Creative Intelligence (SCI) curriculum.

The stated goal of the SCI curriculum is "to provide understanding and experience of creative intelligence and thereby develop the physiology and psychology of every student for full expression of creative intelligence in practical life . . . [The curriculum] unfolds in a sequence of themes that expand the student's awareness to encompass the entire range of life." Deepening the students' understanding of themselves and their natural environment is accomplished in the SCI class by focusing on universal principles and qualities of creative intelligence, stated in language that is appropriate to the students' grade level.

Students discover these universal principles and qualities in their own lives, in their community and traditions, in the natural environment, in their cultural tradition, in the lives of great men and women of their culture, in the different subjects of study, and in the practice of Transcendental Meditation. The materials, language, and learning activities of the SCI curriculum are suited to each age level. The curriculum for preadolescent levels is less abstract than the adolescent level, and uses more interactive materials.

Once per month a teacher or other expert will be invited to discuss with the class these qualities of creative intelligence as they are expressed in the community, traditions, cultural values, legends, or lives of great women and men of the culture to which the participants belong.

Through discussions, creative activities, and group projects, the students discover that these principles unify all subjects of study, and connect the students with each other, with all people, and with their environment. This deepening connection with everything and everyone expresses itself in increasingly mature, responsible, and compassionate behavior.

Examples of SCI principles. Here are some examples of SCI principles and qualities taught at different grade levels.

Grades 7-9: The Nature of Life is to Grow; Outer Depends on Inner; Life is Found in Layers; Order is Present Everywhere; Wholeness is Contained in Every Part; Purification Leads to Progress; Knowledge is Gained from Inside and Outside; Thought Leads to Action, Action Leads to Achievement, Achievement Leads to Fulfillment; Harmony Exists in Diversity; Rest and Activity are the Steps of Progress.

Grade 10: Students study seemingly opposite qualities that are found complementary when life is progressing to higher levels of integration: Stable/Adaptable; Traditional/Innovative; Strong/Tender; Harmonizing/Diversifying; Independent/Helpful; Liberating/Responsible.

Grade 12: Introduction to the different disciplines of study, interconnected and made relevant to the student's daily life through the application of the SCI principles.

Examples of lessons. A series of lessons for tenth graders on the "stable and adaptable" qualities of creative intelligence, for example, might ask students to find examples and write about these two complementary qualities in their own community–what structures and traditions provide stability? What customs enable the community to adapt to new ideas that are useful?

The coexistence of stability and adaptability could also be found in the students' relationships with others: on the ground of stable friendships, they more easily accommodate to each other's needs and differences. These complementary qualities can be found in great sports figures, whose stable repertoire of skills allows them to adapt to any unpredictable situation; or in the way plants adapt to changing environmental conditions on the basis of stable biological structures. Finally, the class would typically discuss how these qualities are more fully expressed in the students' own lives as they develop their creative intelligence through their practice of Transcendental Meditation: as they become stabilized in the deepest, most alert and silent level of their own consciousness, they are more resilient and more easily adapt to the changing and unexpected circumstances of everyday life.

Two treatment/class groups. The students participating in the special TM treatment program should be divided into two treatment/class groups: preadolescents (12-14) and adolescents (15-18).

Length of classes. During the school year, the treatment/class meeting, which includes 15 minutes of group meditation, will be one hour in length. The summer treatment/classes, will last 75 minutes. The added 15 minutes will be discussion of the students' experiences during and after meditation, since they will not be having daily meetings during these months.

Teachers and Supervisors of Meditation

The treatment instructor of the students will be a trained professional teacher of the Transcendental Meditation program, who also has had extensive classroom teaching experience. If he or she has not taught the SCI curriculum at the preadolescent and adolescent levels, he or she will be trained in an intensive 3-5 day seminar at Maharishi School of the Age of Enlightenment in Fairfield, Iowa. This school (enrollment 650 K-12 students) is responsible for developing and testing SCI curriculum materials for elementary and secondary levels, for use in schools throughout the world. The Director of Curriculum and Instruction structures these training sessions for professionals, and will individualize the training for this specific project.

The supervisors of the 20-minute after-care treatment program in the afternoon after school can be adults from the community who have learned Transcendental Meditation and received simple training from the professional TM teacher on how to conduct the after-care treatment meetings held after school.

Parent meetings. The parents or guardians of the participating students, who have themselves learned TM, will participate in two 1-hour meetings per month, during which they will have their meditation checked, discuss their impressions of their children's progress, and receive more intellectual understanding about the principles and effects of the treatment program.

Treatment Procedures Relevant to the Unique Needs of Juvenile Populations

Supervised practice of meditation. This is particularly important for this group of students, since these children generally have not established orderly, positive routines of daily living. Supervised meditation will ensure that they are practicing the technology regularly. Then the benefits will automatically ensue.

Immediate and cumulative results. Students will notice the benefits as soon as they begin practicing, which will be immediately gratifying, and help motivate them to continue the practice.

Positive, personal content of the weekly treatment/class. Students gain an appreciation of the orderliness and underlying unity of nature and the universe, and how their lives can express that orderliness and growth. The course also brings out stages of growth toward the highest levels of human development, based on scientific research and traditional records. Students are inspired when they see that they are developing the qualities associated with these highest states of development. The course also gives them opportunities to express their individuality in creative, positive ways through a variety of learning activities, including writing and art projects, oral presentations, and group projects.

Treatment/class curriculum adapted to this target population. The center for SCI curriculum development for elementary and secondary levels is Maharishi School of the Age of Enlightenment in Fairfield, Iowa. The curriculum professionals, all of whom are experienced classroom teachers, are experienced in adapting the learning activities of the lessons to different populations of students. This group, with the advice of local project leaders, will adapt some of the lesson materials for the target population, focusing on the most elevating aspects of the participants' culture, traditions, history, and great women and men.

Positive peer groups and adult role models. The after-care treatment meeting and treatment/class provide much-needed peer group and adult role models who are positive, supportive, and nourishing; whose own lives are steadily increasing in creativity, vitality, compassion, and achievement as they continue to participate in the program.

Evaluation

Outcome Evaluation

Participants. Participants in the project will be youth from 12 to 18 years of age, and members of their families. These youth will have been referred to the project from one of the sources described in the previous section. Thus, the participants will have been previously identified as having a problem with the use of alcohol or drugs, and at high risk for development of chronic addiction. Both boys and girls will be accepted into the program, both preadolescents (12-14 or middle school) and adolescents (15-18 or high school). Data should be analyzed separately for preadolescents and adolescents.

Design. All youth will pass initial screening and volunteer for admission into the project, and all will participate in the ongoing treatment program. Half of the participants will be randomly selected to also participate in a special extended treatment program that implements the Transcendental Meditation technique and Maharishi Amrit Kalash, as described above.

Schedule and procedures for data collection. Each participant should be pretested at the time of entry into the program (after initial screening and before assignment to treatment group). Participants should also be retested each six months for one year after beginning the program (two posttests). The exception is self-report questionnaires on alcohol and drug use, which should be completed monthly. Because participants may enter the program at different times due to referrals, the project administrator will be responsible for testing of participants at the appropriate time either individually or in small group administration. Tests will be standardized tests, administered according to instructions, and self-report questionnaires. Archival behavioral data will be collected from the appropriate source, and will cover the entire six-month period (e.g., number of school absences during the period).

Measurement instruments. Based upon the holistic model of protective and risk factors outlined in the introduction, those evaluating the effects of the TM and Maharishi Amrit Kalash treatment program can choose among measures of the following variables: reduced depression (e.g., IPAT Depression Scale) reduced anxiety (e.g., "trait anxiety" scale of the State-Trait Anxiety Inventory), reduced hostility (e.g., hostility subscale of the Profile of Mood States), increased self-esteem (e.g., Culture-Free Self-Esteem Inventory), increased field independence (e.g., Embedded Figures Test), improved family relationships (e.g., Family Environment Scale), improved school performance (archival records of grade point average, absenteeism, and disciplinary problems and also teacher ratings of behavior).

The most important outcomes, in addition to any of the above indicators, are measures of alcohol and drug consumption (self-report questionnaires and also archival measures of behavioral problems related to alcohol and drug consumption, such as arrests or hospitalizations). Previous research has shown that monthly self-reports of alcohol consumption are more accurate than six-month self-reports (Taub et al., this volume).

Data analysis plan. There would be four groups for the purpose of data analysis: two major treatment conditions–standard treatment and standard treatment plus TM treatment, and two age groups within each treatment condition (12-14 and 15-18). The major analysis procedure to assess whether the TM treatment program has a significant effect on improving questionnaire outcomes would be analysis of variance, with treatment (TM and standard treatment) and age (12-14 and 15-18) as between-subject factors, and pre and posttestings as a repeated measures or within-subjects factor. The potential influences of gender can be assessed as a covariant in the analysis. With 80 subjects in each of two treatment groups, the analysis will have sufficient power to discriminate effects comparable to those found in previous research.

In the case that there is a high intercorrelation between the various questionnaire measures, the measures may be combined and simplified by principal components analysis based on pre-test data (e.g., Stevens, 1986). The major analysis would then be performed on these simplified component variables.

Behavioral data on grade point average and number of school absences will be analyzed in the same way as the questionnaire data. For archival behavioral variables that have only an infrequent occurrence (e.g., arrests, hospitalizations, or school behavioral problems), a chi-square or log-linear analysis can be performed separately for each age group.

Process Evaluation

A process evaluation of the implementation of the treatment program is recommended. It should be focused primarily on the various factors necessary to ensure the success and standardization of the treatment program for future application in other settings.

Progress Evaluation Report. The first major aspect of the process evaluation would be a monthly progress evaluation report. This report can be generated by a monthly group meeting among all of the major project personnel: the on-site project leaders, the treatment instructors, and the after-care treatment group leaders in each school site. At this meeting, personnel would together review each of the following items on a checklist, to assess any potential improvements or problems:

1. Referral and entry of new participants into the program, and their integration into the ongoing group;
2. Attendance at the after-school after-care treatment group each afternoon;
3. Regularity of morning practice of the TM program, reported by participants in the afternoon meeting;
4. Satisfaction with the weekly treatment/class meetings;

5. Appropriateness of the materials for the treatment/class meetings;
6. Retention of participants in the program;
7. Progress of participating parents or significant others in their own practice of the TM program;
8. Support of parents or significant others for the student participants;
9. Integration of the special treatment program with the standard treatment program;
10. Staffing and program support issues.

Other items can be added to the checklist for monthly review as needed by the members of the project personnel. The minutes from the meeting, including new steps of action taken as needed on the basis of any of the items, would be used to prepare a monthly progress evaluation. The monthly progress evaluation would be available for hospital and school personnel associated with the treatment program, and would be retained as source documents for preparation of an annual progress report on the treatment process.

Implementation Manual and Curriculum Materials

A project manual and curriculum materials for implementing the treatment program should be prepared by the treatment instructors and the on-site project coordinator. The manual should include guidelines on the following areas:

1. Determination of goals and objectives appropriate for a specific site;
2. Procedures for recruiting participants;
3. Procedures for initial organization and implementation of the program;
4. Structure of the treatment program;
5. Administration of the treatment program;
6. Conducting of treatment/class meetings;
7. Development of further needed curriculum materials;
8. Training of staff;
9. Parental involvement in the program;
10. Interacting with schools and other treatment programs;

11. Providing infrastructure support for the success of the program;
12. Coordinating activities in various sites of the program;
13. Conducting process evaluation;
14. Conducting data collection for outcome evaluation;
15. Procedures for cost accounting.

Other areas to be included in the manual can be determined on the basis of the monthly evaluation reports.

Curriculum materials for the weekly treatment/class group should be collected and incorporated into the manual to facilitate further implementation of the program. Notes on the process of designing curriculum materials specific to the particular population should be included, as well as how to generalize this experience to the design of materials specific to other populations.

CONCLUSION

Maharishi's Transcendental Meditation technique has been found by previous research to alleviate the risk factors predisposing individuals to alcohol and drug abuse, and to enhance the protective factors that guard against addiction. Regular twice-daily practice of this technique has also been found to reduce usage of alcohol and drugs of all kinds in a natural way. Maharishi Amrit Kalash has been found to be an effective scavenger of free radicals and reactive oxygen species and a powerful inhibitor of lipid peroxidation, all of which are implicated in the extensive tissue damage caused by alcohol abuse. M-5 has also been found to inhibit brain opioid receptor activity in vitro, which may prove useful in the prevention and treatment of substance abuse. We have designed a treatment program, with Transcendental Meditation and Maharishi Amrit Kalash as the central elements, which, if implemented carefully, will ensure a significant and enduring preventive effect for young people who have previously shown evidence of problems of alcohol or drug abuse. We have also suggested a possible research design for evaluating the effects of the program. We would encourage all those who are working to prevent alcohol and drug abuse problems among juveniles to examine carefully this treatment program and implement it for the long-term benefit of the young people who are entrusted to their care.

REFERENCES

Alexander, C. N., Davies, J. L., Dixon, C. A., Dillbeck, M. C., Druker, S. M., Oetzel, R. M., Muehlman, J. M., & Orme-Johnson, D. W. (1990). Growth of higher states of consciousness: Maharishi Mahesh Yogi's Vedic psychology of human development. In C. N. Alexander & E. J. Langer (Eds.), *Higher stages of human development: Perspectives on adult growth* (pp. 286-340). New York: Oxford University Press.

Aron, E. N., & Aron, A. (1982). Transcendental Meditation program and marital adjustment. *Psychological Reports, 51*, 887-890.

Bangert-Drowns, R. L. (1988). The effects of school-based substance abuse education: A meta-analysis. *Journal of Drug Education, 18*, 243-264.

Baumrind, D. (1985). Familial antecedents of adolescent drug use: A developmental perspective. In C. Jones & R. Battjes (Eds.), *Etiology of drug abuse: Implications for prevention*. National Institute on Drug Abuse Research Monograph Number 56 (pp. 13-44). DHHS Pub. No. (ADM) 85-1335. Washington, DC: U.S. Government Printing Office.

Benard, B. (1986). Characteristics of effective prevention programs. *Prevention Forum, 6*(4), 3-8.

Bielefeld, M. (August, 1981). *Transcendental Meditation: A stress reducing self-help support system*. Cleveland V.A. Medical Center, Cleveland, Ohio, U.S.A. Paper presented at the Annual Convention of the American Psychological Association, Los Angeles, California, U.S.A.

Bleick, C. R., & Abrams, A. I. (1987). The Transcendental Meditation program and criminal recidivism in California. *Journal of Criminal Justice, 15*, 211-230.

Brautigam, E. (1977). Effects of the Transcendental Meditation program on drug abusers: A prospective study. In D.W. Orme-Johnson & J.T. Farrow (Eds.), *Scientific research on the Transcendental Meditation program: Collected papers, Volume 1*. Rheinweiler, W. Germany: Maharishi European Research University Press.

Brooks, J. S., & Scarano, T. (1985). Transcendental Meditation in the treatment of post-Vietnam adjustment. *Journal of Counseling and Development, 64* 212-215.

Chalmers, R. A., Clements, G., Schenkluhn, H., & Weinless, M. (Eds.) (1989). *Scientific research on Maharishi's Transcendental Meditation and TM-Sidhi programme: Collected papers, Volumes 2-4*. Vlodrop, the Netherlands: Maharishi Vedic University Press.

Chen, M. E. (1984). A comparative study of dimensions of healthy functioning between families practicing the TM program for five years or for less than a year. *Dissertation Abstracts International, 45*(10), 3206B.

Cranson, R. (August, 1989). *Increased general intelligence through the Transcendental Meditation and TM-Sidhi program*. Abstract of a paper presented at the Annual Meeting of the American Psychological Association, New Orleans.

Dileepan, K. N., Patel, V., Sharma, H. M., & Stechschulte, D. J. (1990). Priming of splenic lymphocytes after ingestion of an Ayurvedic herbal food supplement: Evidence for an immunomodulatory effect. *Biochemical Archives, 6,* 267-274.

Dillbeck, M. C., & Alexander, C. N. (1989). Higher states of consciousness: Maharishi Mahesh Yogi's Vedic psychology of human development. *The Journal of Mind and Behavior, 10,* 307-334.

Dillbeck, M. C., Clayborne, B. M., & Dillbeck, S. L. (August 1990). *Effects of the Transcendental Meditation program with low-income inner-city children.* Paper presented to the annual meeting of the American Psychological Association, Boston, Massachusetts.

Dillbeck, M. C., & Orme-Johnson, D. W. (1987). Physiological differences between Transcendental Meditation and rest. *American Psychologist, 42,* 879-881.

Drejer, K., Theilgaard, A., Teasdale, T.W., Schulsinger, F., & Goodwin, D.W. (1985). A prospective study of young men at high risk for alcoholism: Neuropsychological assessment. *Alcoholism: Clinical and Experimental Research, 9,* 498-502.

Dryfoos, J. G. (1990). *Adolescents-at-risk: Prevalence and prevention.* New York: Oxford University Press.

Dwivedi, C., Sharma, H. M., Dobrowski, S., & Engineer, F. N. (1991). Inhibitory effects of Maharishi-4 and Maharishi-5 on microsomal lipid peroxidation. *Pharmacology Biochemistry and Behavior, 39,* 649-652.

Emrick, C. D. (1975). A review of psychologically oriented treatment of alcoholism: II. The relative effectiveness of different treatment approaches and the effectiveness of treatment versus no-treatment. *Journal of Studies on Alcoholism, 36,* 534-549.

Eppley, K., Abrams, A., & Shear, J. (1989). Differential effects of relaxation techniques on trait anxiety: A meta-analysis. *Journal of Clinical Psychology, 45,* 957-974.

Evand, R. I., Rozelle, R. M., Berry, W. B., & Havis, J. (1978). Determining the onset of smoking in children: Knowledge of immediate physiological effects and coping with peer pressure, media pressure, and parents modeling. *Journal of Applied Social Psychology, 8,* 126-135.

Fink, R., Clemens, M. R., Marjot, D. H., Patsalos, P., Cawood, P., Norden, A. G., Iversen, S. A., & Dormandy, T. L. (1985). Increased free-radical activity in alcoholics. *Lancet, 2,* 291-294.

Geisler, M. (1978). Therapeutische Wirkungen der Transzendentalen Meditation auf den Drogenkonsumenten. *Zeitschrift für klinische Psychologie, 7,* 235-255.

Gelderloos, P., Walton, K. G., Orme-Johnson, D. W., & Alexander, C. N. (1991). Effectiveness of the Transcendental Meditation program in preventing and treating substance misuse: A review. *International Journal of the Addictions, 26,* 293-325.

Jessor, R., & Jessor, S. L. (1978). Theory testing in longitudinal research on marijuana use. In D. Kandel (Ed.), *Longitudinal research on drug use.* Washington, DC: Hemisphere.

Jones, C., & Battjes, R. (Eds.) (1985). *Etiology of drug abuse: Implications for prevention*. National Institute on Drug Abuse Research Monograph Number 56 (pp. 13-44). DHHS Pub. No. (ADM) 85-1335. Washington, DC: U.S. Government Printing Office.

Jones, M. C. (1968). Personality correlates and antecedents of drinking patterns in adult males. *Journal of Consulting and Clinical Psychology, 26,* 1-15.

Kalliopuska, M. (1982). Field dependence in alcoholics. *Psychological Reports, 51,* 963-968.

Kember, P. (1985). The Transcendental Meditation technique and postgraduate academic performance. *British Journal of Educational Psychology, 55,* 164-166.

Lafferty, P., & Kahn, M. W. (1986). Field dependency or cognitive impairment in alcoholics. *International Journal of the Addictions, 21,* 1221-1232.

Lieber, C.S. (1988). Biochemical and molecular basis of alcohol-induced injury to liver and other tissues. *New England Journal of Medicine, 319,* 1639-1650.

Long, J. V. F., & Scherl, D. J. (1984). Developmental antecedents of compulsive drug use: A report on the literature. *Journal of Psychoactive Drugs, 16,* 169-182.

Marcus, S. V. (1977). The influence of the Transcendental Meditation program on the marital dyad. *Dissertation Abstracts International, 38*(8), 3895B.

Margulies, R. Z., Kessler, R. C., & Kandel, D. B. (1977). A longitudinal study of onset of drinking among high-school students. *Journal of Studies on Alcohol, 38,* 897-912.

Miller, W. R., & Hester, R. K. (1986). Inpatient alcoholism treatment. Who benefits? *American Psychologist, 41,* 794-805.

Niwa, Y. (1991). Effect of Maharishi 4 and Maharishi 5 on inflammatory mediators–with special reference to their free radical scavenging effect. *Indian Journal of Clinical Practice, 1*(8), 23-27.

Niwa, Y., Kasama, T., Miyachi, Y., & Kanoh, T. (1989). Neutrophil chemotaxis, phagocytosis and parameters of reactive oxygen species in human aging: Cross-sectional and longitudinal studies. *Life Sciences, 44,* 1655-1664.

Orme-Johnson, D. W., & Farrow, J. T. (Eds.) (1977). *Scientific research on the Transcendental Meditation program: Collected papers, Volume 1*. Rheinweiler, W. Germany: Maharishi European Research University Press.

Panganamala, R. V., & Sharma, H. M. (1991). Anti-oxidant and antiplatelet properties of Maharishi Amrit Kalash (M-4) in hypercholesterolemic rabbits. International Atherosclerosis Society, Ninth International Symposium on Atherosclerosis, Rosemont, Illinois, U.S.A., October 6-11, 1991, Abstract No. 111.

Patel, V. K., Wang, J., Shen, R. N., Sharma, H. M., & Brahmi, Z. (1992). Reduction of metastases of Lewis Lung Carcinoma by an Ayurvedic food supplement in mice. *Nutrition Research, 12,* 51-61.

Paton, S., Kessler, R., & Kandel, D. (1977). Depressive mood and adolescent illicit drug use: A longitudinal analysis. *Journal of Genetic Psychology, 131,* 267-289.

Patterson, G. R. (1982). *A social learning approach, Vol. 3: Coercive family process*. Eugene: Castalia.

Pelletier, K. R. (1974). Influence of Transcendental Meditation upon autokinetic perception. *Perceptual and Motor Skills, 39,* 1031-1034.

Penner, W. J., Zingle, H. W., Dyck, R., & Truch, S. (1974). Does an in-depth Transcendental Meditation course effect change in the personalities of the participants? *Western Psychologist, 4,* 104-111.

Richards, R. T., & Sharma, H. M. (1991). Free radicals in health and disease. *Indian Journal of Clinical Practice, 2*(7), 15-26.

Robins, L. (1978). Sturdy childhood predictors of adult anti-social behavior: Replications from longitudinal studies. *Psychological Medicine, 8,* 611-622.

Roth, R. (1987). *Transcendental Meditation.* New York: Donald I. Fine.

Schenkluhn, H., & Geisler, M. (1977). A longitudinal study of the influence of the Transcendental Meditation program on drug abuse. In D. W. Orme-Johnson & J. T. Farrow (Eds.), *Scientific research on the Transcendental Meditation program: Collected papers, Volume 1.* Rheinweiler, W. Germany: Maharishi European Research University Press.

Sharma, H. M., Dwivedi, C., Satter, B. C., & Abou-Issa, H. (1991). Antineoplastic properties of Maharishi Amrit Kalash, an Ayurvedic food supplement, against 7,12-dimethylbenz(a)anthracene-induced mammary tumors in rats. *Journal of Research and Education in Indian Medicine, 10*(3), 1-8.

Sharma, H. M., Dwivedi, C., Satter, B. C., Gudehithlu, K. P., Abou-Issa, H., Malarkey, W., & Tejwani, G.A. (1990). Antineoplastic properties of Maharishi-4 against DMBA-induced mammary tumors in rats. *Pharmacology Biochemistry and Behavior, 35,* 767-773.

Sharma, H. M., Feng, Y., & Panganamala, R. V. (1989). Maharishi Amrit Kalash (MAK) prevents human platelet aggregation. *Clinica and Terapia Cardiovascolare, 8,* 227-230.

Sharma, H. M., Hanissian, S., Rattan, A. K., Stern, S. L., & Tejwani, G.A. (1991). Effect of Maharishi Amrit Kalash on brain opioid receptors and neuropeptides. *Journal of Research and Education in Indian Medicine, 10*(1), 1-8.

Sharma, H. M., Hanna, A. N., Kauffman, E. M., & Newman, H. A. I. (1991). Inhibition in vitro of human LDL oxidation by Maharishi Amrit Kalash (M-4 and M-5), Maharishi Coffee Substitute (MCS) and Men's Rasayana (MR). International Atherosclerosis Society, Ninth International Symposium on Atherosclerosis, Rosemont, Illinois, U.S.A., October 6-11, 1991, Abstract No. 112.

Sharma, H. M., Triguna, B. D., & Chopra, D. (1991). Maharishi Ayur-Veda: Modern insights into ancient medicine. *Journal of the American Medical Association, 265,* 2633-2637.

Shecter, H. (1978). A psychological investigation into the source of the effect of the Transcendental Meditation technique. *Dissertation Abstracts International, 38,* 3372B-3373B.

Steffenhagen, N. R. (1980). Self-esteem theory of drug use. In D. Lettieri, M. Sayers, & H. Pearson (Eds.), *Theories of drug abuse.* Washington, DC: National Institute on Drug Abuse.

Stevens, J. (1986). *Applied multivariate statistics for the social sciences*. Hillsdale, NJ: Lawrence Earlbaum.

Suarez, V. W. (1976). *The relationship of the practice of Transcendental Meditation to subjective evaluations of marital satisfaction and adjustment*. Master's thesis, School of Education, University of Southern California, Los Angeles, California, U.S.A.

Swaim, R., Oetting, E., Edwards, R., & Beauvais, F. (1989). Links from emotional distress to adolescent drug use: A path model. *Journal of Consulting and Clinical Psychology, 57*, 227-231.

Tartar, R. E., Jacob, T., Hill, S., Hegedus, A.M., & Carra, J. (1986). Perceptual field dependency: Predisposing trait or consequence of alcoholism? *Journal of Studies on Alcohol, 47*, 498-499.

Taub, E., Steiner, S. S., Smith, R. B., Weingarten, E., & Walton, K. G. (this volume). Effectiveness of broad spectrum approaches to relapse prevention: A long-term, randomized, controlled trial comparing Transcendental Meditation, muscle relaxation and electronic neurotherapy in severe alcoholism. *Alcoholism Treatment Quarterly.*

Tennant, F. S. (1985). *Primer on neurochemistry of drug dependence*. Westcovina, California: Veract.

Tobler, N. S. (1986). Meta-analysis of 143 adolescent drug prevention programs: Quantitative outcome results of program participants compared to a control or comparison group. *Journal of Drug Issues, 16*, 537-568.

Wallace, R. K. (1970). Physiological effects of Transcendental Meditation. *Science, 167*, 1751-1754.

Wallace, R. K., Orme-Johnson, D.W., & Dillbeck, M. C. (Eds.) (1990). *Scientific research on Maharishi's Transcendental Meditation and TM-Sidhi program: Collected papers, Volume 5*. Fairfield, Iowa: Maharishi International University Press.

Wills, T. A., & Shiffman, S. (1985). Coping and substance abuse: A conceptual framework. In S. Shiffman & T. A. Wills (Eds.), *Coping and substance abuse*. Orlando, FL: Academic Press.

Possessing the Self: Maharishi Ayur-Veda and the Process of Recovery from Addictive Diseases

David F. O'Connell, PhD, AAPTA

> Being established in the Self means being established unshakably in the wholeness of life. Health, therefore, means possession of the Self. He who possesses the Self is described as one who is healthy. (Maharishi Mahesh Yogi, quoted in Wallace, 1986, p. 156)

OVERVIEW

The introduction of the technologies of Maharishi Ayur-Veda into the rehabilitation plan for recovering alcoholics and addicts can have a dramatic impact on the nature and course of the patient's recovery from addictive diseases. Maharishi Ayur-Veda has over twenty approaches to promoting health, including the Transcendental Meditation technique. This paper is an exploration of how the technologies of Maharishi Ayur-Veda can profoundly increase

David F. O'Connell has a private practice in West Lawn, PA and is Consulting Psychologist for The Caron Foundation and Attending Psychologist at St. Joseph's Hospital, Reading, PA.

[Haworth co-indexing entry note]: "Possessing the Self: Maharishi Ayur-Veda and the Process of Recovery from Addictive Diseases." O'Connell, David F. Co-published simultaneously in the *Alcoholism Treatment Quarterly* (The Haworth Press, Inc.) Vol. 11, No. 3/4, 1994, pp. 459-495; and: *Self-Recovery: Treating Addictions Using Transcendental Meditation and Maharishi Ayur-Veda* (ed: David F. O'Connell and Charles N. Alexander) The Haworth Press, Inc., 1994, pp. 459-495. Multiple copies of this article/chapter may be purchased from The Haworth Document Delivery Center [1-800-3-HAWORTH; 9:00 a.m. - 5:00 p.m. (EST)].

the effectiveness and quality of recovery from addictive diseases. The presentation of its approaches for addictions recovery will be offered in the context of the developmental model of recovery from chemical dependency (Brown, 1985) and in relationship to self-psychology therapeutic approaches to addictions treatment (Levin, 1987). Both of these approaches represent important previous advances in our understanding of addictions treatment. Consideration will also be given to the spiritual aspect of the recovery process and the role of Ayurvedic technologies in the cultivation of spiritual experiences.

The theory and techniques of treatment for addictive diseases have been developed and refined over the past three decades. Although there is certainly no uniform or preferred approach to addictions treatment, the elements of effective treatment for addictions have become increasingly realized and built into inpatient and outpatient approaches (Nace, 1987).

Many in the addiction fields feel that we now have treatments of choice for alcoholism and drug addiction. However, as both Gorski (1979) and Marlatt and Gordon (1985) have noted, even our best therapeutic solutions are far outweighed by the complexity and severity of addictive disorders, and relapse rates remain unacceptably high.

The Transcendental Meditation technique and other approaches of Maharishi Ayur-Veda, offer a radically new approach to the management and resolution of addictive diseases. The alcoholic or addict who becomes involved in an Ayurvedic program of recovery can experience a qualitative and quantitative improvement in his or her psychological well-being, physical comfort, and spiritual growth in recovery.

A massive amount of theory and research has accumulated on Maharishi Ayur-Veda, particularly the TM technique (Orme-Johnson & Farrow, 1977; Chalmers, Clements, Schenkluhn and Weinless, 1989a,b,c). The unequivocal conclusion of this research is that the practice of Transcendental Meditation results in a psychophysiologically distinct state of restful alertness described as transcendental or pure consciousness and that the regular experience of this state, alternating with activity, cultures the nervous system to function in such a way that the state of pure consciousness is eventually co-experienced along with the other states of consciousness–walking, dreaming, and sleeping. This is a unique style of functioning with profound implications for the chemically dependent patient who begins the practice of meditation. Large scale meta-analyses have shown that TM leads to a marked reduction in psychological distress (Eppley, Abrams, and Shear, 1989) and to striking growth in psychological health and well-being compared to other practices of meditation and relaxation (Alexander, Rainforth, and Gelderloos, 1991).

Although there have been over 25 studies on the positive psychological effects of Transcendental Meditation and enhanced recovery from substance dependence, there is considerably less information available on how TM interfaces with psychotherapy and the clinical management of chemically dependent patients. However, there have been several studies on these themes (Brooks, 1993). Shafii (1973) provided a case study on the psychoanalytic therapeutic process with a drug addicted young man who began the TM technique. Carter and Meyer (1989) have written on the use of TM with severely disturbed psychiatric patients. All of these researchers have concluded that the practice of TM can dramatically accelerate recovery from both psychiatric and addictive diseases and offer the clinician some guidelines and direction on the therapeutic management of patients practicing TM. Thus this approach of Maharishi Ayur-Veda to understanding and treating addictions provides an extremely useful alternative paradigm for understanding the source, course, manifestation and treatment of addictive diseases. An appreciation and understanding of the nature and scope of such changes brought about by this and other Ayurvedic approaches is important for clinicians whose practice would benefit from their introduction, as well as for those who may be already treating patients involved in an Ayurvedic program for recovery.

It has been shown previously that a patient's experience is distinctly different in various stages of recovery from addiction (Gorski, 1989). In general, treatment professionals need to have a developmental perspective to understand what the patient is going through at various phases of recovery and to shape therapeutic interventions appropriately. When a patient takes up the practice of Transcendental Meditation, he or she begins to experience his or her own awareness in an entirely different fashion than was previously possible. Thus, the meditating alcoholic or addict will have vastly different experiences of the self in recovery, both in and out of meditation at each phase of recovery depending on the regularity and length of practice of TM. Because of this often dramatic change in phenomenology, it is essential that addictions professionals have a solid conception of stages of growth in consciousness that patients may experience when they engage in the practice of TM and other approaches of Maharishi Ayur-Veda. Otherwise, counselors may experience less success with the therapeutic management of meditating patients. This paper provides a framework for such an understanding. Also, Ayurvedic approaches to addictions treatment offer new and useful ways to conceptualize and treat addictions that can supplement the clinicians' existing knowledge and motivate them to pursue further education and training in Ayurvedic approaches. Moreover, clinicians who themselves take up the practice of these programs can experience profound personal benefits which can relieve the stress often associated with this profession and lead to greater professional effectiveness.

The Developmental Model of Recovery and the TM Technique

It has long been held in the addictions field that there is a developmental nature to recovery from addictive diseases (for example, Johnson, 1980). Just as the onset of an addictive disease results in a predictable, sequential breakdown in the individual's life, so researchers and clinicians have observed that recovery from an addictive disease likewise occurs in a sequence of developmental phases (Gorski, 1989; Freyer-Rose, 1991; Brown, 1985). Brown (1985, p. 55), in particular, notes that the process of recovery from alcoholism is one of "construction and reconstruction." The recovery process necessitates a fundamental change in the patient's identity and conception of reality. As this author notes, the learning involved in recovery from addictive diseases is "accomplished through behavioral change, cognitive reorganization and restructuring and object substitution and replacement. It involves parallel, simultaneous, and/or reciprocal interactions between behavioral, cognitive, and affective components" (p. 55). With this presupposition, the developmental tasks for the patient in recovery and the interventions by treatment professionals have been delineated. In this section, the role of the TM technique and other Ayurvedic technologies in accelerating and increasing the effectiveness of the developmental processes in recovery will be considered.

Detoxification and Stabilization

This is considered the first therapeutic stage of recovery. The therapeutic tasks of the patient involve recognizing that there is a problem with uncontrollable drinking or drug use, interrupting the pathological preoccupation with alcohol and drugs, developing hope and motivation for sobriety and learning non-chemical means to manage stress and normalize moods. The individual in this phase of recovery comes into it experiencing a great deal of social isolation and alienation and a profound constriction of interest in activities. At this phase, the individual is preoccupied with the ingestion of drugs or alcohol. The patient has been experiencing an intense internal battle to control alcohol and drug use. The personal acceptance of the failure of this struggle for control marks the point of turn towards sobriety.

This phase normally begins with the detoxification of the patient from psychoactive substances. Patients in this phase of recovery often suffer profound psychological and physiological distress and dysfunction. Patients' bodies have frequently fallen into serious disrepair. The withdrawal process from drug and alcohol abuse can be particularly uncomfortable for the patient and at times can be life threatening, underscoring the importance of appropriate medical interventions.

Introducing the TM technique can profoundly accelerate the healing process in this phase of recovery. In this writer's clinical experience, patients frequently report reduced urges and cravings to use drugs and often feel immediate relief from physiological and psychological stresses. Dr. Frank Staggers, Medical Director of the Haight-Ashbury Medical Clinic in California, has noted that the TM technique can play a valuable role in the management of withdrawal symptoms (F. Staggers, personal communication, 1992). Dr. Staggers notes that patients who learn TM during detoxification often report reduced feelings of irritation and agitation and less physical pain. As an adjunct to other medical interventions, the TM technique provides deep and profound rest which can accelerate the removal of physiological impurities brought on by the lengthy abuse of substances.

How does the TM technique impart such changes? A large amount of data has accumulated on the metabolic, hormonal and biochemical changes brought about by the profound rest produced by the TM technique (summarized in Wallace, 1986, and Gelderloos, Walton, Orme-Johnson, and Alexander, 1991). These include:

- significant decreases in respiration rate and heart rate,
- significant decrease in arterial blood lactate,
- restful alertness as indicated by EEG changes showing an increase and spreading of alpha and theta wave spindle activity in the central and frontal areas of the brain,
- significant increases in phenylalanine concentration,
- significant decreases in plasma and urinary free cortisol levels during meditation,
- higher levels of serotonin metabolite 5-HIAA,
- significant increases in galvanic skin responses.

The profound state of restful alertness brought on by the practice of the TM technique may be responsible for the reduction in physical and psychological distress that patients undergoing detoxification have reported. Although these observations of detoxifying patients are based on clinical, anecdotal report and as yet have not been substantiated by controlled research, they are encouraging and suggest an important role for TM and other approaches of Maharishi Ayur-Veda in the management of withdrawal symptoms.

Early Recovery

In this phase of recovery, the tasks of the patient include a full conscious recognition of the presence of the addictive disorder, acceptance of the belief that he or she cannot control alcohol use and a shift in identity to that of being an alcoholic. The patient begins to interact with others without alcohol and the early feelings of helplessness and hopelessness are replaced with a sense of relief and anticipation of a healthier lifestyle. The patient is now usually more physically comfortable than in the previous phase, but can continue to experience symptoms of what is known as the subacute withdrawal syndrome. This is a constellation of psychological and physical symptoms brought about by the neurotoxic effects of prolonged alcohol and drug use. The patient typically experiences a great deal of emotional sensitivity and stress sensitivity, has difficulty with attention and concentration, shows a high level of physical tension, and in general, shows a tenuous psychological and emotional adjustment. During this phase of development, the patient typically develops a strong reliance on Twelve Step programs. Early recovery is the almost exclusive focus of most inpatient treatment programs for alcoholism and chemical dependency. Conventional treatments usually involve the use of addictions education, group therapy, exercise, and AA/NA involvement.

The TM technique can maximize the patient's functioning in this phase of recovery and allow the patient to take full advantage of available therapeutic programs. It is this writer's experience that regular meditation can reduce the emotional and physical discomfort associated with the subacute withdrawal syndrome and reduce pathological defenses, such as denial, projection, and rationalization, which are particularly strong in early phases of recovery. It can also assist the addict in developing clearer thinking and perception so that involvement in educational programs can be maximized and can provide the patient with a growing sense of inner stability.

As the patient continues to practice TM, there is a deepening in experiences during TM practice and consequently more benefit from the practice in activity. In this writer's clinical experience patients commonly report that they feel calmer, less stressed, and less moody and are more open to sharing personal experiences and considering others' points of view on the management of their lives. This reduction in defensiveness and greater cognitive and affective flexibility is particularly important for patients involved in group therapy. A common complaint by addictions clinicians is that patients are often too rigid and guarded to take advantage of what the clinician has to offer. The patient who practices TM regularly appears to be less threatened by the treatment process and is more open to treatment directives (Shafii, 1988). In this writer's clinical experience, patients who had learned TM while undergoing inpatient treatment for chronic relapse, reported a much more satisfying treatment experience and a greater sense of openness to recommendations from the treatment staff and other patients.

Middle Recovery

In this phase of recovery, the patient is expected to internalize a recovery program and become more responsible for formulating and continuing it. The therapeutic tasks involve the patient developing the capacity to manage change in his or her life and establish a balance in lifestyle. The patient also begins the work of repairing damaged social relationships brought about by the active phase of addiction. Therapeutic interventions in this phase are often focused on resolving deep feelings of demoralization associated with the status of being an alcoholic or addict.

Regular TM practice can provide much-needed support during this important developmental phase. Research has shown that individuals who practice TM develop greater internal locus of control (Hjelle, 1974) and become more field independent and, in general, more responsible individuals.

While there is natural personality growth when the patient is free from the presence of psychoactive substances in his or her system, the TM technique can profoundly facilitate this growth and provide a more rapid evolution of personality and self-concept (Alexander, 1982). In addition, the twice-daily practice of TM naturally and effortlessly restores emotional and behavioral balance in the patient's lifestyle. This lifestyle balance may be dramatically improved by the addition of other techniques of Maharishi Ayur-Veda. The aim of these techniques is to maximize and balance the patient's mood, physiology, and behavior. Like the TM technique, they are extremely pleasant and can cultivate a sense of well-being and comfort in both mind and body. With such an experience, the alcoholic can appreciate a life of abstinence much more clearly and fully. For example, one patient seen by the author enjoyed her twice-daily TM practice, but had continuing difficulty managing her daily affairs, dealing with the stress of her job as a hospital administrator, and in general, taking care of her physical and psychological needs. She asked if there was anything more that she could do. After hearing about Maharishi Ayur-Veda, she attended an outpatient program and went through a five-day physiological purification procedure known as *Maharishi Panchakarma* (see Glaser, this volume, for a discussion of Panchakarma and other approaches of Maharishi Ayur-Veda). Immediately after the treatment, she felt an effortlessness and ease in her daily functioning. She stated she felt more "finely tuned" and felt more fluid and balanced in her daily functioning. The patient began getting more pleasure from her job and her relations with family and friends and began to experience more joy in her recovery program.

Late Recovery

This phase is reached after one to several years of drug and alcohol free functioning. When it is achieved, the patient is ready to deal with psychological conflicts and trauma which may have contributed to the development of his or her addiction. In psychotherapy, patients are expected to address childhood trauma and dysfunctional relationships in the family of origin, and to continue to work on removing or reducing pathological behaviors, attitudes, and feelings. Formal psychotherapy is usually most effective in this phase of recovery. As Brown (1985) indicates, during this phase of recovery, the patient begins to integrate internal needs with external demands. Individual awareness is expanded and there is greater receptivity to the environment. This period is also marked by a growing interest in the integration of the spiritual aspect of the patient's life. This interest in a higher power results in a move away from a self-centered view of the world to one which places the individual in a much larger context as he or she begins to see his or her place in the universe.

The TM technique has been shown to be extremely effective in accelerating the psychotherapeutic process (Brooks, 1993). It has also been seen to be quite useful in cultivating the patient's spiritual life (Maharishi Mahesh Yogi, 1963, 1969, 1986a,b; Smith, 1983).

Late recovery is a life-long process. Maintaining long-term abstinence from psychoactive substances results in the development of newer, more flexible and adaptive inner psychological structures. The patient's ego becomes more functional and flexible. Pathological defenses are reduced to a minimum. If sobriety is maintained, the opportunity for full self-actualization unfolds and the potential for development at this phase is theoretically limitless.

The usefulness of the TM technique and other techniques of Maharishi Ayur-Veda can perhaps be most dramatically realized at this phase of recovery. In a seminal paper, Dr. Charles Alexander and his colleagues (Alexander et al. 1990), explore Maharishi Mahesh Yogi's description of higher states of consciousness which can be achieved through Transcendental Meditation, and discuss their relationship with development as described in contemporary psychology (a more complete account of Maharishi's explanation of growth to higher states of consciousness is considered in a later section). Previous research has shown (for example, Taub, Steiner, Smith, Weingarten, & Walton, this volume) that profound and dramatic enhancement of development can occur with TM in even the most dysfunctional populations such as brain damaged alcoholics. By including the TM program in the rehabilitation process, the recovering alcoholic has the opportunity to fulfill the ultimate goal of sobriety and achieve the highest levels of human development. The TM technique appears able to dramatically extend the developmental achievements reported by Brown (1977; 1985) in her study of addicts in late and ongoing recovery. As Alexander and his colleagues (1990) note, at higher levels of individual development brought on by the practice of Transcendental Meditation, the ego and emotions become increasingly flexible. Multiple antithetical feelings, for example, can coexist without the individual experiencing distress or dysfunction. Ambiguity is better tolerated and emotional conflicts are no longer experienced as a threat to the self. Eventually, in higher states of consciousness, the individual is beyond suffering and experiences a continual state of well-being. As consciousness further develops, one gains the experience of the profound unity of subjective and objective existence.

The enormously practical benefits of the TM program in late recovery are captured in the following statement by a patient practicing TM reported by Dr. Catherine Bleick of the Institute for Social Rehabilitation in California:

> I have been meditating regularly twice daily for over nine years. TM has removed on numerous occasions overwhelming urges for me to "just have one drink" or only one Valium to calm

> down. I go to many AA meetings and I see what I call toxic stress messes–individuals who are haggard, tired, worn out, living off coffee, cigarettes, lack of sleep and compulsive attendance at AA meetings, forever searching for a scrap of serenity, relief and release–and I must state emphatically that most of this type of misery in sobriety is nothing but stress and TM removes the stress, giving refreshing rest, and thereby allows anyone to act from fullness and serenity. TM greatly diminishes my physical pain from debilitating medical conditions and has also melted much of the ice around my heart. I feel compassion and love and I am able to listen to the hurt of others without being overwhelmed, judgmental, or condemnatory. (Bleick, 1990, p. 2)

The alcoholic who practices TM in late recovery has an unprecedented opportunity to develop his or her self to the highest levels possible. With this possibility alcoholism can truly be seen as an opportunity for the development of health and happiness that many alcoholics sincerely seek.

Self Psychology Approaches to the Treatment of Addiction

Both modern psychology and Maharishi's Vedic Psychology (the psychological approach associated with Maharishi Ayur-Veda) investigate the nature and experience of the self, although their conceptualization and treatment of disorders of the self differ dramatically. Modern psychological concepts of the individual self have emerged from the ego psychology, object relations, and self psychology systems of thought. The self has also been the focal point of many Eastern traditions of knowledge (Muzika, 1990). Primary among these is the Vedic tradition, which originated in ancient India and is the source of Maharishi's Vedic Psychology. Recently, Maharishi Mahesh Yogi has offered a comprehensive account of his Vedic Psychology which includes precise knowledge of the nature of the self (Orme-Johnson, 1988). In the following sections, self psychology, especially in relation to addictions treatment, will be considered from both a focus on the most dominant modern system of self psychology and the viewpoint of Maharishi's Vedic Psychology.

Self Psychology

A body of psychoanalytic theory and therapeutic technique generated by Heinz Kohut (1971, 1977, 1978, 1984) and his followers forms a subfield within the domain of psychoanalysis known as self-psychology. Initially based on Kohut's experiences in the treatment of narcissistic personality disorders, he later expanded it into a general theory of self-development and utilized his theory and technique to understand psychological processes involved in sexual perversions, delinquent behavior, and addictive diseases. Kohut viewed patients with these disorders as suffering from profound psycho-developmental arrest which he construed as a failure to develop a normal sense of self. These patients were, in his mind, contradistinguished from neurotic patients who suffered from unresolved intrapsychic conflicts but who had established a cohesive sense of self. Earlier, Rogers (1951, 1961) developed his own theory and treatment of the self which he termed Client-centered therapy. These separate schools of thought and practice shared a common focus: the goal of psychotherapy was the development of a coherent, cohesive, actualized self. Kohut was the more prolific of the two writers and developed a much more complex, sophisticated, detailed theory of the self and the treatment of self deficits. Because of this, his name has become synonymous with self-psychology. Levin (1987), in an important work, has developed Kohut's ideas on self psychology and addiction and applied them to the field of alcoholism treatment.

Kohut conceptualized alcoholics and addicts as suffering from a central weakness in the core of their personality. He termed this as a defect in the self. Alcoholics were viewed as lacking a stable, cohesive sense of self, which manifested in self-absorption, self-destructiveness, and a diminished capacity to maintain self-esteem and self-care. This central defect was seen as showing great explanatory power in understanding the many symptoms and pathological manifestations in diverse diagnostic groups of patients, such as those mentioned above. For Kohut, the addict craves the drug because he comes to believe that a psychoactive substance is capable of correcting his self-deficiencies. The drug becomes a kind of substitute for the validation and confirmation he failed to receive from primary care-givers in his early formative years. The ingestion of a drug is seen as a way to provide psychological power; for a brief time the addict feels powerful, validated, and in control of his internal and external world. The drug provides him with self-esteem that he or she does not possess. The pharmacological effects of the drug create a kind of false sense of self-acceptance and self-confidence allowing the patient to feel worthwhile and, more importantly, giving him or her a distinct feeling of being alive. These attempts at self-cure, however, are by nature impermanent and abortive. The drug experience needs to be continually repeated because the central defect in the self continues. The self remains in an enfeebled state and, due to the deteriorating effects of alcohol and drugs, becomes progressively more damaged and deficient.

Self psychology views addiction from a psychological perspective. Alcoholism and addiction are seen to arise because of the addict's pathological experience of the self. Alcoholics are seen as suffering from narcissistic deficits; that is, they have never developed a satisfactory way of caring for and loving themselves. Inwardly they feel fragmented and incomplete. There is a basic insecurity and sense of inadequacy; a feeling that something fundamental is missing. Self psychologists would say that these patients have never developed a cohesive sense of self.

Self Psychology Therapy Approaches

Self psychologists view the self as developing in stages. In the first stage, the infant experiences a primitive or fragmented sense of self devoid of clear boundaries between self and environment. In the next stage, an archaic or nuclear self is formed. This stage of self is enduring and cohesive, but as yet not firmly established. If conditions are auspicious, the development of what is known as the mature self eventually takes place. The alcoholic patient is seen as either fixated in or regressed to the archaic or primitive self. At this stage of development, the self is unable to regulate tension, self-soothe or regulate self-esteem. The individual is seen as lacking those psychic structures that subserve these functions.

In self psychology, the therapy relationship is conceived as a way to build psychic structure. This is accomplished by providing, in the context of the therapeutic relationship, what the patient never received from primary care givers in his or her early psychological development. The tasks of the therapist are to unconditionally accept the patient, provide a model of psychological health through his or her own sobriety and mental stability, and offer an informed understanding of the patient based on the therapist's knowledge of the patient's predicament. As Kohut notes, the patient's self needs validation and confirmation of its ideals, goals and ambitions. In short, the patient needs to become the "gleam in his therapist's eye" which provides the experience of unconditional support that was lacking from the patient's own mother or father. Through the process of therapy, split-off, repressed, disavowed aspects of the patient's self are brought together. The goal of therapy is to bring about what Freud termed a "unification of the ego." The patient's experience of self moves from a fragmented, incomplete experience to a cohesive one. For Kohut, the most central curative factor in therapy is the analysis of the transference between the patient and therapist. One of his greatest contributions to self-psychology is his study and exploration of transference phenomena in narcissistically disturbed patients. The transference or the reenactment in the therapeutic relationship of early relationships with others (primarily the mother or father) was viewed by Kohut as developing in very specific ways with patients with self-deficits (see Levin, 1987 for a comprehensive treatment of such transferences). Levin (1987) views the working through of the transference as the most important therapeutic task in psychotherapy with the stably sober alcoholic or addict.

For the self psychologist, therapy is seen as successful with alcoholic patients when they are able to provide for themselves what formerly drugs and alcohol provided, that is, the capacity to regulate tension, anxiety, and maintain self-esteem.

The treatments generated by self psychology are psychoanalytic or psychodynamically derived. Other writers, such as Khantzian, Halliday and McAuliffe (1990) and Wurmser (1977) have emphasized the need for depth psychology approaches to the treatment of addicts and alcoholics. Psychodynamic therapy, however, can be extremely time-consuming and expensive, and it is not practical for most patients in chemical dependency treatment centers. It is this writer's opinion that it is probably not being practiced very frequently in the addictions field other than by a few select, well-trained psychoanalysts and psychotherapists who possess an understanding of addictive disorders. Additionally, patients who do become involved in self psychology therapy often cannot complete it due to disruptions in the therapeutic relationship such as anger at the therapist or inability to handle the transference. Practical considerations such as geographical moves, intercurrent illnesses and other life developments that can interfere with the successful completion of lengthy therapy work also reduce the practicality of this approach.

Theories of the Self in Modern Psychology and Maharishi's Vedic Psychology

The theories and practices of self psychology have provided an important dimension in understanding the inner emotional life of patients who suffer from addictive diseases. Unlike some schools of thought in psychology, which rejected the idea of the self as unscientific and therefore unworthy of scientific investigation, the concept of the self assumes central importance in self psychology for the understanding and treatment of psychopathology associated with addictive diseases. However, in contrast to the approach to understanding the self in Maharishi's Vedic Psychology, the concept of self as described in self psychology would be viewed as an accurate, yet incomplete understanding of the self. Modern psychologists would define the self as the inner subjective experience of continuity and identity which endures in space and time. According to Levin (1987), an individual experiences the self as both a coherent whole and also as a disparate assembly of disjunctive feelings and experiences. As we shall see in the next section, this description corresponds to what Vedic Psychology would view as the relative aspect of the self, or lower self. In addition to this difference in defining and describing the self, Maharishi's Vedic Psychology utilizes mental and physical approaches, including the TM technique and related procedures of Maharishi Ayur-Veda for bringing about a correction of self-deficits, as opposed to the primarily psychological approach of self psychology. The success of self psychology approaches to addictions treatment depends on the building and refining of psychic structure, which is lacking or exists only in a rudimentary form in the addict or alcoholic. This is accomplished through the analysis of the transference between patient and therapist. The development of our understanding of the nature and manifestation of the transference in patients with self deficits has been one of the greatest contributions of self-psychology. The approach of Maharishi's Vedic Psychology provides a radically different technology for rapidly and effectively healing self-deficits, and like self-psychology is providing an important additional dimension in our understanding of patients with addictive diseases.

In Maharishi's Vedic Psychology, the self is not limited to the conceptualization offered by modern psychological investigation. Maharishi makes clear the distinction between the "lower self" and the "higher Self" (1969, p. 339):

> Self has two connotations: lower self and higher Self. The lower self is that aspect of the personality which deals only with the relative aspect of existence. It comprises the mind that thinks, the intellect that decides, the ego that experiences. This lower self functions only in the relative states of existence–waking, dreaming, and deep sleep . . . The higher Self is that aspect of the personality which never changes, Absolute being [pure consciousness] which is the very basis of the entire field of relativity, including the lower self.

In Maharishi's analysis, the Self is actually the underlying universal reality of life–pure consciousness. The term "pure consciousness" refers to the silent, unseen, non-changing, unified field of consciousness which is at the basis both of all the diverse, active phases of consciousness ordinarily experienced in individual consciousness (Orme-Johnson, 1988), and of all forms and phenomena in the universe (Hagelin, 1987, 1989). Pure consciousness is at the basis of all mental processes such as thinking, perception, feeling, and behaving, but due to the build-up of stresses in the nervous system the experience of it is blocked in most persons. All mental and behavioral phenomena are localized specific manifestations of the non-local underlying, unmanifest reality of pure consciousness.

In the absence of the experience of pure consciousness, in the normal waking state, one's attention is gripped by the localized nature of mental processes. There is an artificial division between the subject and the object, as well as between these two and the process of perceiving which links them: in other words, as Maharishi (1986a) explains, the knower, the process of knowing, and the object of knowledge (the known) are experienced as separate entities. In the state of pure consciousness, however, which is experienced through Transcendental Meditation and other related techniques, one experiences the Self as the unified state of the knower, the process of knowing, and the known. In this state, known as *Samhita* in Maharishi's Vedic Psychology, the artificial division between the subject and the object, as well as between these and the process of knowing, is dissolved. Maharishi refers to this state as "self-referral" because the knower is the sole object of its own knowing: pure consciousness (the knower) knows itself, pure consciousness (the known) through the instrumentality of pure consciousness (the process of knowing).

According to Maharishi's Vedic Psychology, through the practice of Transcendental Meditation, one's awareness becomes identified with pure consciousness and experiences its true nature as the Self. The state of transcendental consciousness is one of clear inner wakefulness. It is the experience of pure Self without any object of awareness other than itself in its own unbounded nature. This is clearly not a pathological state. Research has shown that it is, in fact, a highly coherent, orderly higher state of consciousness (Kesterson, 1986; Farrow & Hebert, 1982; Wallace, 1986).

Higher States of Consciousness

For recovering addicts, the regular experience of pure consciousness through the practice of Transcendental Meditation can greatly accelerate growth in recovery and sobriety. This process ultimately leads to the development of higher states of consciousness promoted through TM. According to Maharishi's Vedic Psychology, when an individual's awareness is opened to and, through repeated experience, established in pure consciousness, life becomes full of bliss and wholeness. Maharishi explains that as the practice of the TM program continues, the pure Self begins to be experienced not only deep within the mind during TM, but as the basis of all one's activity, and eventually of everything in the environment. The transformation in the experience of the Self unfolds in a predictable, orderly, sequential fashion through a series of well-defined higher states of consciousness (Maharishi Mahesh Yogi, 1969; Alexander & Boyer, 1989). Growth to higher states of consciousness is effortless and spontaneous and is propelled along by the desire of the human psyche to know itself fully.

With regular experience of the field of pure consciousness, an individual gains strength and stability as he or she experiences a profound purification of all aspects of functioning-spiritual, emotional, physical, and psychological (Maharishi Mahesh Yogi, 1963, 1969). Deeply rooted stresses and impurities dissolve. The individual's nervous system becomes increasingly capable of supporting more refined, advanced states of mental clarity and activity. On the level of feelings and behavior, a substantial amount of research has demonstrated that individuals who practice Transcendental Meditation and other technologies of Maharishi Ayur-Veda experience profound improvements in mental and physical health (Orme-Johnson, 1988; Dillbeck, 1988; Wallace, 1993).

Through the regular alternation of pure consciousness in TM with daily activity, Maharishi (1969) explains that the state of pure consciousness eventually becomes permanently established and coexists along with the ordinary cycles of waking, dreaming, and sleeping. This is an indelible state which is qualitatively and quantitatively distinct from previous states of consciousness and is termed *cosmic consciousness*. At this stage in development, the individual experiences his or her unbounded Self on a continual basis. This is a state of constant well-being entirely free from stress. An individual in this state experiences a deep silence, even in the midst of the most dynamic activity, and an unshakable strength of personality. There is a profound sense of inner freedom, happiness, and fulfillment. The individual becomes more skillful in activities, and desires are achieved in an effortless fashion.

Maharishi also explains that in this state the Self has become separate from the field of activity:

> When, through constant practice, complete integration of the Self with the mind is achieved, the pure status of Being [pure consciousness] gained by the mind is not in any way overshadowed even though the mind occupies itself with activity in the

> relative field. This is the state of cosmic consciousness where the Self has separated itself completely from the field of activity. In this state, where absolute [unchanging] Being and the relative world of activity are lived simultaneously, the Self is said to have been permanently freed from all stain. It has achieved absolute purity. (1969, pp. 338-339)

At this point, the Self becomes fully differentiated, non-attached, and no longer identifies with any passing experience or boundary. At this stage of development, the realized Self appears as radically separate from everything and everyone around it. Although the individual may feel separate from the environment in this state, the experience is one of deep inner contentment and blissfulness.

This is not, however, the final phase of development. The process of psychophysiological refinement continues, and the gap between the individual and the environment begins to dissolve. With this further development, the experience of inner bliss begins to extend to the environment. Maharishi (1969) explains, "The heart in its state of eternal contentment begins to move, and this begins to draw everything together and eliminate the gulf of separation between the Self and activity" (p. 307).

As the process of development continues, activity involving the most refined qualities of feeling–reverence, service, and love–results in perceptual refinement and a greater sense of intimacy between the Self and the objects of perception: one begins to perceive finer levels of the objects in the environment (Maharishi Mahesh Yogi, 1969, p. 315). This state is known as *refined cosmic consciousness* or *God consciousness*. Maharishi has termed this stage God consciousness because the individual who has attained it experiences the world as permeated by the glory of the divine. One naturally and spontaneously comes to appreciate the beauty and divine quality of the most refined levels of creation, and thus naturally appreciates the glory of its Creator; one feels a sense of universal love and a perfect sense of harmony in life. For the recovering alcoholic or addict, this may represent the fulfillment of the Twelve Steps program to develop a state of deep intimacy with a "higher power."

In the highest state of consciousness described in Maharishi's Vedic Psychology, *unity consciousness*, a complete unification between the Self and the objective world is achieved. Everything in the objective world is experienced as an expression of the same Self which underlies one's own individual life. The gap between the "relative" and "absolute" aspects of life, which was nearly dissolved in the previous state of God consciousness, is completely eliminated in unity consciousness. This is the goal of life, the ultimate state of human functioning. The Bhagavad-Gita, one of the central aspects of the Vedic literature, describes how in this state, one "sees the Self in all beings and all beings in the Self" (Maharishi Mahesh Yogi, 1969, p. 441). In the state of unity consciousness, everything is experienced in terms of the unbounded Self. The individual experiences infinite dynamism and self-sufficiency. For the spiritual seeker, this is the state to which he or she ultimately aspires.

Maharishi Ayur-Veda and the Theory of Addictions

It is interesting to note that the therapeutic transformations Kohut (1971) noted in patients completing a lengthy analysis to cure self disturbances occur to varying degrees in patients who have been practicing Transcendental Meditation for only a brief period of time (Eppley, Abrams & Shear, 1989). According to Kohut, these changes include an increase and expansion in love for others, greater empathy for others, greater passion and interest in life, and an increase in humor and wisdom. Such changes are reflective of a growing sense of maturity in the self. With the application of the TM program and Maharishi Ayur-Veda to the rehabilitation process, the patient can more rapidly and easily experience higher levels of self-development. In higher levels of development, addictive substances are no longer necessary to maintain balance and esteem.

According to Maharishi Ayur-Veda, the basis for the transformation these chemically dependent patients experience is the regular experience of pure consciousness. The Transcendental Meditation technique, the advanced TM-Sidhi program, and other procedures of Maharishi Ayur-Veda are all designed to permanently and fully establish the experience of pure Self. The empirical research reviewed and summarized in the opening chapter of this volume by Dr. Alexander and his colleagues attests to the effectiveness of the Maharishi Ayur-Veda approach to treating addictions. Maharishi

Ayur-Veda provides the technologies for the self to experience its own self-referral state and thus heal itself and begin to experience the true nature of life in bliss consciousness.

Both the disease model and medical model of alcoholism and addictions emphasize the genetic and physical basis for addictive diseases. Ongoing research into the genetic etiology of addictions has provided mounting evidence for the explanatory power of these models. Developing evidence for a biological marker, and thus a physical basis for the more severe forms of alcoholism and addiction has emerged over the past decade from family, twin, and adoption studies (Parsian, & Cloninger, 1991) and has been made possible through developments in technology such as DNA sequencing and recombinant DNA. Research has implicated the dopamine receptor gene Al allele (DRG2) and a reduction of dopamine released in reward centers in the brain with drug-seeking and drug-craving behavior (Blum, Noble, & Sheridan, 1990). Parsian and Cloninger report that alcoholics show lowered MAO platelet activity and lowered adenylate cyclase activity as compared to non-alcoholic controls. Comings (1991) has established an association between a mutation in the human tryptophan oxygenase gene which can affect serotonin production and the development of Tourettes Syndrome, attention deficit hyperactivity disorder and addictive diseases.

Although the researchers involved in these studies stress that their findings are preliminary and that they are understandably cautious in the interpretation of their results, the addictions field is becoming more and more accepting of viewing at least some forms of chemical dependency as physical diseases with genetic etiologies. This confirms the beliefs of adherents to the medical model of alcoholism and chemical dependency who have used this model as the basis for treatment programs for well over a decade.

Like the medical model of addictions, Maharishi Ayur-Veda involves a focus on the physiological basis for addictive diseases. Gelderloos and his colleagues (1991) have provided initial efforts to understand the Maharishi Ayur-Veda framework or model for understanding the development and treatment of addictive diseases. In commenting on the biochemical effects of Transcendental Meditation for example, the authors note that the effects of TM "suggest it normalizes abnormal conditions and fosters the development of a balanced state of the key neurotransmitters most directly involved in psychological functioning" (p. 316). Research indicates that the practice of TM results in enhanced serotonin function (Bujatti and Rieder, 1976), a normalization of catecholamine activity (Subrahmanyam & Porkodi, 1980), and an increase in the effectiveness of melatonin in the prevention and elimination of stress. Research also indicates that the practice of TM results in increased mood elevation, enhanced psychological status, and increased ability to cope with stressors (Mills, Schneider, Hill, Walton, & Wallace, 1987). Gelderloos et al. conclude, based on a review of research on TM and addictions, that "neurochemical and neuroendocrine research appears to be uncovering plausible mechanisms by which TM could produce both short and long-term benefits in the treatment of drug use" (p. 317). These authors note that although a comprehensive understanding of the psychophysiological mechanisms involved in the development and manifestation of addictive diseases is not currently available, the practice of TM and other procedures of Maharishi Ayur-Veda address the suggested causal factors in substance abuse, for example psychological distress, lack of coping abilities, and neurotransmitter imbalances. The authors note that TM can provide a natural way to achieve the experiences that a drug user is looking for, such as relief from stress, increased self-esteem, enhancement of well-being, self-sufficiency, and a sense of personal power and meaning in life. The practice of TM is seen as resulting in a psychophysiological state of maximum integration and balance. "Resetting" the nervous system through regular practice of TM creates a more orderly style of functioning that "directly counteracts the deteriorating effects of addictive behaviors" (Gelderloos et al., 1991, p. 318).

Both Walton and Levitsky (this volume) and Glaser (1988) have investigated an Ayurvedic understanding of addictive diseases. According to Walton and Levitsky, the practice of Transcendental Meditation, the primary mental approach of Maharishi Ayur-Veda, increases the availability of serotonin and decreases cortisol levels in the body. This leads to a reduction of psychological distress and an increase in the body's adaptive mechanisms. Through these processes, the practice of Transcendental Meditation can interrupt the drug use cycle in addictive behaviors. Within this model, stress is seen as the primary cause of addictive disorders, although a genetic predisposition to addictive behavior is acknowledged. Maharishi Ayur-Veda emphasizes the importance of bringing about a stable state of homeostasis for the body through its twenty-plus approaches, and this renders the process of recovery much more effective and the possibility of long-term sobriety within easier reach for the addict.

Sands (this volume) notes that addiction, like other disorders, is caused by specific predispositions in one's individual constitution (*prakriti*), which are exacerbated by one's lifestyle. Drug use is conceptualized as an inappropriate means to restore a disturbance in the balance of mind and body. The predisposition towards drug use is based in part on a distorted, incomplete view of the Self.

According to Maharishi Ayur-Veda, addiction like other diseases arises from the "mistake of the intellect," known as *pragyaparadha*, in which one perceives one's self not in terms of the wholeness of pure consciousness (the Self), but rather as a highly limited individual personality burdened with conflicting impulses and feelings, cut off from the wholeness of pure consciousness. Pragyaparadha arises in the absence of the experience of pure consciousness, and the consequence for the addict is that his or her identity shrinks from its universal status to a localized one in which well-being is replaced by pain, suffering, and guilt. The techniques of Maharishi Ayur-Veda are designed to restore balance in the mind and physiology, creating a style of psychophysiological functioning that supports the experience of pure consciousness, eliminates pragyaparadha, and thus does not support the expression of an addictive disorder.

Maharishi Ayur-Veda is not just fanciful or mystical theorizing. There is a growing and impressive body of empirical evidence to support both gains in self-development and the experience of higher states of consciousness (Alexander, Rainforth, & Gelderloos, 1991). A large amount of data has accumulated on the positive effects of the Transcendental Meditation technique on mental health and addiction rehabilitation and personality development. A study by Eppley, Abrams and Shear (1989) documents significant reductions in both state and trait anxiety in meditators. The effects of TM on the positive development of personality have been reported by Nidich,

Seeman & Dreskin (1973) and Hjelle (1974), while Turnbull and Norris (1982) have demonstrated the effect of TM on improving self-concept. The systematic practice of TM and related techniques of Maharishi Ayur-Veda has resulted in the following:

- increased emotional stability and maturity
- increased ability to handle stress and tension
- significant improvements in depression, psychosomatic disorders, schizophrenia, and neurotic disorders
- improvements in bipolar disorder
- improvements in addictive disorders including alcoholism, drug addiction, gambling, and cigarette smoking
- improvements in personality disorders
- improvements in aggressive psychiatric patients resulting in decreased frequency and severity of attacks of assaultive behavior.

(Summarized in Orme-Johnson & Farrow, 1977; Chalmers, Clements, Schenkluhn, & Weinless, 1989a,b,c.)

Cross-sectional and longitudinal studies reviewed by Alexander and Boyer (1989) indicate that the practice of Transcendental Meditation accelerates the rate of development of higher states of consciousness compared to control groups. The increased frequency of experiences of higher states of consciousness was found to be correlated with such measures as: increased alpha and theta EEG coherence, Hoffman reflex recovery, periods of respiratory suspension indicating a qualitatively distinct state of restful alertness; increased self-actualization, attentional focus, creativity, fluid intelligence, and cognitive perceptual abilities; and increased mind-body coordination as evidenced by refinement of sensory thresholds.

To the seasoned alcoholism counselor, the idea that life in sobriety can be a supremely blissful experience and that the alcoholic or addict can rise to the highest level of human development may indeed seem impossible. However, indications that this may be so can be found in the early writings of the founders of Alcoholics Anonymous, who viewed sobriety as an open-ended process of development and recovery from alcoholism as a gateway to spiritual fulfillment (AA World Services, 1984). Embracing the approaches of Maharishi Ayur-Veda as viable treatments for addictive diseases will require professionals in the addictions treatment field to let go of preconceived notions and ideas about the source, course, and treatment of addictive diseases. With the advent of Maharishi Ayur-Veda, spiritual and self-realization can become a reality.

The TM Program and Psychotherapy

When a patient begins the practice of Transcendental Meditation, the counselor or therapist needs to be aware of the patient's experiences both within and outside of meditation, the significance of these and how they should be addressed in the context of the therapy relationship. Most of the literature on meditation techniques and psychotherapy has emerged from the transpersonal school of therapy (for example, see Borstein, 1991). In general, the insights and experiences of the patient during these types of meditation techniques are used as material for exploration in the therapeutic hour by the transpersonal therapist. The patient may even be "guided" through the meditation experience by a knowledgeable therapist who employs various other types of meditation techniques in treatment.

In the case of the Transcendental Meditation technique, the situation is quite different. During TM, the mind settles down to quieter and quieter levels of functioning and thoughts are experienced at increasingly subtler levels until eventually all thoughts are transcended and left behind (Maharishi Mahesh Yogi, 1963, pp. 52-56). The meditator, at this point, experiences pure consciousness, which is not a particular thought, but rather the source of all thoughts. In the process of learning TM, the meditator is instructed not to be concerned with any particular thought, sensation or experience that may occur during meditation. TM is a systematic procedure to experience pure consciousness, and any particular insight, realization, or other mental experience is viewed as a by-product of the practice of meditation. Thus, the therapist should not directly interfere during a meditation and should not encourage the patient to attempt to analyze or understand experiences during meditation. The patient's innocence must be maintained during the practice of TM. It is important to note that the positive effects of the TM technique on mental and physical functioning arise completely effortlessly. Neither the patient nor the therapist can provide or directly influence the positive changes experienced by the patient during the process of TM. Unlike the situation with other meditation techniques, the therapist or TM teacher does not become involved in directing the practice of meditation. Although the TM technique is very simple, natural, and easy to learn, because it is also a delicate practice, and because individual experiences with the technique may vary, it is important for the therapist to understand that TM must be learned from a qualified TM instructor who has received extensive training (Maharishi Mahesh Yogi, 1963, pp. 56-59).

The primary curative factor for the patient who begins the practice of TM is the experience of pure consciousness and not the psychotherapeutic relationship. What then is the therapist's role with a recovering chemically dependent patient who practices the TM technique? The use of TM in psychotherapy has been addressed by Rigby (1989) and Brooks (1993), who have provided guidelines and information to therapists with patients who are practicing the TM technique and the other twenty-some approaches of Maharishi Ayur-Veda.

In general, the therapist's role with a patient who practices TM is to provide support and stability while TM and related techniques purify and stabilize the patient's neuropsychological and neurophysiological functioning. Therapists of various therapeutic persuasions can assist patients in dealing with the problems and demands of day-to-day life while encouraging and supporting the patient's regular TM practice. In this writer's clinical experience, chemically dependent patients carry a great deal of shame and guilt and can become overly concerned with their shortcomings when engaged in psychotherapy. Liberal use of "reframing" can be helpful here. Both the use of substances and other self-destructive behaviors should be reframed as attempts to heal the self, however inappropriate. The therapist can then emphasize that the practice of TM is providing the healing function that the patient looked to drugs to provide. In general, the focus should be on the patient's health and development. This emphasis on evolution rather than on psychopathology and limitations is important because the patient, once he or she begins to practice TM regularly, begins experiencing rapid changes in his or her psychological and physiological functioning. Deeply rooted stresses and traumas can dissolve very quickly. A focus on the patient's health is necessary to keep pace with these changes and to assist the patient in letting go of his or her attachment to past stresses and traumas. Many recovering patients are often preoccupied with their psychopathology and this, unfortunately, may be unwittingly reinforced by involvement in Twelve Step programs. By reframing pathological behaviors and keeping the focus on the patient's health and growth, the patient can be inspired and can avoid obsessive rumination and brooding about past setbacks.

In addition to this, it is important to encourage spiritual exploration in the context of the patient's own concept of spirituality and especially in his or her religion. The patient can also be introduced to literature on Maharishi Ayur-Veda. The books of Maharishi Mahesh Yogi can be particularly useful in deepening patients' spiritual awareness and expanding their concept of spirituality. (See resources section of this book.) In addition, case studies in Maharishi Ayur-Veda, such as the Bhagavad-Gita (Maharishi Mahesh Yogi, 1969), can be very useful in cultivating an understanding of the patient's spiritual and psychological predicament. In this writer's experience, this literature is extremely uplifting and insightful.

It is also important to spend some time each session focusing on the patient's physical health. Patients should be encouraged to practice the natural health-promoting techniques of Maharishi Ayur-Veda. The most useful text for patients to read in this area is *Freedom from Disease* (Sharma, 1993). This book provides a wealth of information on the care of the body through Maharishi Ayur-Veda. Extremely useful companions to this are the educational materials and videotape on the *Fundamentals of Maharishi Ayur-Veda* (Averbach & Rothenberg, 1989). These resources can work in a complementary fashion in guiding the patient's daily routine and behavior. The focus on maintaining physical health is important for chemically dependent patients, especially to assist them in avoiding relapse and maximizing discomfort due to the post-acute withdrawal syndrome which can last up to as much as a year following detoxification and stabilization.

The TM Program and Spirituality

Most modern approaches to alcoholism treatment incorporate the Twelve Steps of Alcoholics Anonymous; these steps have as their basis a spiritual awakening. This involves a conversion to a new life and an entirely different way of functioning for the alcoholic. However, it is this writer's experience that the spiritual aspect of recovery is often a major stumbling block for patients.

This is particularly true for the relapse prone alcoholic or addict. As indicated in earlier works (O'Connell, 1990, 1991), many recovering patients report that they have never experienced a spiritual conversion and have difficulty understanding the whole concept. The concept of spirituality is indeed elusive to many recovering patients and can be a source of great frustration and consternation.

Most chemically dependent patients who present for counseling with a psychologist or alcoholism therapist will have been exposed to Twelve Step programs and many will be deeply involved in them. In this writer's experience, and in the experience of many drug and alcohol therapists, such patients often have questions about spirituality and pursuing a spiritual program in recovery. The therapeutic relationship is often the context for discussion of spiritual issues. Because of this and because spirituality is a difficult subject to deal with, a psychotherapist who incorporates the Transcendental Meditation program should be in a position to intelligently and effectively handle spiritual concerns as they arise.

First of all, it must be emphatically stated that the TM program is not a form of prayer, worship, or religious ritual and does not constitute a system of religious beliefs or doctrine. The practice of TM requires no changes in values, beliefs, attitudes or behaviors on the part of the meditator. However, even though TM is not a religious practice per se, it can have profound practical implications for an individual's own spiritual pursuits or religious practices.

Maharishi explains (1969) that the practice of TM, by purifying both mind and body, allows the individual to rise to the highest level of spiritual development. In his book *Science of Being and Art of Living* (1963), he describes how the practice of TM supports and strengthens any path to spiritual fulfillment. Nystul and Garde (1977) report on empirical evidence for these principles and note that regular practitioners of the TM program report an upsurgence of love and devotion in their daily lives and a greater appreciation of their sense of spirituality.

O'Brien (1983), a theologian and teacher of Transcendental Meditation, has written on the effects of the TM program on spiritual growth and development. He has found, as Maharishi describes, that the practice of TM, by providing deep rest, helps eliminate the psychological and physical obstacles that block the natural development of one's spirituality. He also notes that persons who regularly practice Transcendental Meditation report a greater appreciation of their own religion and a clearer understanding of the tenets of their faith. Bleick (in this volume), in her detailed case analyses of Twelve Step participants who began the TM program, notes that many of these patients report that the practice of TM had a profound impact on their spiritual programs in AA/NA and that TM gave them a sense of peace and well-being they could not find through other approaches to recovery from addiction.

The ultimate goal of the TM program is the complete unfoldment of the Self in the state of unity consciousness. This is life in complete integration, wholeness and freedom and, doubtless, an aspiration shared by all spiritual seekers regardless of religious preference.

For therapists who employ the TM program in clinical practice with alcoholics, there are two important points to consider:

1. The practice of TM is completely effortless; it provides direct experience of the transcendental field of pure consciousness at the basis of all existence, and facilitates the infusion of pure consciousness into the nature of the mind.

2. The practice of TM removes deeply ingrained stresses in the nervous system that impede the patient's spiritual growth, promoting development in all spheres of life.

These two points are considered in the following section.

How the TM Program Promotes Spiritual Development

How does the TM technique bring about spiritual development? It must be emphasized that TM is both a *mental* and *physiological* approach to spiritual growth and development. As was seen in previous sections, there are profound biochemical and structural changes in the nervous system brought on by the regular practice of TM and other technologies of Maharishi Ayur-Veda. Maharishi (1963, 1969) has always contended that when the nervous system of a human being is free from all stresses and physical and psychological abnormalities, then the Self is experienced in all its purity and spiritual realization will become an effortless, living reality.

Ultimately, Maharishi explains (1969), it is the Self that unfolds its own nature. In this context, he uses the analogy of the wind and sun to explain the mechanics of how the practice of TM removes the obstacles to experiencing the Self:

> Meditation does not unfold the Self–the Self, it must be repeated, unfolds Itself by Itself to Itself. The wind does nothing to the sun; it only clears away the clouds and the sun is found shining by its own light. The light of the sun is self-effulgent. Meditation only takes the mind out of the clouds of relativity. The absolute state of the Self ever shines in its own glory. (p. 396)

Some rare individuals in the Western spiritual tradition have recognized the necessity of purification in spiritual development. The great sixteenth-century contemplative and mystic St. John of the Cross wrote movingly about the value of meditation and other similar practices in purifying oneself to reveal the ultimate divine nature of life within:

> A ray of sunlight shining upon a smudgy window is unable to illume that window completely and to transform it into its own light. It could do this if the window were cleaned and polished. The less film and stain are wiped away, the less the window will be illumed and the cleaner the window is, the brighter will be its illumination. The extent of illumination is not dependent upon the ray of sunlight, but upon the window. If the window were totally clean and pure, the sunlight would so transform and illume it, that to all appearances the window would be identical with the ray of sunlight . . . . The soul upon which the Divine light of God's being is overshining or better in which it is always dwelling by nature, is like this window . . . . A man makes room for God by wiping away all the smudges and smears of creatures by uniting his will perfectly to God . . . . When this is done, the soul will be illumed by and transformed in God . . . . (Kavanaugh & Rodriguez, 1979, p. 117)

There are many forms of meditation available to recovering addicts and alcoholics. Most types of meditation involve some effort on the part of the aspirant and can be experienced by the practitioner as fatiguing or unpleasant. In contradistinction, the TM technique requires no effort whatsoever and is extremely pleasant. This is an important point: the effortlessness of the TM technique lies at the heart of its effectiveness as a spiritual program. Other techniques tend to keep the mind busy at the surface level of thinking with devotional or inspirational thoughts. However, as Maharishi (1969, p. 471) has explained, such a style of functioning of the mind will not promote the direct experience of pure consciousness, the most settled, simple state of awareness. The technique of Transcendental Meditation allows the mind to effortlessly settle down and directly experience this state (Maharishi Mahesh Yogi, 1963, pp. 53-59).

In the practice of TM, the mind experiences increasingly more subtle levels of thought until thought is completely transcended. Thus, the mind has gone from experiencing a surface-level thought of spirituality and God to directly experiencing the transcendental field of absolute, pure divine Being at the basis of all existence. As described earlier, this experience is a fundamental prerequisite to developing higher states of consciousness. Maharishi (1969) emphasizes the necessity of directly experiencing this field:

> Therefore, let the mind transcend thought and enter the realm of absolute purity which is the abode of God. Thinking about it is wasting time in the surface of life. A thought keeps the mind away from that blessed realm. A thought of bread neither gives the taste of bread, nor fills the stomach. If you want bread, go to the kitchen and get it instead of sitting outside thinking about it. (p. 444)

The following quote by the German theologian and philosopher Meister Eckert (quoted in Aubrey, 1983) also notes the importance of direct experience:

> We ought not to have or let ourselves be satisfied with a God we have thought of. For when the thought slips from the mind, the thought of God slips with it. What we want rather, is the reality of God exulted far above any human thought or creature. (p. 97)

Many inpatient and outpatient facilities draw heavily on inspirational and meditative readings to assist alcoholics in the recovery process. Such practices, however, are quite different from the practice of TM. This fundamental difference is important for a therapist to understand when providing guidance and counseling about spiritual concerns for patients. However, the TM program can act in a complementary fashion with other treatment procedures.

The importance of a daily spiritual program in recovery cannot be overemphasized. The sense of spirituality is perhaps the most intimate experience a person can have. The founders of AA intuitively realized the importance of spirituality and erected their entire program upon the necessity of a spiritual awakening. If an alcoholic is to remain sober, then he or she must experience a fundamental change within. No amount of surface behavior change, conscious self-affirmations or good works, however selflessly offered, can bring about the fundamental internal changes necessary for spiritual awakening and development. O'Brien (1983, p. 72) has written on the effects of TM on spirituality: "It is only by throwing ourselves into the inner presence, by surrendering to the indwelling source of divine love, that we can find that happiness, that identity, which as creatures in God's image is our birthright."

Maharishi (1986b) explains that when the individual experiences and imbibes the nature of the transcendental field of life (pure consciousness) every area of life blossoms. As a result, instead of being cut off from one's spiritual origin, all one's thinking and activity are brought in accord with one's ultimate inner nature, which is the nature of life itself:

> Spiritual life means life in direct communication with the primordial power of Being, with the cosmic life energy, and man has to be bright and energetic in every field of life–in thought, speech, and action–no retardation or one-sided way of life; he has to be an all-round full-bloomed flower.
>
> Freedom grows in life with spiritual development; intelligence grows, energy grows, happiness grows, peace grows. The man comes out of all these small bits of life, comes out of bondage of all types. That is spiritual life. Whatever he is, he is in accordance with nature. Not that he has to think about right

> and wrong, but whatever he does, it's in accordance with the laws of nature, and this is only when the mind gets surcharged with the primordial life power, which is the source of the entire creation, the basis of all the natural laws.
>
> Such a natural life in freedom is the life that we call spiritual life, and that comes directly with the infusion of the transcendental Being into the nature of the mind. (pp. 420-421)

The practice of TM allows the individual to experience his or her higher Self as the nervous system is cleared of all abnormalities. When this "natural life in freedom" and fulfillment that Maharishi describes is achieved, the aim of the spiritual program in recovery is fulfilled.

CONCLUSION

Maharishi Ayur-Veda provides the necessary understanding and procedures to bring about the highest level of development of the self: the possession of the Self. The chemically dependent individual now has the opportunity to experience a more blissful recovery process and achieve a life of sobriety and spiritual fulfillment. These achievements are supported by a growing body of experimental and clinical evidence, as well as the subjective reports of alcoholics and addicts practicing the TM technique and other modalities of Maharishi Ayur-Veda.

In the final analysis, the recovering alcoholic aspires to what we all desire–complete freedom and fulfillment in life. And sadly, for the majority of humanity, this supreme desire is rarely attained.

Alcoholism and addiction are complex, insidious, devastating diseases that continue to create enormous mental and physical suffering despite our best efforts to eliminate them. With the advent of Maharishi Ayur-Veda technologies, we now have in place a therapeutic program as powerful in a positive direction as addiction is in a negative one. Hopefully, addictions professionals and patients alike will take advantage of this program. As Maharishi concludes in his book *Science of Being and Art of Living:*

> A formula exists to take care of the very root of individual life. To maintain and restore health on all levels of mind, body and

surroundings, we offer this formula in no spirit of competition or challenge, but out of love for man and with all good will towards those people all over the world who are endeavoring to alleviate suffering by whatever means they have found useful.

REFERENCES

Alcoholics Anonymous World Services (1984). *Pass it on: The story of Bill Wilson and how the AA message reached the world.* New York: Author.

Alexander, C. N. (1982). Ego development, personality, and behavioral change in inmates practicing the Transcendental Meditation technique or participating in other programs: A cross-sectional and longitudinal study. *Dissertation Abstracts International, 43*, 539B.

Alexander, C., & Boyer, R. (1989). Seven states of consciousness: Unfolding the full potential of the cosmic psyche in individual life through Maharishi's Vedic Psychology. *Modern Science and Vedic Science*, 2(4), 325-371.

Alexander, C. N., Davies, J. L., Dixon, C. A., Dillbeck, M. C., Oetzel, R. M., Druker, S. M., Muehlman, J. M., & Orme-Johnson, D. W. (1990). Growth of higher stages of consciousness: The Vedic psychology of human development. In C. N. Alexander & E. J. Langer (Eds.), *Higher stages of human development: Perspectives on adult growth* (pp. 286-340). New York: Oxford University Press.

Alexander, C. N., Rainforth, M. V., & Gelderloos, P. (1991). Transcendental Meditation, self-actualization and psychological health: A conceptual overview and statistical meta-analysis. *Journal of Social Behavior and Personality*, *6*(5), 189-247.

Aubrey, B. (1983). Rediscovering ancient springs: TM and the Christian mystical tradition. In A. Smith (Ed.), *TM: An aide to Christian growth.* Great Wakering, Essex, England: Mayhew McCrimmon.

Averbach, R. & Rothenberg, S. (1989). *Fundamentals of Maharishi Ayurveda: Natural health care for the mind and body.* Lancaster, MA: Maharishi Ayur-Veda Products International.

Bleick, C. R. (this volume). Case histories: Using the Transcendental Meditation program with alcoholics and addicts. *Alcoholism Treatment Quarterly.*

Bleick, C. R. (1990, Autumn). *Los Angeles Area Report.* Los Angeles: Institute of Social Rehabilitation.

Blum, K., Noble, E., & Sheridan, P. (1990). Allelic association of human dopamine D2 receptor gene in alcoholism. *Journal of the American Medical Association, 263*,2055-2060.

Borstein, S. (Ed.). (1991). *Transpersonal psychotherapy.* Stanford, CA: JTP Books.

Brooks, J. (1993). *Peace of mind: An Ayurvedic guide to total mental and emotional health.* (Unpublished book manuscript).

Brown, S. (1977). *Defining a process of recovery in alcoholism.* Doctoral Dissertation. California School of Professional Psychology. Berkeley, April.

Brown, S. (1985). *Treating the alcoholic: A developmental model of recovery.* New York: John Wiley & Sons.

Bujatti, M., & Riederer, P. (1976). Serotonin, noradrenaline, dopamine metabolites in Transcendental Meditation technique. *Journal of Neuronal Transmission, 39*, 257-262.

Carter, R., & Meyer, J. (1989). The use of the Transcendental Meditation technique with severely disturbed psychiatric patients. In R. Chalmers, G. Clements, H., Schenkluhn & M. Weinless (Eds.), *Scientific Research on Maharishi's Transcendental Meditation and TM-Sidhi Programme: Collected papers,* Vol. 3 (pp. 2112-2115). Vlodrop, The Netherlands: Maharishi Vedic University Press.

Chalmers, R., Clements, G., Schenkluhn, H., & Weinless, M. (Eds.). (1989a, 1989b, 1989c). *Scientific Research on Maharishi's Transcendental Meditation and TM-Sidhi Programme: Collected papers*, Vols. 2-4. Vlodrop, the Netherlands: Maharishi Vedic University Press.

Comings, D. (1991). The genetics of addictive behaviors: The role of childhood behavioral disorders. *Addiction and Recovery, 11*(6), 13-16.

Dillbeck, M. (1988). The self-interacting dynamics of consciousness as the source of the creative process in nature and in human life. *Modern Science and Vedic Science*, 2, 245-278.

Eppley, K. R., Abrams, A., & Shear, J. (1989). Differential effects of relaxation techniques on trait anxiety: A meta-analysis. *Journal of Clinical Psychology, 45*(6), 957-974.

Farrow, J., & Hebert, J. (1982). Breath suspension during the Transcendental Meditation technique. *Psychosomatic Medicine, 44*(2), 133-153.

Freyer-Rose, K. E. (1991). Late recovery: A process of integration. *Addiction and Recovery, 11*(6), 20-23.

Gelderloos, P., Walton, K., Orme-Johnson, D., & Alexander, C. (1991). Effectiveness of the Transcendental Meditation program in preventing and treating substance misuse: A review. *International Journal of the Addictions*, 26(3), 293-325.

Glaser, J. (1988). Maharishi Ayurveda: An introduction to recent research. *Modern Science and Vedic Science*, 2(1), 89-108.

Gorski, T. (1979). *Counseling for relapse prevention.* Hazelcreste, IL: Alcoholism Systems Associates.

Gorski, T. (1989). *Passages through a recovery.* Center City, MN: Hazelden Educational Materials.

Hagelin, J. S. (1987). Is consciousness the unified field? A field theorist's perspective. *Modern Science and Vedic Science, 1*(1), 29-87.

Hagelin, J. S. (1989). Restructuring physics from its foundation in light of Maharishi's Vedic Science. *Modern Science and Vedic Science, 3*(1), 3-72.

Hjelle, L. (1974). Transcendental Meditation and psychological health. *Perceptual and Motor Skills, 39*, 623-628.

Johnson, V. (1980). *I'll quit tomorrow: A practical guide to alcoholism treatment.* New York: Harper and Row.

Kavanaugh, K., & Rodriguez, O. (1979). *The collected works of St. John of the Cross* (2nd ed.). Washington, DC: ICS Publications.

Kesterson, J. B. (1986). Changes in respiratory control pattern during the practice of the Transcendental Meditation technique. *Dissertation Abstracts International, 47*, 4337B.

Khantzian, E., Halliday, K., & McAuliffe, W. (1990). *Addiction and the vulnerable self.* New York: Guilford.

Kohut, H. (1971). *The analysis of the self: A systematic approach to the psychoanalytic treatment of narcissistic personality disorders.* New York: International Universities Press.

Kohut, H. (1977). *The restoration of the self.* New York: International Universities Press.

Kohut, H. (1978). Thoughts on narcissism and narcissistic rage in the search for the self. In P. Ornestein (Ed.), *Search for the Self, Vol. 2* (pp. 615-658). New York: International Universities Press.

Kohut, H. (1984). *How does analysis cure?* Chicago: University of Chicago Press.

Levin, J. (1987). *Treatment of alcoholism and other addictions: A self-psychology approach.* Northvale, NJ: Jason Aronson.

Maharishi Mahesh Yogi. (1963). *Science of being and art of living.* New York.

Maharishi Mahesh Yogi. (1969). *On the Bhagavad Gita: A translation and commentary (Chapters 1-6).* New York: Penguin.

Maharishi Mahesh Yogi. (1986a). Life supported by natural law: Fairfield IA: Maharishi International University Press.

Maharishi Mahesh Yogi. (1986b). *Thirty years around the world–Dawn of the age of enlightenment.* Vlodrop, the Netherlands: Maharishi Vedic University.

Marlatt, G., & Gordon, J. (Eds). (1985). *Relapse prevention: Maintenance strategies in the treatment of addictive behaviors.* New York: Guilford.

Mills, P., Schneider, R., Hill, D., Walton, K., & Wallace, R. (1987). Lymphocyte beta-adrenergic receptors and cardiovascular responsivity in TM participants and Type A behavior [Abstract]. *Psychosomatic Medicine, 49*, 211.

Muzika, E. (1990). Object relations theory, Buddhism and the self: Synthesis of eastern and western approaches. *International Philosophical Quarterly, 30*(1), 59-74.

Nace, E. (1987). *The treatment of alcoholism.* New York: Brunner/Mazel.

Nystul, M., & Garde, M. (1977). Comparison of self concepts of Transcendental Meditators and non-meditators. *Psychological Reports, 41*, 303-306.

Nidich, S., Seeman, W., & Dreskin, T. (1973). Influence of Transcendental Meditation: A replication. *Journal of Counseling Psychology, 20*, 565-566.

O'Brien, A. (1983). Sin, center, and self. In A. Smith (Ed.), *TM: An aide to Christian growth.* Great Wakering, Essex, England: Mayhew McCrimmon.

O'Connell, D., (Ed.). (1990). *Managing the dually diagnosed patient: Current issues and clinical approaches.* New York: The Haworth Press, Inc.

O'Connell, D. (1991). The use of Transcendental Meditation in relapse prevention counseling. *Alcoholism Treatment Quarterly, 8*(1), 53-68.

Orme-Johnson, D.W. (1988). The cosmic psyche–An introduction to Maharishi's

Vedic Psychology: The fulfillment of modern psychology. *Modern Science and Vedic Science, 2*, 113-163.

Orme-Johnson, D., & Farrow, J. (Eds). (1977). *Scientific research on Maharishi's Transcendental Meditation program: Collected papers, Vol. 1.* New York: Maharishi International University Press.

Parsian, A., & Cloninger, C. (1991). Genetics of high risk populations. *Addiction, and Recovery, 11*(6), 9-12.

Rigby, B. (1989). Enlightenment in world psychiatry: The Transcendental Meditation technique–New light on consciousness. In R. Chalmers, G. Clements, H. Schenkluhn, & M. Weinless (Eds.), *Scientific Research on Maharishi's Transcendental Meditation and TM-Sidhi programme: Collected papers,* Vol. 2 (pp. 1389-1420). Vlodrop, the Netherlands: Maharishi Vedic University Press.

Rogers, C. (1951). *Client-centered therapy: Its current practice, implications and theory.* Boston: Houghton Mifflin.

Rogers, C. (1961). *On becoming a person: A therapist's view of psychotherapy.* Boston: Houghton Mifflin.

Sands, D. (this volume). Introducing Maharishi Ayur-Veda into clinical practice. *Alcoholism Treatment Quarterly.*

Shafii, M. (1973). Adaptive and therapeutic aspects of meditation. *International Journal of Psychoanalytic Psychotherapy. 2,* 264-382.

Shafii, M. (1988). *Freedom from the self: Sufism, meditation and psychotherapy.* New York: Human Sciences Press.

Sharma, H. (1993). Freedom from disease. Toronto: Veda Publishing.

Smith, A. (Ed). (1983). *TM: An aide to Christian growth.* Great Wakering, Essex, England: Mayhew McCrimmon.

Subrahmanyam, S., & Porkodi, K. (1980). Neurohumoral correlates of Transcendental Meditation. *Journal of Biomedicine, 1,* 73-88.

Taub, E. Steiner, S. S., Smith, R. B., Weingarten, E., & Walton, K. G. (this volume). Effectiveness of broad spectrum approaches to relapse prevention in severe alcoholism: A long-term randomized, controlled trial of Transcendental Meditation, EMG biofeedback and electronic neurotherapy. *Alcoholism Treatment Quarterly.*

Turnbull, M., & Norris, H. (1982). Effects of Transcendental Meditation on self-identity indices and personality. *British Journal of Psychology, 73*, 57-68.

Wallace, R. K. (1986). *The Maharishi Technology of the Unified Field: The neurophysiology of enlightenment.* Fairfield, IA: Maharishi International University Press.

Wallace, R. K. (1993). *The physiology of consciousness.* Fairfield, IA: MIU Press

Walton, K. G., & Levitsky, D. (this volume). Role of Transcendental Meditation in reducing drug use and addictions: Neurochemical evidence and a theory. *Alcoholism Treatment Quarterly.*

Wurmser, L. (1977). Mr. Pecksniff's horse? Psychodynamics in compulsive drug use. In J. Blaine & D. Julius (Eds.), *Psychodynamics of drug dependence.* National Institute on Drug Abuse Research Monograph 12. DHEW, No. ADM 77-470. Washington DC: U.S. Government Printing Office.

Resources on the Transcendental Meditation Program and Maharishi Ayur-Veda

A growing number of educational resources are available to health care professionals interested in gaining greater knowledge of the Transcendental Meditation program and the approaches of Maharishi Ayur-Veda. A list of recommended resources follows:

BOOKS ON THE TRANSCENDENTAL MEDITATION AND MAHARISHI AYUR-VEDA PROGRAMS

Books by the founder of the Transcendental Meditation program, Maharishi Mahesh Yogi:

- *Science of Being and Art of Living.* New York, NY: Signet. 1968.
- *Enlightenment and Invincibility.* Rheinweiler, Germany: Maharishi European Research University (MERU) Press. 1978.
- *Life Supported by Natural Law.* Fairfield, IA: Maharishi International University (MIU) Press. 1986.
- *Maharishi Mahesh Yogi on the Bhagavad-Gita: A Translation and Commentary (Chapters 1-6).* New York NY: Penguin. 1988.
- *Thirty Years Around the World–Dawn of the Age of Enlightenment: Volume One 1957-1964. Vlodrop, Netherlands: Maharishi Vedic University Press.*

[Haworth co-indexing entry note]: "Resources on the Transcendental Meditation Program and Maharishi Ayur-Veda." Co-published simultaneously in the *Alcoholism Treatment Quarterly* (The Haworth Press, Inc.) Vol. 11, No. 3/4, 1994, pp. 497-502; and: *Self-Recovery: Treating Addictions Using Transcendental Meditation and Maharishi Ayur-Veda* (ed: David F. O'Connell and Charles N. Alexander) The Haworth Press, Inc., 1994, pp. 497-502. Multiple copies of this article/chapter may be purchased from The Haworth Document Delivery Center [1-800-3-HAWORTH; 9:00 a.m. - 5:00 p.m. (EST)].

- *Maharishi's Absolute Theory of Government.* (1993). Vlodrop, Netherlands: Maharishi Vedic University Press.

Other books on the Transcendental Meditation program:

- Alexander, Charles N., & Langer, Ellen J. (Eds.). (1990). *Higher Stages of Human Development: Perspectives on Adult Growth.* New York, NY: Oxford University Press.
- Denniston, Denise (1986). *The TM Book–How to Enjoy the Rest of Your Life,* 2nd Edition. Fairfield, IA: Fairfield Press.
- Ellis, George (1983). *Inside Folsom Prison: Unified Field Based Rehabilitation.* Burlington, VT: Accord Books.
- Lonsdorf, Nancy; Butler, Veronica and Brown, Melanie. (1993). *A Women's Best Medicine: Health, Happiness, and Long Life through Ayur-Veda.* New York, NY: Tarcher/Putnum.
- Marcus, Jay B. (1990). *Success from Within: Discovering the Inner State that Creates Personal Fulfillment and Business Success.* Fairfield, IA: MIU Press.
- Nidich, Sanford I. & Nidich, Randi J. (1990). *Growing up Enlightened.* Fairfield, IA: MIU Press.
- Oates, Robert (1990). *Creating Heaven on Earth: The Mechanics of the Impossible.* Fairfield, IA: Heaven on Earth Publications.
- Roth, Robert (1987). *Maharishi Mahesh Yogi's Transcendental Meditation.* New York: Donald I. Fine, Inc.
- Sharma, Hari (1993). *Freedom from Disease.* Toronto: Veda Publishing.
- Swanson, Gerald & Oates, Robert (1989). *Enlightened Management: Building High Performance People.* Fairfield, IA: MIU Press.
- *The Maharishi Unified Field Based Integrated System of Rehabilitation in Senegalese Prisons.* (1988). Vlodrop, Netherlands: Maharishi Vedic University Press.
- *Total Rehabilitation: The Theoretical Basis and Practical Application of Maharishi's Integrated system of Rehabilitation* (in

press). Vlodrop, Netherlands: Maharishi Ayur-Veda University Press.

- Wallace, Robert Keith (1986). *The Neurophysiology of Enlightenment.* Fairfield, IA: MIU Press.
- Wallace, Robert Keith (1993). *The Physiology of Consciousness.* Fairfield, IA: MIU Press.

AUDIO AND VIDEO CASSETTE TAPES ON TRANSCENDENTAL MEDITATION AND MAHARISHI AYUR-VEDA

- Maharishi Mahesh Yogi: *Love* (side 1) and *The Untapped Source of Power that Lies Within* (side 2). (Audio). Fairfield, IA: MIU Press.
- Maharishi Mahesh Yogi: *Deep Meditation* and *Healing Powers of Deep Meditation.* (Audio). Fairfield, IA: MIU Press.
- Maharishi Mahesh Yogi: *The Seven States of Consciousness.* , (Audio). Fairfield, IA: MIU Press.
- TM: Success without Stress. (VHS). Fairfield, IA: Age of Enlightenment Press.
- Averbach, Richard, and Rothenberg, Stuart: *Fundamentals of Maharishi Ayur-Veda.* (VHS) Available through Maharishi Ayur-Veda Products International (MAPI), Colorado Springs, CO.
- *Blissful Baby: Natural Healthcare for Pregnancy and Post Partum Care.* (VHS) Available through MAPI, Colorado Springs, CO.

JOURNALS/REFERENCE BOOKS

- *Modern Science and Vedic Science* (Journal). Available through MIU Press, Fairfield, IA.
- David Orme-Johnson and John T. Farrow (Eds.). (1977). *Scientific Research on the Transcendental Meditation Programme: Collected Papers, Volume 1.* West Germany: MERU Press.

- Roger Chalmers, Geoffrey Clements, Hartmut Schenkluhn, and Michael Weinless (Eds.). (1989). *Scientific Research on Maharishi's Transcendental Meditation and TM-Sidhi Programme: Collected Papers, Volumes 2-4. Vlodrop,* Netherlands: Maharishi Ayur-Veda University Press.
- Robert Keith Wallace, David Orme-Johnson, and Michael Dillbeck (Eds.) (1990). *Scientific Research on Maharishi's Transcendental Meditation and TM-Sidhi Program: Collected Papers, Volume 5* Fairfield, IA: MIU Press.
- *The Maharishi Effect* (1990). Fairfield, IA: MIU Press.
- *Scientific Research on Maharishi's Transcendental Meditation and TM-Sidhi Program: A Review.* (1992, 1993). Fairfield, IA: MIU Press.

Except where noted, the resources listed above are available through:

MIU Press
1000 North 4th Street
Department Box 1115
Fairfield, IA, 52557-1115
(515) 472-1101 (Telephone & Fax)

or

Maharishi Ayur-Veda Products International (MAPI)
P.O. Box 49667
Colorado Springs, CO 80949-9667
FAX: (719) 260-7400
Toll Free Telephone: 1-800-ALL-VEDA (255-8332)
For orders from outside the USA: (719) 260-5500.

MAPI is also the only US distributor of the full range of Maharishi Ayur-Veda herbal food supplements, including Maharishi Amrit Kalash. To inquire about these products, call the MAPI Information Service, 1-800-843-8332.

Instruction in the Transcendental Meditation Program

Instruction in Transcendental Meditation is available through Maharishi Vedic Universities (or schools), located in most major cities worldwide. To locate the nearest Maharishi Vedic University call toll free (in USA): 800-843-8332. If you are phoning from outside the USA, call (719) 260-5500 or write to MAPI Information Service, P.O. Box 49967, Colorado Springs, CO 80949-9667, USA.

A 33-lesson course on the theoretical principles underlying TM–called the Science of Creative Intelligence–is also available both in-residence at MIU and through the local Maharishi Vedic Universities to those who begin TM.

Maharishi Ayur-Veda Treatment

Maharishi Ayur-Veda Universities (or schools) and Maharishi Ayur-Veda Medical Centers throughout the world provide prevention-oriented health education programs and comprehensive Ayurvedic medical care. Some centers provide care on an inpatient as well as outpatient basis. To locate a Maharishi Ayur-Veda University or Medical Center near you, call 1-800-843-8332, or contact

College of Maharishi Ayur-Veda
Maharishi International University
1603 N. 4th Street
P.O. Box 282
Fairfield, IA 52556
(515) 472-8477

PROFESSIONAL TRAINING IN MAHARISHI AYURVEDIC MEDICINE: PHYSICIANS' TRAINING PROGRAM

Training for physicians in Maharishi Ayurvedic diagnosis and treatment is provided in-residence on a regular basis. This course is offered in two blocks, each one week long, and includes both theoretical knowledge and clinical training to equip physicians to treat a broad range of symptoms and diseases. For information contact the College of Maharishi Ayur-Veda at the address and phone number listed above.

MAHARISHI INTERNATIONAL UNIVERSITY

Maharishi International University, accredited through the doctoral level by the North Central Association of Colleges and

Schools, integrates the study of traditional academic disciplines with the technologies of consciousness for unfolding the full potential of every student. MIU offers 15 undergraduate majors, including a BA in Maharishi Ayur-Veda which includes training as an Ayur-Veda technician, 14 master's programs, and 6 PhD programs in Neuroscience of Human Consciousness, Management and Public Affairs, Physics, Physiology and Molecular and Cell Biology, Psychology, and Science of Creative Intelligence.

RESEARCH AND POLICY IMPLICATIONS

The Institute of Science, Technology, and Public Policy at MIU was established to identify, scientifically evaluate, and promote through public policy the most up-to-date, life supporting solutions to problems facing the nation. One division of the Institute focuses on crime prevention, rehabilitation, and drug abuse.

For more information on programs and research on the Transcendental Meditation technique and Maharishi Ayur-Veda, contact:

Institute of Science, Technology, and Public Policy
Maharishi International University
1000 North 4th Street, DB 1137
Fairfield, IA 52557
(515) 472-1200
(515) 472-1165 FAX

Index

Numbers followed by "f" indicate figures; "t" following a page number indicates tabular material.

COSTS: Please figure your cost to order quality copies of an article.

1. Set-up charge per article: $8.00
   ($8.00 × number of separate articles) ________
2. Photocopying charge for each article:
   - 1-10 pages: $1.00 ________
   - 11-19 pages: $3.00 ________
   - 20-29 pages: $5.00 ________
   - 30+ pages: $2.00/10 pages ________
3. Flexicover (optional): $2.00/article ________
4. Postage & Handling: US: $1.00 for the first article/
   $.50 each additional article ________
   Federal Express: $25.00 ________
   Outside US: $2.00 for first article/
   $.50 each additional article ________
5. Same-day FAX service: $.35 per page ________
6. Local Photocopying Royalty Payment: should you wish to copy the article yourself. Not intended for photocopies made for resale. $1.50 per article per copy
   (i.e. 10 articles x $1.50 each = $15.00) ________

GRAND TOTAL: ________

METHOD OF PAYMENT: (please check one)

❑ Check enclosed ❑ Please ship and bill. PO # ________
(sorry we can ship and bill to bookstores only! All others must pre-pay)

❑ Charge to my credit card: ❑ Visa; ❑ MasterCard; ❑ American Express;

Account Number: ________ Expiration date: ________

Signature: X ________ Name: ________

Institution: ________ Address: ________

City: ________ State: ________ Zip: ________

Phone Number: ________ FAX Number: ________

MAIL or *FAX* THIS ENTIRE ORDER FORM TO:

Attn: **Marianne Arnold**
Haworth Document Delivery Service
The Haworth Press, Inc.
10 Alice Street
Binghamton, NY 13904-1580

or FAX: (607) 722-1424
or CALL: 1-800-3-HAWORTH
(1-800-342-9678; 9am-5pm EST)